# TNM
# Supplement

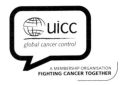

Union for International Cancer Control
www.uicc.org

# TNM Supplement

## A Commentary on Uniform Use

**FIFTH EDITION**

EDITED BY

**Christian Wittekind**
Leipzig, Germany

**James D. Brierley**
Toronto, ON, Canada

**Anne Lee**
Hong Kong, China

**Elisabeth van Eycken**
Brussels, Belgium

## WILEY Blackwell

This edition first published 2019 © 2019 UICC
Published 2019 by John Wiley & Sons Ltd

This work is a co-publication between the UICC and John Wiley & Sons, Ltd

*Edition History*
ISBN 3-540-56556-6 Springer-Verlag Berlin Heidelberg New York 1993
ISBN 0-387-56556-6 Springer-Verlag New York Berlin Heidelberg 1993
ISBN 0-471-37939-5 Wiley-Liss New York 2001
ISBN 0-471-46666-2 Wiley-Liss New York 2003
ISBN 978-1-4443-3243-8 John Wiley & Sons, Ltd Oxford 2012

The right of Christian Wittekind, James D. Brierley, Anne Lee and Elisabeth van Eycken to be identified as the authors of the editorial material in this work has been asserted in accordance with law.

*Registered Offices*
John Wiley & Sons, Inc., 111 River Street, Hoboken, NJ 07030, USA
John Wiley & Sons, Ltd, The Atrium, Southern Gate, Chichester, West Sussex, PO19 8SQ, UK

*Editorial Office*
9600 Garsington Road, Oxford, OX4 2DQ, UK

For details of our global editorial offices, customer services and more information about Wiley products visit us at www.wiley.com.

Wiley also publishes its books in a variety of electronic formats and by print-on-demand. Some content that appears in standard print versions of this book may not be available in other formats.

*Library of Congress Cataloging-in-Publication Data*

Names: Wittekind, Ch. (Christian), editor. | Brierley, James, editor. | Lee, A. W. M. (Anne W. M.), editor. |
  Eycken, E. van, editor. | Union for International Cancer Control, issuing body.
Title: TNM supplement : a commentary on uniform use / edited by Ch. Wittekind,
  J.D. Brierley, Anne Lee, Elisabeth van Eycken.
Other titles: Tumour-node-metastasis supplement
Description: Fifth edition. | Hoboken, NJ : Wiley-Blackwell ; [Geneva, Switzerland] : UICC, 2019. |
  Includes bibliographical references and index. |
Identifiers: LCCN 2019003455 (print) | LCCN 2019005429 (ebook) | ISBN 9781119263944
  (Adobe PDF) | ISBN 9781119263920 (ePub) | ISBN 9781119263937 (pbk.)
Subjects: | MESH: Neoplasms–classification
Classification: LCC RC258 (ebook) | LCC RC258 (print) | NLM QZ 15 | DDC 616.99/40012–dc23
LC record available at https://lccn.loc.gov/2019003455

Cover image: © UICC
Cover design by Wiley

Set in 9.25/13pt Frutiger Light by SPi Global, Pondicherry, India
Printed and bound in Singapore by Markono Print Media Pte Ltd

10  9  8  7  6  5  4  3  2  1

# CONTENTS

## Chapter 3 SITE-SPECIFIC REQUIREMENTS FOR pT AND pN

## Chapter 4 NEW TNM CLASSIFICATIONS RECOMMENDED FOR TESTING AND OTHER CLASSIFICATIONS

## Chapter 5 OPTIONAL PROPOSALS FOR TESTING NEW SUBCATEGORIES OF TNM

## Chapter 6 FREQUENTLY ASKED QUESTIONS

# PREFACE

First published in 1987 [1], and revised in 1992 [2], the fourth edition of the *TNM Classification of Malignant Tumours* was the result of a push from all national TNM committees towards the establishment of a uniform classification system that could be used worldwide. It was, therefore, the first edition of the text in which the featured classification criteria were identical to those detailed in the fourth edition of the AJCC's *Manual for Staging of Cancer of the American Joint Committee on Cancer* [3].

Although the classification system was, by 1987, widely accepted, medical professionals had pointed out that some of its definitions and rules for staging were imprecise and could lead to inconsistency in its application. Discrepant understandings of organ classifications, general rules and, in particular, the requirements of pathological classification (pT, pN) were all potential risks.

In an effort to address these concerns, the TNM Project Committee of the UICC collected and reviewed criticisms and suggestions from the national TNM committees, as well as from registries, oncological associations and individual users. The solution that they found was to complement the fourth edition of the *TNM Classification* [1, 2] with the publication of a new book: the *TNM Supplement* [4]. Designed to provide guidance on the uniform use of the classification system, the first edition of this new text was published in 1993.

By 1997, the *TNM Classification* was in its fifth edition [5], though most descriptions of tumour sites had remained largely unchanged, with only minor additions made so as to reflect new data on prognosis and new methods of outcome assessment. The TNM Project Committee of the UICC was aware that not all classification proposals and updates received could be included in this fifth edition and so the decision was made to produce another *TNM Supplement* within which they may be accommodated [6]. The second edition of the *TNM Supplement* therefore comprised, for the most part, of the first edition's contents, amended to include a number of new items.

Retaining much of its predecessor's content, the sixth edition of the *TNM Classification* [7] again featured only small revisions but was elaborated upon in a third edition of the *TNM Supplement* [8].

The *TNM Classification*'s seventh edition [9] saw the inclusion of several novel tumour classifications. While comments on the new entities and modifications concerned had been published elsewhere [10], it was nevertheless deemed important to highlight and examine these with a fourth edition of the *TNM Supplement* [11].

In the current, eighth edition of the *TNM Classification* [12], the featured tumour sites are much the same as those found in the book's previous edition. Some hitherto unexamined tumour entities and anatomic sites have, however, been introduced, while others have seen their analyses modified and revised to take account of new data on prognosis and prognosis assessment [13]. This strategy is in accord with the core philosophy of maintaining the classification system's stability over time.

A new approach was adopted in the *TNM Classification*'s seventh edition [9] that helped to distinguish stages from prognostic groupings. This has been expanded upon in the eighth edition, which introduces new clinical and pathological stages for some tumour entities. Additionally, a helpful overview of prognostic factors for different tumour entities has been given. These prognostic factor grids are based on former publications of the UICC and have been expanded to reflect new data [14–16].

This fifth edition of the *TNM Supplement* contains a number of changes. While the previous edition's contents have been largely preserved, feedback from users of the TNM classification and the TNM Help Desk (https://www.uicc. org/tnm-help-desk) has helped to refine and clarify certain elements. Two chapters of 'Explanatory Notes' have, for example, been reworked so that anatomical sites and subsites, regional lymph nodes, and T, N and M categories are more precisely defined. Elsewhere, a chapter discussing 'Pending Questions and Problems' has been added, while the minimum requirements for the pathological classification of individual tumour sites and entities are now described in a chapter on 'Site-Specific Requirements for pT and pN'.

Since the publication of the eighth edition of the *TNM Classification*, the UICC TNM Project Committee has reviewed several recommended changes and amendments, the details of which are outlined in this *TNM Supplement*'s fourth and fifth chapters, entitled 'New TNM Classifications Recommended for Testing and Other Classifications' and 'Optional Proposals for Testing New Subcategories of TNM', respectively. Relevant references have been included wherever data exist to support these recommendations. Where they do not, it may be assumed that such proposals are based on either anecdotal experience or more general considerations. All proposals included are based on the principle of ramification, whereby the T, N and M categories featured in the *TNM Classification*, eighth edition, remain unchanged but optional subdivisions are provided within specific categories. After classifying according to these subdivisions, one may determine to what extent a change of the present categories improves the classification process with respect to prognostic statements or the choice of treatment.

In light of the development of new techniques in molecular biology, the most important and widely used methods of enhancing the accuracy of the TNM classification system have also been presented here. Furthermore, several authors have emphasized that, in the current era of evidence-based medicine, future amendments must be substantiated with data [13, 17]. Others have raised questions regarding the use and interpretation of TNM in specific situations. These, along with informative answers, can be found in the sixth chapter of this supplement: 'Frequently Asked Questions'.

The present stage groupings – as defined in the *TNM Classification*, eighth edition [12] – are generally based on the anatomical extent of disease, represented by T, N and M or pT, pN and pM. For some tumour sites or entities, however, additional factors are included. These are as follows:

| | |
|---|---|
| Histologic type | Thyroid |
| Age | Thyroid |
| Grade | Gastrointestinal neuroendocrine tumours |
| | Appendix carcinoma |
| | Bone |
| | Soft tissues |
| Mitotic rate | GIST |
| Tumour markers | Testis |

- For oesophageal carcinoma (excluding the anatomical stage), an additional prognostic grouping is provided to encompass squamous cell carcinoma and adenocarcinoma. This group takes into account grade and – for squamous cell carcinoma – location.
- For gestational trophoblastic tumours, a prognostic grouping is provided that considers T/pT, M/pM and relevant risk factors.
- As more non-anatomic prognostic factors become available, this approach may provide a means of separating extent-of-disease staging from prognostic grouping.

Both the AJCC and the TNM Project Committee of the UICC recognize that, in addition to the anatomical extent of disease pre- and post-initial treatment, the residual tumour status after treatment – i.e. the R (residual tumour) classification – and other non-anatomical factors (e.g. host factors, biochemical markers, DNA analysis, oncogenes, oncogene products) may be important when estimating outcome. TNM and R aside, these prognostic factors are currently under investigation and it can be assumed that their roles in treatment planning, analysis of treatment and design of future clinical trials will grow.

The eighth edition of the *TNM Classification* [12] contains rules of classification and staging that correspond to those in the eighth edition of 2017's AJCC *Cancer Staging Manual* [18] and have approval of all national TNM committees.

Institutions and physicians interested in the further development of the TNM system are encouraged to test the recommendations included in this supplement. These may concern the ramification of existing classifications or the classification of new tumour sites and entities. Equally, they may concern methods of enhancing the accuracy of the TNM system over the years to come. Publication of both retrospective and prospective studies is desired. The TNM Project Committee would appreciate receiving relevant information and is available to provide further details and consultation.

The TNM Prognostic Factors Project welcomes comments from TNM users.

Union for International Cancer Control (UICC)
31–33 Avenue Giuseppe Motta, CH-1202 Geneva, Switzerland
F: +41 22 809 1810     http://www.uicc.org

*Christian Wittekind, Leipzig, Germany*
*James D. Brierley, Toronto, Canada*
*Anne Lee, Hong Kong, China*
*Elisabeth van Eycken, Brussels, Belgium*

# References

[1] UICC (International Union Against Cancer) *TNM Classification of Malignant Tumours*, 4th edn, Hermanek P, Sobin LH (eds). Berlin, Heidelberg, New York: Springer; 1987.

[2] UICC (International Union Against Cancer) *TNM Classification of Malignant Tumours*, 4th edn, 2nd revision, Hermanek P, Sobin LH (eds). Berlin, Heidelberg, New York: Springer; 1992.

[3] American Joint Committee on Cancer (AJCC) *AJCC Manual for Staging of Cancer*, 4th edn, Beahrs OH, Henson DE, Hutter RVP, et al. (eds). Philadelphia: Lippincott; 1992.

[4] UICC (International Union Against Cancer) *TNM Supplement 1993: A Commentary on Uniform Use*, Hermanek P, Henson DE, Hutter RVP, Sobin LH (eds). Berlin, Heidelberg, New York: Springer; 1993.

[5] UICC (International Union Against Cancer) *TNM Classification of Malignant Tumours*, 5th edn, Sobin LH, Wittekind Ch (eds). New York: Wiley; 1997.

[6] UICC (International Union Against Cancer) *TNM Supplement 2001: A Commentary on Uniform Use*, 2nd edn, Wittekind C, Henson DE, Hutter RVP, Sobin LH (eds). New York: Wiley; 2001.

[7] UICC (International Union Against Cancer) *TNM Classification of Malignant Tumours*, 6th edn, Sobin LH, Wittekind Ch. (eds). New York: Wiley; 2002.

[8]　UICC (International Union Against Cancer) *TNM Supplement: A Commentary on Uniform Use*, 3rd edn, Wittekind C, Henson DE, Hutter RVP, Sobin LH (eds). New York: Wiley; 2003.

[9]　Sobin LH, Gospodarowicz MK, Wittekind C (eds), *TNM Classification of Malignant Tumours*, 7th edn. Oxford: Blackwell Publishing Ltd; 2010.

[10]　Sobin LH, Compton CC. TNM seventh edition: what's new, what's changed. *Cancer* 2010; 116:5336–5339.

[11]　UICC (Union for International Cancer Control) *TNM Supplement: A Commentary on Uniform Use*, 4th edn, Wittekind C, Compton CC, Brierley J, Sobin LH (eds). Oxford: Wiley-Blackwell; 2012.

[12]　UICC (Union for International Cancer Control) *TNM Classification of Malignant Tumours*, 8th edn, Brierley JD, Gospodarowicz MK, Wittekind C (eds). Oxford: Wiley-Blackwell; 2017.

[13]　Gospodarowicz MK, Miller D, Groome PA, et al. The process for continuous improvement of the TNM classification. *Cancer* 2004; 100:1–5.

[14]　UICC (Union for International Cancer Control) *Prognostic Factors in Cancer*, Hermanek P, Gospodarowicz MK, Henson DE, et al. (eds). Berlin, Heidelberg, New York: Springer; 1995.

[15]　UICC (Union for International Cancer Control) *Prognostic Factors in Cancer*, 2nd edn, Gospodarowicz MK, Henson DE, Hutter RVP, et al. (eds). New York: Wiley; 2001.

[16]　UICC (Union for International Cancer Control) *Prognostic Factors in Cancer*, 3rd edn, Gospodarowicz MK, O'Sullivan B, Sobin LH (eds). New York: Wiley; 2006.

[17]　Quirke P, Cuvelier C, Ensari A, et al. Evidence-based medicine: the time has come to set standards for staging. *J Pathol* 2010; 221:357–360, correspondence 361–362.

[18]　American Joint Committee on Cancer (AJCC) *Cancer Staging Manual*, 8th edn, Amin MB, Edge SB, Greene FL, et al. (eds). New York: Springer; 2017.

# ORGANIZATIONS ASSOCIATED WITH THE TNM SYSTEM

CDC    Centers for Disease Control and Prevention (USA)
FIGO    International Federation of Gynaecology and Obstetrics
IACR    International Association of Cancer Registries
IARC    International Agency for Cancer Research
IASLC    International Association for the Study of Lung Cancer
ICCR    International Collaboration on Cancer Reporting
WHO    World Health Organization

# NATIONAL COMMITTEES

| | |
|---|---|
| Australia and New Zealand: | National TNM Committee |
| Austria, Germany, Switzerland: | Deutschsprachiges TNM-Komitee |
| Belgium: | National TNM Committee |
| Brazil: | National TNM Committee |
| Canada: | National Staging Steering Committee |
| China: | National TNM Cancer Staging Committee of China |
| Denmark: | National TNM Committee |
| Gulf States: | TNM Committee |
| India: | National TNM Committee |
| Israel: | National Cancer Staging Committee |
| Italy: | Italian Prognostic Systems Project |
| Japan: | Japanese Joint Committee |
| Latin America and Caribbean: | Sociedad Latinoamericana y del Caribe de Oncología Médica |
| Netherlands: | National Staging Committee |
| Poland: | National Staging Committee |
| Singapore: | National Staging Committee |
| Spain: | National Staging Committee |
| South Africa: | National Staging Committee |
| Turkey: | Turkish National Cancer Staging Committee |
| United Kingdom: | National Staging Committee |
| United States of America: | American Joint Committee on Cancer |

## Members of UICC Committees Associated with the TNM System

In 1950, the UICC appointed a Committee on Tumour Nomenclature and Statistics. In 1954, this committee became known as the Committee on Clinical Stage Classification and Applied Statistics and, in 1966, it was renamed the Committee on TNM Classification. With new prognostic factors taken into consideration, the committee was renamed twice more, becoming the TNM Prognostic Factors Project Committee in 1994 and then the TNM Prognostic Factors Core Group in 2003.

### UICC TNM Prognostic Factors Core Group: 2018

| | |
|---|---|
| Asamura, H. | Japan |
| Brierley, J.D. | Canada |
| Brookland, R.K. | USA |
| Gospodarowicz, M.K. | Canada |
| Lee, A. | China |
| Mason, M. | UK |
| O'Sullivan, B. | Canada |
| Van Eycken, E. | Belgium |
| Wittekind, Ch. | Germany |

# ACKNOWLEDGEMENTS

The editors appreciate the advice and assistance received from the members of the UICC TNM Prognostic Factors Core Group, the national TNM Committees and the Surveillance, Epidemiology and End Results (SEER) Program of the National Cancer Institute (USA).

We thank Professor Patti Groome and Ms Colleen Webber for supervising and performing the literature watch from its inception until 2015 and 2016, respectively and subsequently Dr. Malcolm Mason and Ms. Bernadette Coles. The fifth edition of the *TNM Supplement* is the result of a number of consultative meetings organized and supported by the UICC and AJCC secretariats.

This publication was made possible by grants *1U58DP001818* and *1U58DP004965* from the Centers for Disease Control and Prevention (CDC) (USA). Its contents are solely the responsibility of the authors and do not necessarily represent the official views of the CDC.

The authors are grateful for comments, additions and questions from Ramon Rami-Porta, Mary Gospodarowicz and Brian O'Sullivan.

The Union for International Cancer Control (UICC) provided encouragement and support and its secretariat arranged meetings and facilitated communications.

# ABBREVIATIONS

| | |
|---|---|
| a | autopsy, p. 23 |
| c | clinical, p. 1 |
| G | histopathological grading, p. 26 |
| ICD-O | International Classification of Diseases for Oncology, 3rd edition, 2000 |
| ITC | isolated tumour cells, p. 10 |
| L | lymphatic invasion, p. 24 |
| m | multiple tumours, pp. 5 and 20 |
| M | distant metastasis, p. 11 |
| N | regional lymph node metastasis, p. 9 |
| p | pathological, p. 1 |
| Pn | perineural invasion, p. 24 |
| r | recurrent tumour, p. 21 |
| R | residual tumour after treatment, p. 15 |
| sn | sentinel lymph node, p. 11 |
| Stage | anatomical Stage, p. 13 |
| T | extent of primary tumour, p. 7 |
| V | venous invasion, p. 24 |
| y | classification after initial multimodality treatment, p. 20 |

**Substantial changes in the 2019 fifth edition compared with the 2012 fourth edition are marked by a bar at the left-hand side of the page.**

CHAPTER 1

# EXPLANATORY NOTES – GENERAL

## The General Rules of the TNM System

### General Rule No. 1
**All cases should be confirmed microscopically as malignant tumours including histological type. Any cases not so proved must be reported separately.**

Microscopically unconfirmed cases can be staged, but should be analysed separately.

### Examples
Microscopic confirmation of choriocarcinoma is not required if the serum/urine βHCG level is abnormally elevated.
Microscopic confirmation of hepatocellular carcinoma is not required if the serum AFP level is abnormally elevated in the presence of characteristic radiological appearance.

### General Rule No. 2 (Table 1.1)
**Two classifications are described for each site, namely:**
(a) *Clinical classification:* the pre-treatment clinical classification designated TNM (or cTNM) is used to select and evaluate therapy. This is based on evidence acquired before treatment. Such evidence is based on physical examination, imaging, endoscopy, biopsy, surgical exploration and other relevant examinations.
(b) *Pathological classification:* the post-surgical histopathological classification, designated pTNM, is used to guide adjuvant therapy and provides additional data to estimate prognosis and calculate end results. This is based on evidence acquired before treatment, supplemented or modified by additional evidence acquired from surgery and from pathological examination.

*TNM Supplement: A Commentary on Uniform Use*, Fifth Edition.
Edited by Christian Wittekind, James D. Brierley, Anne Lee and Elisabeth van Eycken.
© 2019 UICC. Published 2019 by John Wiley & Sons Ltd.

**Table 1.1** Definitions of various TNM terms

---

**Definitions**

1. **Cancer stage** (a noun) – 'the stage'
   The UICC has defined the term 'stage' as the anatomical extent of disease (UICC 8th edition [2, 3]).

2. **Cancer staging** (a verb) – 'to stage'
   It refers to the process of deriving the 'stage'. This includes the investigational work-up, most usually examination and imaging studies, or, alternatively, verifying or consulting the T, N and M category definitions and combinations.

3. **Stage migration**
   The term 'stage migration' describes a change in the proportion of T, N or M categories following introduction of new means of assessing disease extent in populations of patients rather than in individual patients.

4. **Stage shift**
   The term 'stage shift' describes a change in the pattern of stage distribution within a defined population to a lower stage following the introduction of early detection or screening programs, or to a higher stage when access to care becomes limited.

5. **Downstaging/downsizing/upstaging/understaging**
   - The term 'downstaging' is used to describe a reduction in the T or N category after neoadjuvant therapy.
   - The term 'downsizing' is used to describe a reduction in size of the tumour after neoadjuvant therapy.
   - The terms 'upstaging' and 'understaging' are occasionally used, and typically relate to different diagnostic accuracy of various staging investigations. We do not recommend their use.

---

The pathological assessment of the regional lymph nodes (pN) entails removal of at least one lymph node to validate the absence or presence of cancer. It is not necessary to pathologically confirm the status of the highest N category to assign the pN. The assignment of the regional lymph nodes (pN) requires pathological assessment of the primary tumour (pT), except in cases of an unknown primary (T0).

An excisional biopsy of a lymph node without assessment of the pT category is insufficient to fully evaluate the pN category and is considered a clinical classification.

**Example**
The examination of axillary lymph nodes (sentinel lymph node or non-sentinel lymph nodes) with only a biopsy diagnosis of the primary tumour in the breast is classified as cN, e.g. cN1, if there are metastases in movable ipsilateral level I, II axillary lymph node(s).

**The pathological assessment of distant metastasis (pM1) entails micro-scopic examination.**

TNM is a dual system that includes a clinical (pre-treatment or after neoadju-vant radio-/chemo-/radiochemotherapy but before surgery) and a pathological (post-surgical histopathological) classification. It is imperative to differentiate between them since they are based on different methods of examination and serve different purposes. The clinical classification is designated TNM or cTNM; the pathological, pTNM. When TNM is used without a prefix, it implies the clinical classification (cTNM). Microscopic confirmation does not in itself justify the use of pT. The requirements for pathological classification are described in Chapter 3 on page 157.

Biopsy provides the diagnosis, including histological type and grade (if possible). The clinical assessment of tumour size should not be based on the biopsy.

In general, the cTNM is the basis for the choice of treatment and the pTNM is the basis for prognostic assessment. In addition, the pTNM determines adjuvant treatment. Comparison between cTNM and pTNM can help in evaluating the accuracy of the clinical and imaging methods used to determine the cTNM. Therefore, it is important to retain the clinical as well as the pathological classification in the medical record.

A tumour is primarily described by the clinical classification before treatment or before the decision not to treat. In addition, a pathological classification is performed if specific requirements are met (see Chapter 3, page 157). Therefore, for an individual patient there should be a clinical classification, e.g. cT2cN1cM0 and a pathological classification pT2pN2cM0.

**Note.**
The various T, N and M categories as well as the categories of optional classifications like R, L, V, G should be written as common Arabic numerals, not as subscripts, e.g. T1 (not $T_1$) and N3 (not $N_3$). Stages are designated by Roman numerals.

## General Rule No. 3
**After assigning cT, cN and cM and/or pT, pN and pM categories, these may be grouped into stages. The TNM classification and stages, once established, must remain unchanged in the medical records. The clinical stage is essential to select and evaluate therapy, while the pathological stage provides the most precise data to estimate prognosis and calculate end results.**

The rule that the TNM classification, once established, must remain unchanged in the patient's record applies to the definitive TNM classification determined just before initiation of treatment or before making the decision not to treat.

If, for instance, the initial classification cT2cN0cM0 is made in one hospital and is later updated to cT2cN1cM0 after the patient is referred to another center where special imaging techniques are available, then the latter classification, based on a special examination, is considered the definitive one.

Following two surgical procedures for a single lesion, the pTNM classification should be a composite of the histological examination of the specimens from both operations.

### Example

Initial endoscopic polypectomy of a carcinoma of the ascending colon is classified pT1pNXcM0; the subsequent right hemicolectomy contains two regional lymph nodes with tumour and a suspicious metastatic focus in the liver, later found to be a haemangioma, is excised: pT0pN1cM0. The definitive pTNM classification consists of the results of both operative specimens: pT1pN1bcM0 (Stage IIIA).

If an initial local excision of a rectal carcinoma is performed and the margins are positive the stage may be pT1pNXcM0, R1.

If radiotherapy is given, followed by anterior resection and there is no residual disease, the stage is ypT0pN0cM0, R0.

The definitive classification is ypT0pN0cM0, R0.

### Note.

Assignment of the 'y' as an additional descriptor for cases involving multimodality therapy is described on page 20.

For an estimation of the final stage, clinical and pathological data may be combined when only partial information is available in either the pathological classification or the clinical classification. See examples below.

It is important to note that the category is defined by whether it is determined clinically or pathologically. Stage should not be assigned as is not clinical or pathological.

However, for surveillance purposes stage data are lost if clinical and pathological data are not combined when only partial information is available either in the clinical classification or pathological classification. The term harmonized stage, hTNM, has been proposed.

### Example

A CT scan reveals a bladder cancer but there is no evidence of lymph node metastasis and the clinical stage is cT3bcN0cM0, cStage IIIA. A cystectomy is performed and the pT category is pT2 but there are no lymph nodes in the specimen so the pN category is pNX. The stage is therefore pT2bpNXcM0 and a pathological stage cannot be assigned but a combined harmonized stage group can be assigned as hStage II.

'X' denotes the absence or uncertainty of assigning a given category (T or N) when all reasonable clinical or pathological methods of assessment have been used or are unavailable to assess the patient. 'X' should not be used to simply fill in the blanks when data are unavailable to one individual on the assessment team. For further discussion on the meaning and application of X (e.g. NX) see Greene et al. [1].

## General Rule No. 4
**If there is doubt concerning the correct T, N or M category to which a particular case should be allotted, then the lower (i.e. less advanced) category should be chosen. This will also be reflected in the stages.**

### Example
Sonography of the liver: suspicious lesion but no definitive evidence of metastasis - assign cM0 (not cM1).

If there are conflicting results from different methods, the classification should be based on the most reliable method of assessment.

### Example
Colorectal carcinoma, pre-operative examination of the liver: sonography, suspicious, but no evidence of metastasis; CT, evidence of metastasis. The results of CT determine the classification: cM1. If a biopsy is performed and metastases are confirmed, then it would be classified as pM1. However, if CT were negative, the case would be classified cM0.

## General Rule No. 5
**In the case of multiple simultaneous tumours in one organ, the tumour with the highest T category should be classified and the multiplicity or the number of tumours should be indicated in parentheses, e.g. T2(5) or T2(m). In simultaneous bilateral cancers of paired organs, each tumour should be classified independently. In tumours of the liver (HCC), intrahepatic bile ducts (ICC) as well as ovary and fallopian tube, multiplicity is a criterion of T classification.**

The following apply to *grossly* recognizable multiple primary simultaneous carcinomas at the same site. They do not apply to one grossly detected tumour associated with multiple separate microscopic foci.

1. Multiple synchronous tumours in one organ may be:
   a) Multiple non-invasive tumours
   b) Multiple invasive tumours
   c) Multiple invasive tumours with associated non-invasive tumours (carcinoma in situ)

d) A single invasive tumour with an associated non-invasive tumour (carcinoma in situ)

For (a) the multiplicity should be indicated by the suffix '(m)', e.g. Tis(m).

For (b) and (c) the tumour with the highest T category is classified and the multiplicity or the number of invasive tumours is indicated in parentheses, e.g. T2(4) or T2(m).

For (c) and (d) the presence of an associated carcinoma in situ may be indicated by the suffix '(is)', e.g. T3(m, is) or T2(3, is) or T2(is).

2. For classification of multiple simultaneous tumours in 'one' organ, the tumours at these sites with the highest T category should be classified and the multiplicity of the number of tumours should be indicated in parentheses, e.g. T2(5) or T2(m).

Combining multiple carcinomas of skin should be done only with subsites (C44.5-7 or C63.2) [3]. Carcinomas of the skin of the head and neck should only be combined with carcinomas of the skin of the head and neck. A carcinoma of the skin in subsite C44.3 and a synchronous one in subsites C44.6 and C44.7 should be classified as synchronous tumours.

Examples of sites for separate classifications of two tumours are:
- Oropharynx and hypopharynx
- Submandibular gland and parotid gland
- Urinary bladder and urethra (separate tumours)
- Skin carcinoma of the eyelid and skin carcinoma of the head and neck, since both have their own classifications

Examples for classification of the tumour with the highest T category and indication of multiplicity (m symbol) or numbers of tumours:
- Two separate tumours of the hypopharynx
- Skin carcinoma of the abdominal wall and the back (both part of the trunk)

Cancer Registries have their own rules to decide on multiple tumours in order to improve comparability and uniformity in cancer incidence reporting. These rules should be clearly documented when reporting.

For tumours of the colon or rectum in different localizations it is recommended to classify those tumours separately; e.g. a carcinoma of the ascending colon and one of the sigmoid colon should be classified separately, particularly because the regional lymph nodes are defined differently (see *TNM Classification of Malignant Tumours*, 8th edition [2], pages 73–74).

Second or subsequent primary cancers occurring in the same organ or in different organs after initial treatment are staged independently and are known as metachronuous primary tumours. Such cancers are not staged using the prefix 'y'.

For systemic or multicentric cancers potentially involving many discrete organs, four histological groups – malignant lymphomas, leukemias, Kaposi sarcoma and mesothelioma – are included. They are counted only once in any individual.

A tumour in the same organ with a different histologic type is counted as a new tumour, e.g. lung carcinomas (see page 88).

# The TNM Clinical and Pathological Classifications

## T/pT Classification

1. When size is a criterion for the T/pT category, it is a measurement of the invasive component. If in the breast, for example, there is a large in situ component (e.g. 4 cm) and a small invasive component (e.g. 0.5 cm), the tumour is coded for the invasive component only, i.e. pT1a.

2. Neither in the TNM Classification nor in the 1st [5] to 4th edition [6–8] of the TNM Supplement are there any statements concerning the way to measure tumour size for pT classification. According to the AJCC *Cancer Staging Manual*, 2017 [3], 'pT is derived from the actual measurement of the unfixed tumour in the surgical specimen. It should be noted, however, that up to 30% shrinkage of soft tissues may occur in the resected specimen'. Thus, in cases of discrepancies of clinically and pathologically measured tumour size, the clinical measurement should also be considered for the pT classification.

   In some cases, especially with those tumour entities where size is important for the pT category, it may be necessary to correlate the macroscopic size (fixed or infixed) with the microscopic size. A thorough calculation of the latter should be the basis for the size calculation.

3. Penetration or perforation of visceral serosa is a criterion for the T classification of some tumour sites, e.g. stomach, colon, rectum, liver (HCC and ICC), gallbladder, lung, ovary. It may be confirmed by histological examination of biopsies or resection specimens or by cytological examination of specimens obtained by scraping the serosa overlying the primary tumour.

4. The microscopic presence of a tumour in lymphatic vessels or veins does not qualify as local spread of the tumour and does not affect the cT/pT category (except for liver (HCC and ICC), testis, kidney and penis). It can be recorded separately (*TNM Classification*, 8th edition, page 10 [2]).

5. A tumour in perineural spaces at the primary site is considered part of the T classification, but can also be recorded separately as Pn1 (*TNM Classification*, 8th edition, [2], page 10), as it may be an independent prognostic factor.

**Example**
In carcinoma of the uterine cervix, direct invasion beyond the myometrium of the uterine cervix qualifies as parametrial invasion with T2a/b, but not if based only on the discontinuous presence of tumour cells in lymphatics of the parametrium. The L (lymphatic invasion) and V (venous invasion) symbols (*TNM Classification*, 8th edition [2], page 10) can be used in this case to record lymphatic and venous involvement.

6. Direct spread of tumour into an adjacent organ, e.g. the liver from a gastric primary, is recorded in the T/pT classification and is not considered to be distant metastasis.
   Direct spread of the primary tumour into regional lymph nodes is classified as lymph node metastasis.
7. The very uncommon cases with direct extension into an adjacent organ or structure not mentioned in the T definitions are classified as the highest T category.
8. Tumour spillage during surgery is considered a criterion in the T classification of tumours of ovary, Fallopian tube and primary peritoneal carcinoma. For all other tumours, tumour spillage does not affect the TNM classification or stages.

**Note.**
In tumours of the uterus (endometrium) positive cytology should be reported separately without change of the stage.

## Regional Lymph Nodes

1. If a tumour involves more than one site or subsite, e.g., contiguous extension to another site or subsite, the regional lymph nodes include those of all involved sites and subsites.

**Example**
Carcinoma of the sigmoid colon involving the small intestine (jejunum): the regional lymph nodes are those for the sigmoid colon, i.e. the sigmoid, left colic, superior rectal (haemorrhoidal), inferior mesenteric and rectosigmoid as well as those for the small intestine, i.e. the mesenteric nodes including the superior mesenteric nodes.

2. In rare cases, one finds no metastases in the regional lymph nodes, but only in lymph nodes that drain an adjacent organ directly invaded by the primary tumour. The lymph nodes of the invaded site are considered regional as those of the primary site for N classification.

### Example

Carcinoma of the stomach with direct extension into an adjacent small bowel loop: perigastric lymph nodes are tumour-free, but metastases of 0.5 cm size are found in two mesenteric lymph nodes in the vicinity of the invaded small bowel – this is classified as pT4bpN1M0 (Stage IIIC) for cancer of the stomach.

## N/pN Classification

1. The clinical category N0 ('no regional lymph node metastasis') includes lymph nodes not clinically suspicious for metastasis even if they are palpable or visualized with imaging techniques. The clinical category N1 ('regional lymph node metastasis') is used when there is sufficient clinical evidence, such as firmness, enlargement or specific imaging characteristics. The term 'adenopathy' is not precise enough to indicate lymph node metastasis and should be avoided.

2. Size of lymph nodes: in advanced lymphatic spread, one often finds perinodal tumour and the confluence of several lymph node metastases into one large tumour conglomerate. In the definition of the N classification, the perinodal component should be included in the size for isolated lymph node metastasis; for conglomerates, the overall size of the conglomerate should be considered and not only the size of the individual lymph nodes.

3. Direct extension of the primary tumour into lymph nodes is classified as lymph node metastasis.

4. Tumour deposits (satellites) are discrete macroscopic or microscopic nodules of cancer in the lymph drainage area of a primary carcinoma that are discontinuous from the primary carcinoma and without histological evidence of residual lymph node or identifiable vascular or neural structures. If a vessel is identifiable on H&E, elastic or other stains, it should be classified as venous invasion (V1/2) or lymphatic invasion (L1). Similarly, if neural structures are identifiable, the lesion should be classified as perineural invasion (Pn1). The presence of tumour deposits does not change the T categories of the primary tumour. This rule is to be followed particularly in tumours of the colon and rectum as well as in tumours of the appendix and may be applicable to other tumour sites.

5. The reliability of the pN classification depends on the number of histologically examined regional lymph nodes. Thus, it is recommended to add the number of examined and involved lymph nodes in parentheses to the pN category, e.g. in colorectal tumours pN1b (3/15).

   For the various organs the number of lymph nodes ordinarily included in the lymph node dissection specimen is stated. If the lymph nodes are negative, but the number ordinarily examined is not met, pN0 is classified. The addition of the number of lymph nodes (in colon tumours, e.g. 0/4) characterizes the reliability of the pN classification.

6. Metastasis in any lymph node other than regional is classified as a distant metastasis. If there is doubt concerning the correct category to which a particular case should be allotted, then the lower (i.e. less advanced) category should be chosen.

7. When size is a criterion for pN classification, measurement is made of the metastasis, not of an entire lymph node. However, for the cN classification only, the overall size of the lymph node should be considered.

8. Invasion of lymphatic vessels (tumour cells in endothelium-lined channels, so-called lymphangiosis carcinomatosa or lymphangitic spread) in a distant organ is coded as pM1, e.g. lymphangitic spread in the lung from prostate carcinoma or liver cell carcinoma.

9. Cases with micrometastasis only, i.e. no metastasis larger than 0.2 cm, can be identified by the addition of '(mi)', e.g. pN1(mi) or pN2(mi). If deposits of tumour cells are 0.2 mm or smaller they are likely to be considered isolated tumour cells (see below).

10. Isolated tumour cells (ITC) are single tumour cells or small clusters of cells not more than 0.2 mm in greatest extent that can be detected by routine H and E stains or immunohistochemistry. An additional criterion has been proposed to include a cluster of fewer than 200 cells in a single histological cross-section [10]. The same applies to cases with findings suggestive of tumour cells or their components by non-morphologic techniques such as flow cytometry or DNA analysis. ITCs may be apparent with routine histological stains as well as with immunohistochemical methods. ITCs do not typically show evidence of metastatic activity (e.g. proliferation or stromal reaction) or penetration of lymphatic sinus walls.

The following classification of isolated tumour cells was published in the 6th edition of the TNM booklet [10] following a communication by the UICC in 1999 [11]. These cases with ITC in regional lymph nodes should be analysed separately since the prognostic importance of those ITC cases is not yet clear.

   Cases with ITC cells in lymph nodes or at distant sites should be classified as cN0 or cM0. The exceptions are in malignant melanoma of the skin [12, 13] and in Merkel cell carcinoma, where ITC in a lymph node are classified as N1/pN1 [3]. These cases should be analysed separately.

The classification is as follows:

(p)N0        No regional lymph node metastasis histologically, no examination for isolated tumour cells (ITC)

(p)N0(i–)    No regional lymph node metastasis histologically, negative morphological findings for ITC (p)N0(i+)   No regional lymph node metastasis histologically, positive morphological findings for ITC

(p)N0(mol-)   No regional lymph node metastasis histologically, negative non-morphological findings for ITC

(p)N0(mol+)   No regional lymph node metastasis histologically, positive non-morphological findings for ITC

**Note.**
This approach is consistent with TNM General Rule No. 4.

## Sentinel Lymph Node
*Definition*

The sentinel lymph node is the first lymph node to receive lymphatic drainage from a primary tumour. If it contains metastatic tumour this indicates that other lymph nodes may contain tumour. If it does not contain metastatic tumour, other lymph nodes are unlikely to contain tumour. Occasionally, there is more than one sentinel lymph node.

   The following designations are applicable when sentinel lymph node assessment is attempted following resection of the primary tumour:

(p)NX (sn)   Sentinel lymph node could not be assessed

(p)N0 (sn)   No sentinel lymph node metastasis

(p)N1 (sn)   Sentinel lymph node metastasis

Excisional biopsy of a sentinel node, in the absence of assignment of a pT, is classified as a clinical N, e.g. cN1(sn).

   Cases with or examined for isolated tumour cells (ITC) in sentinel lymph nodes can be classified as follows:

(p)N0 (i-)(sn)   No sentinel lymph node metastasis histologically, negative morphological findings for ITC

(p)N0 (i+)(sn)   No sentinel lymph node metastasis histologically, positive morphological findings for ITC

(p)N0 (mol-)(sn)   No sentinel lymph node metastasis histologically, negative non-morphological findings for ITC

(p)N0 (mol+)(sn)   No sentinel lymph node metastasis histologically, positive non-morphological findings for ITC

## M Classification
The MX category is considered to be inappropriate in the clinical assessment of TNM if metastasis can be evaluated based on physical examination alone. (The use of MX may result in exclusion from staging [2, 3, 14].)

**pM0 is only to be used after autopsies.**
**pMX is not a valid category.**

1. In tumours of the gastrointestinal tract, multiple tumour foci in the mucosa or submucosa ('skip metastasis') are not considered in the TNM classification and should not be classified as distant metastasis. They should be distinguished from synchronous tumours, for example those with obvious mucosal origin. The synchronous tumours are categorized as multiple primary tumours if appropriate, e.g. pT2(m).
2. Metastasis in any lymph node other than regional is classified as distant metastasis.
3. Invasion of lymphatic vessels (tumour cells in endothelium-lined channels, so-called lymphangiosis carcinomatosa or lymphangic spread) in a distant organ is coded as pM1, e.g. lymphangitic spread in the lung from prostatic carcinoma or liver cell carcinoma.
4. Positive cytology using conventional staining techniques from the peritoneal cavity based on laparoscopy or laparotomy before any other surgical procedure is classified as M1, except for primary tumours of the ovary and Fallopian tube, where it is classified in the T category. Data indicate that the worsening of prognosis as indicated by positive lavage cytology may have been overestimated [15–22]. Thus, it seems important to analyse such cases separately. For identification of cases with positive cytology from pleural or peritoneal washings or pleural effusions or ascites as the sole basis for M1, the addition of 'cy+' is recommended, e. g. cM1(cy+). In the R classification R1(cy+) may be used [11, 23, 24]
5. Micrometastasis, i.e. no metastasis larger than 0.2 cm, in viscera (lung, liver, etc.) or bone marrow can be identified by the addition of '(mi)', e.g. pM1(mi).
6. Isolated tumour cells found in bone marrow with morphological techniques are classified according to the scheme for N, e.g. cM0(i+). For non-morphologic findings 'mol' is used in addition to M0, e.g. cM0(mol+).

## Who Is Responsible for TNM Coding?

Data for TNM are derived from a variety of sources, e.g. the examining physician, the radiologist, the gastroenterologist, the operating surgeon and the histopathologist. The final TNM classification and/or stage rest with a designated individual physician who has access to the most complete data.

## The Significance of X

An X classification of an individual component of TNM or pTNM, e.g. TX or pNX, does not necessarily signify inadequate staging [1]. The practical value of staging in the individual situation is to be considered, e.g. in patients with distant metastasis an effort to assess N is without clinical significance. In selected pT1 tumours of the colorectum, pNX may be the result of the correct decision to treat by endoscopic polypectomy or local excision. Also, experience shows that – at least in some sites, e.g. colon and rectum – in T1/pT1 tumours of low grade and without lymphatic invasion (L0) the frequency of regional lymph node metastasis as well as of distant metastasis is exceptionally rare and therefore no supplementary efforts are needed to assess the N category and N0 is appropriate. However, if there is a reasonable possibility of nodal metastases and no nodes have been removed pNX is appropriate (for example a thyroidectomy for thyroid carcinoma with no nodes in the specimen). The M is assessed clinically, cM0.

## Stages

Although the anatomical extent of disease, as categorized by TNM, is a very powerful prognostic indicator in cancer, it is recognized that many other factors can have a significant impact on predicting outcomes (see factors listed in the 'Prognostic Factors Grid' supplied in the 8th edition of *TNM Classification of Malignant Tumours* [2]). Some have been incorporated into stages, as has grade in bone and soft tissue sarcomas and age in thyroid cancer. These classifications will be adapted in this edition according to the changes introduced in the 8th edition [2]. In the newly revised classifications for oesophagus carcinomas, *stage* has been maintained as defining the anatomical extent of disease and new *Pathological Prognostic Groups* that incorporate other prognostic factors, have been proposed.

1. The term 'stage' should be used only for combinations of T, N and M or pT, pN and pM categories. **The expressions 'T stage' and 'N stage' should be avoided**. It is correct to speak of T categories or N categories.
2. The stage can be determined exclusively according to the clinical classification (cTNM), exclusively according to the pathological classification (pTNM) or based on a combination of clinical and pathological findings (e.g. pT, pN and cM or pT, cN and cM or cT, cN and pM). If available, the pathological classifications are to be used for estimating stage.

### Examples

Pedunculated polyp of sigmoid colon discovered endoscopically, superficial biopsy: tubular adenoma with carcinoma in situ, endoscopically, no suspicion of invasion, no regional lymph node or distant metastasis. Clinical classification: cTiscN0cM0.

Endoscopic polypectomy: adenocarcinoma arising in a tubular adenoma invading the superficial stalk, with clear deep stalk. No further treatment. Pathological classification: pT1pNXcM0. Summarizing classification: pT1cN0cM0, stage I. This is justified because experience shows that regional lymph node metastasis and distant metastasis in pT1 are very rare.

*Primary tumour of head and neck:* clinical diagnosis of regional lymph node metastasis by CT, no sign of distant metastasis. Treatment by surgical local excision of the primary tumour and radiotherapy of cervical lymph nodes. Clinical classification – cT1cN1cM0. Pathological classification – pT1pNXcM0. Summarizing classification – pT1cN1cM0, stage III (except oropharynx – p16-positive, nasopharynx and thyroid).

3. In the assessment of distant metastases, the entire situation must be considered. If there is only a clinically determined cM1 in an organ that could not be microscopically examined, this finding must be taken into consideration.

**Example**
Colon carcinoma with multiple lung metastases (by radiography). Resection of the colon carcinoma because of stenosis – pT3pN2cM1a. Simultaneously, also local excision of an area suspicious for metastasis in liver, histologically found to be haemangioma. Final classification pT3pN2cM1a, stage IV.

4. In the definitions of stages 'any T' includes T0 and TX.

**Example**

| | |
|---|---|
| Breast carcinoma | cT0cN3cM0 = stage IIIC |
| Malignant melanoma of skin | pT0cN1cM0 = stage III |

5. If the T or N cannot be determined, stage grouping is possible under the following circumstances:

- Despite TX/pTX, stage can be defined on the basis of N and M or pN and pM findings.
  **Example**
  A firm head of pancreas with one grossly involved peripancreatic lymph node and no signs of distant metastasis at surgery – cTXcN1cM0, stage IIB.

- Despite NX/pNX, stage can be undertaken when M/pM classification is possible.
  **Example**
  A carcinoma of the pancreas with liver metastasis cT1cNXcM1, Stage IV. Cases with cM1 or pM1 are generally classified as stage IV even in cases of T/pTX and N/pNX.

- Despite NX/pNX, stage grouping is possible when a T category and M0 are provided.
  **Example**
  Squamous cell carcinoma of the oesophagus with invasion of trachea, regional lymph nodes not assessable, no signs of distant metastasis – cT4bcNXcM0, clinical stage IVA.

**Note.**

There are different stage proposals for squamous cell carcinomas and adeno-carcinomas of the oesophagus, both having a clinical stage and a pathological stage.

- Cases of Tis (clinical classification based on biopsy) or pTis (pathological classification based on the examination of the resected specimen) can be classified as stage 0, when combined with NX/pNX and cM0, because by definition no metastasis can be present.
- If substages (A, B, etc.) are designated in the list of stages, in most cases a summarizing definition of the stage is not included. If in such a situation a differentiation between the substages is not possible, often an assignment to the stage is possible and should be performed.

6. After neoadjuvant therapy, if the primary tumour has completely disappeared but lymph node metastasis remained, e.g. oesophagus squamous cell carcinoma, ypT0pN1cM0, the stage can be calculated by assuming that T equals the lowest category and the N essentially determines the stage, therefore pathological Stage IIB.

**Note.**

The AJCC introduced specific stages after neoadjuvant therapy for both squamous cell carcinomas and adenocarcinomas [3], where the above-mentioned case would be classified as Stage IIIA.

In the 8th edition of the *TNM Classification* [2], for some tumour entities clinical stages and pathological stages have been introduced with different definitions of the stages. Therefore, it should be clearly documented which stage was calculated. It must be further noted that the clinical stage and the pathological stage may not be comparable for different reasons.

## Residual Tumour (R) Classification

TNM and pTNM describe the anatomical extent of cancer in general without considering treatment. The residual tumour (R) classification deals with tumour status after treatment. It reflects the effects of treatment, influences further therapeutic procedures and is a strong predictor of prognosis.

In the R classification, not only is a local-regional residual tumour to be taken into consideration, but also as it was initially described, a distant residual tumour in the form of remaining distant metastasis. Variation in the clinical application of the R classification in different practice settings is discussed below.

R0 corresponds to clinical remission or resection for cure. It is appropriate for cases in which a residual tumour cannot be detected by any diagnostic means. The R0 status, therefore, does not exclude non-detectable residual tumours, which may give rise to tumour recurrence or metastasis during follow-up. R0, in fact, corresponds to no detectable residual tumour and may not be identical to cure.

R1 and R2 should be annotated to indicate which site is positive, e.g. if a colonic polypectomy margin is microscopically positive for cancer, it is R1 (colon). If the patient's subsequent colectomy margin has no tumour, it would change to R0 (colon) and if a liver metastasis was found at colectomy, and confirmed microscopically (but not removed surgically), it would be R2 (liver).

The R classification can be used following surgical treatment alone, after radiotherapy alone, after chemotherapy alone or following multimodal therapy. After non-surgical treatment, the presence or absence of a residual tumour is determined using clinical methods. Following surgical treatment, the R classification requires close cooperation between the surgeon and pathologist in a two-step process, illustrated in Figure 1.1.

In the R0 group there may be M0 cases as well as M1 cases. In the latter, the distant metastasis as well as the primary tumour must be removed completely.

### Example
pT3pN1cM1a colon cancer with resection for cure of both the primary tumour and a liver metastasis: R0 (colon); R0 (liver).

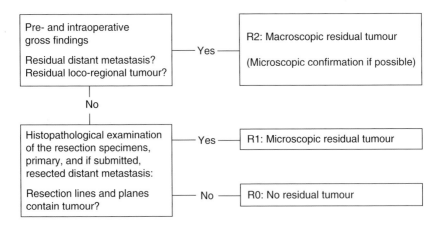

**Figure 1.1** R classification following surgery.

In a tumour specimen with a formal lymphadenectomy the 'marginal' lymph node is the one near the resection line that is most distant from the primary tumour. Involvement of such 'marginal' or 'apical' nodes or of a sentinel node does not influence the R classification unless an involved lymph node has been transected by the surgeon at the margin.

Difficulties may arise in the case of removal of the tumour in two or more parts and not 'en bloc'. Without an exact and reliable topographical orientation the pathologist cannot make a definitive assessment of the resection line. In this case the classification 'RX' (presence of residual tumour cannot be assessed) is appropriate.

The presence of non-invasive carcinoma (in situ) at the resection margin should be indicated by the suffix (is), e.g. R1(is).

### Example
Invasive carcinoma of the breast with associated in situ component. Breast preserving surgery, according to the surgeon, was complete. Histology showed:
(a) Invasive carcinoma at the resection margin: R1.
(b) Invasive carcinoma completely removed, but associated in situ component at the resection margin: R1(is).

'R0-Ablation' after radiofrequency ablation of liver metastasis: if after radiofrequency ablation of liver metastasis no residual tumour is found by clinical (including imaging) techniques, sometimes 'R0-ablation' has been used. Because the diagnosis 'R0' requires histopathological examination of a tumour resection specimen (primary tumour and/or distant metastasis) the correct designation in this situation is 'complete clinical response'.

Patients classified for residual tumour by conventional methods and those classified by new specialized methods cannot be compared. To prevent stage migration by refined diagnostic techniques, the methods used for R classification should be stated in the documentation and be considered in the analysis of treatment results [25].

In the R classification, the serum level of tumour markers is not considered.

Examination of resection specimens is done by conventional methods in histopathological processing of areas marked by the surgeon or areas suspicious by gross inspection. Besides these conventional methods some new techniques have been developed to refine the R classification. Examples of such methods are:

1. Imprint cytology of the resection margin (surface), introduced by Veronesi et al. [9] for breast cancer, but applicable to stomach cancer and other tumour types as well.

2. Cytologic examination of ascites or abdominal lavage fluid to detect metastasis on the peritoneum, which are not grossly recognizable. This was applied to gastric carcinoma [15, 16, 26]. In the R classification R1(cy+) may be used [24, 25].
3. Examination of bone marrow biopsies in patients without evidence of bone metastasis with monoclonal antibodies against cytokeratin. Such investigations have been described by Schlimok et al. [27] for gastric carcinomas and were reviewed by Pantel et al. [28] (see pages 10–12 regarding detection of isolated tumour cells and evidence of tumour by non-morphologic methods).

Although there have been proposals (see below) to code a tumour R1 if the tumour is 1 mm or less from the resection margin, only if the tumour is transected should R1 be used; otherwise it is R0.

According to the data from Erlangen Cancer Center (ECC) and Australia, R1 was only diagnosed if a tumour was demonstrated at the resection margins (tumour transected).

In recent years, an alternative definition of resection margin involvement has gained increasing acceptance, at first for the circumferential resection margin (CRM) in rectal cancer [29–31] but also for other resection margins and other tumour entities. These data strongly supported the following definitions:

1. CRM positive, tumour directly at the CRM or a minimal distance between the tumour and the CRM of $\leq 1$ mm.
2. CRM negative, a minimal distance between the tumour and the CRM $> 1$ mm.

This 'new' definition of tumour involvement has gained general acceptance in the United Kingdom [29–33]. It has been supported in the United States [34, 35].

Following a Total Mesorectal Excision (TME) in the management of rectal cancer it is recognized that the circumferential resection margin (CRM) is of great prognostic importance; hence instead of considering tumour within 1 mm of that margin as being R1, it can be classed as CRM positive.

In some practice settings around the world, particularly the USA [36], Canada and the UK, the R classification has been employed only in application to the primary tumour and its local or regional extent. Others have applied it more broadly to include distant metastasis.

With regard to the overall prognostic relevance of the R classification, distant metastasis should be included. This is in accordance with the original definition in 1977 [37].

Further confusion results from different definitions of resection margin involvement: direct involvement of the resection margin by a tumour or the minimal distance between a tumour and the resection margin of 1 mm or less.

To avoid confusion a proposal for an expanded uniform R classification has recently been published [24]. This proposal differentiated between the following categories:

RX      Presence of residual tumour cannot be assessed

R0>1 mm      No residual tumour, minimal distance between tumour and resection margin>1 mm

R0≤1 mm      No residual tumour, minimal distance between tumour and resection margin≤1 mm

R1-dir      Microscopic residual tumour, tumour directly at the resection margin (tumour transected)

R2a      Local macroscopic residual tumour

R2b      Distant macroscopic residual tumour

R2c      Macroscopic residual tumour in both sites

Further discussion of the R classification, including its application to leukemias and malignant lymphomas and after non-surgical treatment can be found in Wittekind et al. (2002) [23].

Following neoadjuvant therapy in the R classification only a viable tumour at the resection margin is considered. Scars, fibrotic areas, fibrotic nodules, granulation tissue, mucin lakes, etc., occurring at the resection margin do not qualify as R1.

## Definitions of Completeness of Resection

### R0(un)

Concerns have been expressed that the definition of complete resection conferring R0 status is too imprecise and that the application of General Rule No. 4 does not allow one to assess several features that may represent minimal residual disease and have an adverse prognostic influence. The category 'Uncertain resection' has been proposed for testing [38].

A new category, 'R0(un)', is proposed to document those other features that fall within the proposed category 'uncertain resection', i.e. no macroscopic or microscopic evidence of residual disease but any of the following reservations apply:

i) Nodal assessment has been based on less than the number of nodes/stations ordinarily included in a lymphadenectomy specimen.

ii) The highest mediastinal node removed/sampled is positive (for lung cancers).

In a recent paper the above proposals have been validated by another institution [39].

## Additional Descriptors

**For identification of special cases in the TNM or pTNM classification, the m, y, r and a symbols may be used. Although they do not affect the stage grouping, they indicate cases needing separate analysis.**

### m Symbol

The suffix m, in parenthesis, is used to indicate the presence of multiple primary tumours at a single site. See the TNM Rule No. 5 (page 5).

### y Symbol – Classifying Treated Tumours

cTNM is the pre-treatment clinical classification, based on evidence acquired before treatment. pTNM is the post-surgical histopathological classification, based on evidence acquired before treatment, supplemented or modified by additional evidence acquired from surgery and from pathological examination.

After multimodal therapy (neoadjuvant radio- and/or chemotherapy prior to surgery) the pathological assessment may be affected by possible tumour regression or other treatment effects. Thus, such a classification should be identified by the prefix 'y' to indicate that this classification has not the same reliability as the pTNM classification after surgery alone. The ypTNM classification deals with the extent of cancer after neoadjuvant therapy. Therefore, the ypTNM should consider only viable tumour cells and not signs of regressed tumour tissue such as necrotic cell debris, scars, fibrotic areas, fibrotic nodules, granulations tissue, mucin lakes, etc.

In analysing results, one should always differentiate between patients treated with primary surgery (cTNM, pTNM) and those treated by surgery following neoadjuvant treatment (ycTNM, ypTNM). Not only for the TNM categories but also for the stage grouping the 'y' symbol should be used (Stage yI, Stage yII, …; Stage ypI, Stage ypII, …).

After neoadjuvant treatment two additional stages could be used:

Stage y(p)0 = ypT0N0M0 and
Stage y(p)is = ypTisN0M0.

In contrast, after primary surgery, stage 0 is defined as pTisN0M0.

This differentiation is based on:
- the different prognosis of patients with yTNM and ypTNM,
- the different clinical consequences, in particular in the case of yT0, ypT0, stage y0.

After multimodal treatment histological grading may be unreliable and should not be used. It is recommended to add some information on the extent of histologic regression of tumours. For several sites tumour regression scoring systems, mostly semiquantitative, have been published.

Following neoadjuvant therapy, the extent of residual tumour found at resection reflects the response to the preceding therapy. Various proposals of describing the extent of tumour after therapy have been described.

It should be emphasized that there is no generally accepted regression grading system for all tumour entities. Table 1.2 addresses this issue on a site by site basis.

The AJCC has proposed the following to describe the response to neoadjuvant therapy for rectal carcinoma [34]. This scheme in a modified version has been recommended for several tumours of the digestive system.

**Note.**
However, this is a classification of response to treatment and not a stage classification.

| Description | Tumour Regression Score |
|---|---|
| No viable cancer cells | 0 (complete response) |
| Single cells or small groups of cancer cells | 1 (moderate response) |
| Residual cancer outgrown by fibrosis | 2 (minimal response) |
| Minimal or no tumour kill; extensive residual cancer | 3 (poor response) |

## Recurrent Tumour, r Symbol

The prefix 'r' is used for classification of recurrent tumours in terms of T, N and M. The use of stages is not appropriate for recurrent tumours. While TNM and pTNM without the prefix 'r' always characterize the first manifestation of a tumour, recurrences after curative treatment are described by rTNM or rpTNM. In this way a chronological TNM/pTNM documentation of the course of the disease may be created. An example of such a 'Pathogram' is shown in Table 1.3.

For the description of a recurrence in the area of the primary tumour the T categories can be used only in the case of recurrence on the anastomotic suture line after partial or total resection of an organ of the gastrointestinal tract.

It has been suggested that the r symbol can also be used after a period of observation without treatment. For example, it may be described to observe a patient with a cT1ccN0cM0 prostate cancer found on biopsy following identification for an elevated PSA. Subsequently, on restaging after a period of active surveillance, the carcinoma has progressed and now involves more than one half of a single lobe. The classification would be rcT2bcN0cM0.

**Table 1.2**  Proposed regression grading system

| Tumour site | Authors |
| --- | --- |
| Head and neck squamous Cell carcinoma | Braun et al. 1989 [40] Eich et al. 2008 [41] Hermann et al. 2001 [42] Wedemeyer et al. 2014 [43] |
| **For all gastrointestinal sites** | Werner and Höffler 2000 [44] |
| Oesophagus | Japanese Esophageal Society 2017 [45] Mandard et al. 1994 [46] Baldus et al. 2004 [47] Hermann et al. 2006 [48] |
| Stomach | Japanese Gastric Cancer Association 1998 [49] Becker et al. 1997, 2003 [50, 51] |
| Colon and rectum | Dworak et al. 1997 [52] Japanese Society for Classification of Cancer of Colon and Rectum (JSCCR) 1997 [53] Wheeler et al. 2002 [54] Ryan et al. 2005 [34] Williams et al. 2008 [55] Bateman et al. 2009 [56] |
| Anal canal | Klimpfinger et al. 1994 [57] |
| Liver | Adachi et al. 1999 [58] |
| Pancreas (ductal adenocarcinoma) | Evans et al. 1992 [59] |
| Lung | Junker et al. 2001 [60] Langner et al. 2003 [61] |
| Bone tumours/osteosarcoma | Salzer-Kuntschick et al. 1983 [62] Huvos 1991 [63] |
| Soft tissue tumours | Schmidt et al. 1993 [64] |
| Breast | Chevallier et al. 1993 [65] Sinn et al. 1994 [66] Sataloff et al. 1995 [67] Fisher et al. 2002 [68] Ogston et al. 2003 [69] Symmans et al. 2007 [70] (RCB System) |

**Table 1.3**  'Pathogram' of a patient with rectal carcinoma

| Date | Treatment | TNM/pTNM | R |
|---|---|---|---|
| April 2012 | Initial local excision of rectal carcinoma | pT1pNXM0 | R1 |
| July 2012 | Radiotherapy, followed by anterior resection | ypT0pN0M0 | R0 |
| October 2012 January 2013 April 2013 July 2013 | | cT0cN0cM0 | |
| January 2014 April 2014 July 2014 | | cT0cN0cM0 | |
| October 2016 | Liver tumour resection | rcT0cN0cM1 (liver) rcT0cN0pM1 | R0 |
| January 2018 | | cT0cN0cM0 | |
| Last contact March 2018 | | cT0cN0cM0 | |

## Example

Previous total gastrectomy, without remaining local-regional residual tumour. Local recurrence at the oesophagojejunostomy involving mucosa, submucosa, muscularis propria and perimuscular tissue: rT3.

In other cases, the recurrence in the area of the primary tumour may be indicated by 'rT+'.

## Example

Local recurrence after simple mastectomy, 2 cm in greatest dimension, with or without invasion of skin or chest wall: rT+.

## a Symbol

The prefix 'a' indicates that classification is first determined at autopsy. Tumours that have been clinically diagnosed and then classified, based on autopsy findings can be recorded in two ways:

- Recurrence after a disease-free interval: rpTNM
- Other cases: pTNM

It should be emphasized that assignment of pM0 by pathological assessment is possible only at autopsy.

## Optional Descriptors

### Lymphatic Invasion (L Classification)

Lymphatic vessels include those within and at the margins of the primary tumour as well as afferent and efferent lymphatics. Invasion of small lymphatic vessels requires the demonstration of tumour cells (single or groups) within channels that are unequivocally lined with endothelium. If spaces around tumour nests caused by shrinkage during tissue processing cannot be distinguished from lymphatic invasion, L0 is selected (General Rule No. 4). The categories of the L classification are:

LX   Lymphatic invasion cannot be assessed
L0   No lymphatic invasion
L1   Lymphatic invasion

### Venous Invasion (V Classification)

Venous invasion (V1 or V2) can be diagnosed if there is tumour invasion in the vessel wall. V1 or V2 does not necessarily require demonstration of tumour cells in the lumen of the vessels. The categories of the V classification are:

VX   Venous invasion cannot be assessed
V0   No venous invasion
V1   Microscopic venous invasion
V2   Macroscopic venous invasion

**There is no classification for invasion of arteries, which is very rare. These cases should be documented separately.**

### Pn – Perineural Invasion

In the 7th edition of the *TNM Classification* [71] perineural invasion was introduced as a new and optional parameter. The findings of the Pn classification have no impact on the T classification or stage but have been shown to be an additional prognostic factor for many tumour entities [72]. The categories of the Pn classification are:

PnX   Perineural invasion cannot be assessed
Pn0   No perineural invasion
Pn1   Perineural invasion

## Symbols for Describing Methods of Staging

Because of interest in the differentiation between imaging methods such as ultrasound, computerized tomography (CT) and magnetic resonance imaging (MRI), prefixes have been proposed for the clinical staging of rectal carcinoma by Schaffzin et al. 2004 [73] and Moran et al. 2007 [74]:

- Ultrasound: 'u', e.g. uT2 or uN1
- CT: 'ct', e.g. ctT3 or ctN0
- MRI: 'mr', e.g. mrT4 or mrN2

## Unknown Primary

In the absence of a primary tumour, the presence of metastasis can be coded as T0 plus the assessment of the N and M.

In the head and neck a chapter with an unknown primary and the presence of cervical nodes has been introduced assuming that the primary tumour is located somewhere in the head and neck region with regional cervical lymph nodes. In those cases with cervical lymph nodes that are positive with squamous cell carcinoma and no evidence of a primary tumour the coding is cT0cN2cM0, Stage IVA. In cases without a primary and positive cervical lymph node metastasis occurs as well as distant metastasis: cT0cN2cM1, Stage IVC.

If there is evidence of HPV positivity or EB virus positivity the lymph node is staged as if the primary is from the oropharynx or nasopharynx, respectively.

If the lung contains multiple nodules of malignant melanoma with no primary site identified, the coding would be cT0cNXcM1, Stage IV.

## Staging of Tumours for Which No TNM Classification is Provided

Staging according to the rules of the SEER Program [75] is recommended if no TNM classification is provided (see website link: https://training.seer.cancer.gov/staging/systems/summary/).Staging is based on the concept of local, regional and distant.

- In situ (non-invasive, intraepithelial)
- Localized (confined to the organ of origin)

- Regional, direct extension
- Regional, lymph nodes
- Regional, direct extension and lymph nodes
- Distant, direct extension or metastasis
- Distant, lymph nodes

These cases should be analysed separately.

In addition, the 8th edition of *TNM Classification of Malignant Tumours* [2] offers an essential TNM for cancer registries in low- and middle-income countries frequently having insufficient information to determine complete TNM data. In view of this, the UICC TNM Project has developed with the International Agency for Research in Cancer and the National Cancer Institute a new classification system 'Essential TNM' that can be used to collect stage data when complete information is not available. Essential TNM schemes have been developed for breast, cervix, colon and prostate cancer, and are presented in the 8th edition and are available for download at www.uicc.org.

## Histopathological Grading

The following applies only to the TNM classification and not to the ICD-O morphology code.

Histopathological grading of tumours of the same histological type is performed to provide some indication of their aggressiveness, which may in turn relate to prognosis or treatment. Grading should follow the recommendations of the WHO Classification of Tumours. For histopathological grading of invasive breast carcinoma see Elston and Ellis [76].

For most sites, histopathological grading consists of four grades:

G1   Well differentiated
G2   Moderately differentiated
G3   Poorly differentiated
G4   Undifferentiated

In the event that there are different degrees of differentiation in a tumour, one should assign the tumour to the least favourable grade of G1–G4.

**Example**
Partially well differentiated, partially moderately differentiated adenocarcinoma of the colon – G2.

G1 and G2 may be grouped together as low grade (G1–G2) and G3 and G4 as high grade (G3–G4). In some tumour sites, no differentiation is made between

G3 and G4 and therefore the category G3–G4 is used. This is valid for carcinomas of the penis, renal pelvis, ureter, urinary bladder and urethra.

In prostate carcinomas the use of the WHO grade group has been introduced as below:

| WHO grade group | Gleason score | Gleason pattern |
|---|---|---|
| 1 | ≤6 | ≤3+3 |
| 2 | 7 | 3+4 |
| 3 | 7 | 4+3 |
| 4 | 8 | 4+4, 3+5, 5+3 |
| 5 | 9–10 | 4+5, 5+4, 5+5 |

In the 7th edition, special staging criteria have been introduced with the TNM classification of gastrointestinal stromal tumour (GIST). Grading for GIST is dependent on the mitotic rate [71] and has been kept in the 8th edition [2].

A grading system has been proposed for well-differentiated neuroendocrine tumours (carcinoids) and well-differentiated neuroendocrine carcinomas. The grading system depends on the mitotic count and Ki-67 index [2].

Only three grades (G1–G3) are used for all gynaecological sites except gestational trophoblastic tumours.

Grading is not applicable for the following tumour entities:

- Malignant melanoma of the upper aerodigestive tract
- Carcinoma of the thyroid
- Pleural mesothelioma
- Thymic tumours
- Malignant melanoma of the skin
- Merkel cell carcinoma
- Uterine sarcomas
- Gestational trophoblastic tumours
- Germ cell tumours of the testis
- Adrenal gland carcinoma
- Malignant melanoma of the uvea
- Retinoblastoma

For undifferentiated carcinomas of the oesophagus, stomach, small intestine, colorectum, gallbladder and pancreas the category G4 is appropriate. By definition, an adenocarcinoma of these organs can be classified only as G1, G2 or G3. When, in an adenocarcinoma of these organs, there are undifferentiated areas next to areas with glandular differentiation, the tumour is classified as a poorly differentiated adenocarcinoma. The same applies for squamous cell carcinoma with undifferentiated areas.

In some sites the WHO classification does not list 'undifferentiated carcinoma' as a specific tumour type, e.g. in the lung and breast. In those cases the category G4 is not applied [77].

In the absence of an assigned grade the following can be considered G4:

- Undifferentiated carcinoma
- Small cell carcinoma
- Large cell carcinoma of the lung
- Ewing sarcoma of bone and soft tissue
- Rhabdomyosarcoma of soft tissue

In grading, different methods may be appropriate for the various tumour entities (type and site). For example, in gastrointestinal adenocarcinomas the growing edge of a tumour should not be assessed as it may appear to be of a high grade [78, 79]. In contrast, grading that considers the histologically invasive edge is appropriate for predicting the prognosis of oral squamous cell carcinoma [80].

The pathologist should indicate the grading system used in the report.

Grading is generally performed by a combined evaluation of various histological and cytological features, including similarity to tissue of origin, cell arrangement, cellularity, differentiation, cellular and nuclear pleomorphism, mitotic activity and necrosis. Grading is a semiquantitative, sometimes subjective procedure, which requires considerable experience by the pathologist. To reduce individual variability and to increase reproducibility of grading, semiquantitative methods have been proposed. Various morphological parameters have been scored from 1 to 3 or 1 to 4, with the scores for each variable added into a total malignancy score for each tumour. A high malignancy score suggests a poorly differentiated tumour.

# References

[1]   Greene FL, Brierley JD, O'Sullivan B, et al. On the use and abuse of X in the TNM Classification. *Cancer* 2005; 103:647–649.

[2]   UICC (Union for International Cancer Control) *TNM Classification of Malignant Tumours*, 8th edn, Brierley JD, Gospadarowicz MK, Wittekind C (eds). Oxford: Wiley Blackwell; 2017.

[3]   American Joint Committee on Cancer (AJCC) *Cancer Staging Manual*, 8th edn, Amin MB, Edge SB, Greene FL, et al. (eds). New York: Springer; 2017.

[4]   Fritz A, Percy C, Jack A, et al. *International Classification of Diseases for Oncology (ICD-O)*, 3rd edn. Geneva: WHO; 2000.

[5] UICC (Union for International Cancer Control) *TNM Supplement 1993. A Commentary on Uniform Use*, Hermanek P, Henson DE, Hutter RVP, Sohin LH (eds). Berlin, Heidelberg, New York: Springer; 1993.

[6] UICC (Union for International Cancer Control) *TNM Supplement 2001. A Commentary on Uniform Use*, 2nd edn, Wittekind C, Henson DE, Hutter RVP, Sobin LH (eds). New York: Wiley; 2001.

[7] UICC (Union for International Cancer Control) *TNM Supplement. A Commentary on Uniform Use*, 3rd edn, Wittekind Ch, Henson DE, Hutter RVP, Sobin LH (eds). New York: Wiley; 2003.

[8] UICC (Union for International Cancer Control) *TNM Supplement. A Commentary on Uniform Use*, 4th edn, Wittekind Ch, Compton CC, Brierley JD, Sobin LH (eds). Oxford: Wiley Blackwell; 2012.

[9] Veronesi U, Farante G, Galimberti V, et al. Evaluation of resection margins after breast conservative surgery with monoclonal antibodies. *Eur Surg Oncol* 1991; 17:338–341.

[10] UICC (Union for International Cancer Control) *TNM Classification of Malignant Tumours*, 6th edn, Sobin LH, Wittekind Ch (eds). New York: Wiley; 2002.

[11] Hermanek P, Hutter RVP, Sobin LH, Wittekind Ch. Communication of the UICC (Union for International Cancer Control) Classification of isolated tumour cells and micrometastasis. *Cancer* 1999; 86:2668–2673.

[12] van Akkoi AC, de WiltJH, Verhoef C, et al. Clinical relevance of melanoma micrometastasis (<1.1 mm) in sentinel nodes: Are these nodes to be considered negative? *Ann Oncol* 2006; 17:1578–1585.

[13] Scheri RP, Essner R, Turner RR, et al. Isolated tumour cells in the sentinel node affect long-term prognosis of patients with melanoma. *Ann Surg Oncol* 2007; 14:2861–2866.

[14] American Joint Committee on Cancer (AJCC) *Cancer Staging Manual*, 7th edn, Edge SB, Byrd DR, Compton CC, Fritz AG, Greene FL, Trotti A (eds). New York: Springer; 2009.

[15] Jaehne J, Meyer HJ, Soudah B, et al. Peritoneal lavage in gastric carcinoma. *Dig Surg* 1989; 6:26–28.

[16] Martin JK Jr, Goellner JR. Abdominal fluid cytology in patients with gastrointestinal malignant lesions. *Mayo Clin Proc* 1986; 61:467–471.

[17] Maruyama K. Diagnosis of invisible peritoneal metastasis: cytologic examination by peritoneal lavage. In *Staging and Treatment of Gastric Cancer*, Cordine C, de Manzoni G (eds). Padua: Piccin Nuova Libraria; 1991, pp. 180–181.

[18] Warshaw AL. Implications of peritoneal cytology for staging of early pancreatic cancer. *Am J Surg* 1991; 161:26–30.

[19] Zeng Z, Cohen AM, Haydu S, et al. Serosal cytologic study to determine free mesothelial penetration by intraperitoneal colon cancer. *Cancer* 1992; 70:737–740.

[20] Ang CW, Tan LC. Peritoneal cytology in the staging process of gastric cancer: Do or don't? *J Gastroint Dig Syst* 2013; 3:156. Doi: 10.4172/2161-069X.1000156.

[21] Frattini F, Rausei S, Chiappa C, et al. Prognosis and treatment of patients with positive peritoneal cytology in advanced gastric cancer. *World J Gastrointest Surg* 2013; 27:135–137.

[22] Mezhir JJ, Posner MC, Roggin KK. Prospective clinical trial of diagnostic peritoneal lavage to detect positive peritoneal cytology in patients with gastric cancer. *J Surg Oncol* 2013; 107:794–798.

[23] Wittekind C, Compton CC, Greene FL, Sobin LH. TNM residual tumour classification revisited. *Cancer* 2002; 94:2511–2519.

[24] Wittekind C, Compton CC, Quirke P, et al. A uniform residual tumour (R) classification. Integration of the R classification and the circumferential margin status. *Cancer* 2009; 115: 3483–3488.

[25] Hermanek P, Wittekind C. The pathologist and the residual tumour (R) classification. *Path Res Pract* 1994; 190:115–123.

[26] Nakajima T, Harashima S, Hirata M, Kajitani T. Prognostic and therapeutic values of peritoneal cytology in gastric cancer. *Acta Cytol* 1978; 22:225–229.

[27] Schlimok G, Funke I, Pantel K, et al. Micrometastatic tumour cells in bone marrow of patients with gastric cancer: methodological aspects of detection and clinical significance. *Eur J Cancer* 1991; 27:1461–1465.

[28] Pantel K, Coste RJ, Fodstad O. Detection and clinical importance of micrometastatic disease. *J Natl Cancer Inst* 1999; 91:113–1124.

[29] Quirke P, Dudley P, Dixon MF, Williams NS. Local recurrence of rectal adenocarcinoma due to inadequate surgical resection. Histopathologic study of lateral tumour spread and surgical resection. *Lancet* 1986; 2:996–999.

[30] Quirke P, Dixon MF. The prediction of the local recurrence in rectal adenocarcinoma by histopathological examination. *Int Colorectal Dis* 1988; 3:127–131.

[31] Quirke P. The pathologist, the surgeon and colorectal cancer – get it right because it matters. *Progress in Pathology* 1998; 4:201–213.

[32] Jass JR, O'Brien MJ, Riddell RH, Snover DC, on behalf of the Association of Directors of Anatomic and Surgical Pathology (ADASP). Recommendation for reporting of surgically resected specimens of colorectal carcinoma. *Hum Pathol* 2009; 38:537–545.

[33] Quirke P, Cuvelier C, Ensari A, et al. Evidence-based medicine: the time has come to set standards for staging. *J Pathol* 2010; 221:357–360, correspondence 361–362.

[34] Ryan R, Gibbons D, Hyland JMP, et al. Pathological response following long-course neoadjuvant chemoradiotherapy for locally advance rectal cancer. *Histopathology* 2005; 47:141–146.

[35] Compton CC, Fenoglio-Preiser CM, Pettigrew N, Fielding LP. American Joint Committee on Cancer Prognostic Factors Consensus Conference: Colorectal Working Group. *Cancer* 2000; 88:1739–1757.

[36] Compton CC. Pathologic prognostic factors in the recurrence of rectal cancer. *Clin Colorect Cancer* 2002; 2:149–160.

[37] American Joint Committee for Cancer Staging and End Results Reporting. *Manual for Staging of Cancer 1977*. Chicago, Illinois: American Joint Committee on Cancer; 1977.

[38] Rami-Porta R, Wittekind Ch, Goldstraw P for the International Association for the Study of Lung Cancer (IASLC) Staging Committee. Complete resection in lung cancer surgery: proposed definitions. *Lung Cancer* 2005; 49:25–33.

[39] Galiasso M, Migliaretti G, Ardissone F. Assessing the prognostic impact of the International Association for the Study of Lung Cancer proposed of complete, uncertain, and incomplete resection in non-small cell lung cancer surgery. *Lung Cancer* 2017; 111:124–136.

[40] Braun OM, Neumeister B, Neuhalod N, et al. Histological grading of therapy induced regression in squamous cell carcinomas of the oral cavity. A morphological and immunohistochemical study. *Pathol Res Pract* 1989; 186:368–372.

[41] Eich HAT, Löscheke M, Scheem, et al. Neoadjuvant radiochemotherapy and radical resection for advanced squamous cell carcinoma of the oral cavity. *Strahlentherapie und Onkologie* 2008; 184:23–29.

[42] Hermann RM, Krech R, Hartlapp J, et al. Wertigkeit eines qualitativen Regressionsgrading als prognostischer Faktor für das Überleben bei präoperativ radiochemotherapierten Patienten mit fortgeschrittenen Kopf-Hals-Karzinomen. *Strahlenther Onkol* 2001; 177:277–282.

[43] Wedemeyer I, Kreppel M, Scheer M, et al. Histopathological assessment of tumour regression, nodal stage and status if resection margin determines prognosis in patients with oral squamous cell carcinoma treated with neoadjuvant radiochemotherapy. *Oral Dis* 2014; 20:e81–e89.

[44] Werner M, Höffler H. Pathologie. In *Therapie gastrointestinaler Tumoren*, Roder JD, Stein HJ, Fink U (Hrsg). Berlin, Heidelberg, New York: Springer; 2000, pp. 45–63.

[45] Japan Esophageal Society. Japanese Classification of Esophageal Cancer, 11th edition: part I, part II, part III. *Esophagus* 2017; 14:1–65.

[46] Mandard A-M, Dalibard F, Mandard JC, et al. Pathologic assessment of tumour regression after preoperative chemoradiotherapy of oesophageal carcinoma. *Cancer* 1994; 73:2680–2696.

[47] Baldus SE, Mönig SP, Schröder W, et al. Regression von Ösophaguskarzinomen nach neoadjuvanter Therapie. *Pathologe* 2004; 25: 421–427.

[48] Hermann RM, Horstmann O, Haller F, et al. Histomorphological tumour regression grading of oesophageal carcinoma after neoadjuvant radiochemotherapy: Which score to use? *Dis Esophag* 2006; 19: 329–334.

[49] Japanese Gastric Cancer Association (JGCA). Japanese Classification of Gastric Carcinoma. 2nd English edition. *Gastric Cancer* 1998; 1:10–24.

[50] Becker K, Müller J, Fink U, et al. The interpretation of pathologic changes in the resection specimen following multimodal therapy for gastric adeno-carcinoma. In *Progress in Gastric Cancer Research*, Siewert JR, Roder JD (eds). Bologna: Monduzzi; 1997, pp. 1275–1280.

[51] Becker K, Müller JD, Schumacher C, et al. Histomorphology and grading of regression in gastric carcinomas treated with neoadjuvant chemotherapy. *Cancer* 2003; 98:1521–1530.

[52] Dworak O, Keilholz L, Hoffmann A. Pathological features of rectal cancer after preoperative chemotherapy. *Int J Colorect Dis* 1997; 12:19–32.

[53] Japanese Society for Classification of Cancer of the Colon and Rectum (JSCCR). *Japanese Classification of Colorectal Carcinoma*, 1st English edn. Tokyo: Kanehara & Co.; 1997.

[54] Wheeler JMD, Warren BF, Mortensen NJMC, et al. Quantification of histologic regression of rectal cancer after irradiation. *Dis Colon Rectum* 2002; 45:1051–1056.

[55] Williams GT, Quirke P, Shepherd NA on behalf of the RC Path Cancer Services Working Group. *Royal College of Pathologists Dataset for Colorectal Cancer*, 2nd edn 2007. www.rcpath.org, access December 02, 2009.

[56] Bateman AC, Jaynes E, Bateman AR. Rectal cancer staging post neoadjuvant therapy – How should the changes be assessed? *Histopathology* 2009; 54:713–721.

[57] Klimpfinger M, Hauser H, Berger A, Hermanek P. Aktuelle klinischpathologische Klassifikation von Karzinomen des Analkanals. *Acta Chir Aust* 1994; 26:345–351.

[58] Adachi E, Marsumata T, Nishizaki T, et al. Effects of preoperative transcatheter hepatic arterial chemoembolisation for hepatocellular carcinoma. *Cancer* 1999; 72:3593–3598.

[59] Evans DB, Rich TA, Byrd DR, et al. Preoperative chemoradiation and pancreatectomy for adenocarcinoma of the pancreas. *Arch Surg* 1992; 127:1335–1339.

[60] Junker K, Langner K, Klinke F, et al. Grading of tumor regression in non-small cell lung cancer: morphology and prognosis. *Chest* 2001; 120:1584–1591.

[61] Langner K, Thomas M, Klinke F, et al. Neoadjuvant therapy in non-small cell lung cancer. Prognostic impact of mediastinal downstaging. *Chirurg* 2002; 74:42–48.

[62] Salzer-Kuntschik M, Delling G, Beron G, et al. Morphological grades of regression in osteosarcoma after polychemotherapy – Study Coss 80. *J Cancer Res Clin Pract* 1993; 106, Suppl:21–24.

[63] Huvos AG. *Bone Tumours. Diagnosis, Treatment and Prognosis*, 2nd edn. Philadelphia, London, Toronto: Saunders; 1991.

[64] Schmidt RA, Conrad EU, Collins C, et al. Measurement and prediction of short-term response of soft tissue sarcomas to chemotherapy. *Cancer* 1993; 72:2593–2601.

[65] Chevalier B, Roche H, Olivier JP, et al. Inflammatory breast cancer: pilot study of intensive induction chemotherapy (FEC-HD) results in a high histologic response rate. *Am J Clin Oncol* 1993; 16:223–228.

[66] Sinn HP, Schmid H, Junkermann H, et al. Histologische Regression des Mammakarzinoms nach primärer (neoadjuvanter) Chemotherapie. *Geburtsh Frauenheilk* 1994; 34:332–338.

[67] Sataloff DM, Mason BA, Prestipino AJ, et al. Pathologic response to induction chemotherapy in locally advanced carcinoma of the breast: a determinant of outcome. *J Am Coll Surg* 1995; 180:297–306.

[68] Fisher ER, Wang J, Bryant J, et al. Pathobiology of preoperative chemotherapy: findings from the National Surgical Adjuvant Breast and Bowel (NSABP) Protocol B-18. *Cancer* 2002; 95:681–695.

[69] Ogston KN, Miller ID, Pyne S, et al. A new histological grading system to assess the response of breast carcinomas to primary chemotherapy: prognostic significance and survival. *Breast* 2003; 12:320–327.

[70] Symmans WF, Peintinger F, Hatzis C, et al. Measurement of residual breast cancer burden to predict survival after neoadjuvant chemotherapy. *J Clin Oncol* 2007; 25:4414–4422.

[71] UICC (Union for International Cancer Control). *TNM Classification of Malignant Tumours*, 7th edn, Sobin LH, Gospodarowicz MK, Wittekind Ch (eds). New York: Wiley Blackwell; 2010.

[72] Liebig C, Ayala G, Wilks J, et al. Perineural invasion is an independent predictor of outcome in colorectal cancer. *J Clin Oncol* 2009; 27:5131–5137.

[73] Schaffzin DM, Wong DE. Endorectal ultrasound in the preoperative evaluation of rectal cancer. *Clin Colorect Cancer* 2004; 4:124–133.

[74] Moran B, Brown G, Cunningham D, et al. Clarifying the TNM staging of rectal cancer in the context of modern imaging and adjuvant treatment: 'y', 'u' and 'p' need 'mr' and 'ct'. *Colorectal Dis* 2007; 10:242–243.

[75] *SEER Program: Code Manual*, Cunningham I, Ries L, Hankey B, et al. (eds), NIH Publication No. 92–1999. Bethesda: National Cancer Institute; 1992.

[76] Elston CW, Ellis LO. Pathological prognostic factors in breast cancer. The value of histological grade in breast cancer: experience from a large study with long-term follow-up. *Histopathology* 1991; 19:403–410.

[77] Henson DE, Ries L, Freedman LS, Carriaga M. Relationship among outcome, stage of disease, and histologic grade for 22,616 cases of breast cancer. *Cancer* 1991; 68:2142–2149.

[78]   Jass R, Sobin LH. *Histological Typing of Intestinal Tumours*, 2nd edn, WHO International Histological Classification of Tumours. Berlin, Heidelberg, New York: Springer; 1989.

[79]   Bosman F, Carneiro F, Hruban RH, Thiese ND. *WHO Classification of Tumours of the Digestive System*. Lyon: IARC; 2010.

[80]   Bryne M, Koppang HS, Lilleng R, et al. New malignancy grading is a better prognostic indicator than Broder's grading in oral squamous cell carcinoma. *J Oral Pathol Med* 1989; 18:432–437.

# CHAPTER 2

# EXPLANATORY NOTES – SPECIFIC ANATOMICAL SITES

## Head and Neck Tumours

### General

In the 8th edition of the *TNM Classification* for all sites (except tumours of the nasopharynx, malignant melanoma of the upper aerodigestive tract, tumours of the thyroid), there are now separate classifications for clinical and pathological neck lymph nodes. In addition, depth of invasion has been incorporated into the definition of the T/pT category in oral cavity tumours. There is a new classification for p16 positive oropharyngeal cancers. The classification for nasopharyngeal cancers and thyroid cancers has been modified. There is a new classification for squamous cell carcinoma of the skin in the head and neck region. There is a new classification for cervical nodal involvement with an unknown primary.

### *Anatomy*

A uniform topographic terminology should be used for classification, and the 'sites, subsites, adjacent sites and adjacent structures' should be used as defined in the text.

Tumours involving two anatomical sites are classified according to the site in which the greater part of the tumour is located. In invasive tumours with an associated carcinoma in situ only the invasive component is considered for classification.

### Example

A carcinoma with two thirds in the hypopharynx and one third in the supraglottis is classified as a hypopharynx carcinoma.

*TNM Supplement: A Commentary on Uniform Use*, Fifth Edition.
Edited by Christian Wittekind, James D. Brierley, Anne Lee and Elisabeth van Eycken.
© 2019 UICC. Published 2019 by John Wiley & Sons Ltd.

## Definition of Masticator Space

The masticator space (MS) is the lateral anatomic region below the middle cranial fossa and is defined by distinct fascial planes (Plate 2.1). The main fascial boundary is related to the superficial layer of the deep cervical fascia. This is also known as the investing fascia. The investing fascia is formed when the superficial layer of the deep cervical fascia splits at the lower margin of the body of the mandible and rises to enclose the muscles of mastication. Medially the fascia combines with another fascia, the interpterygoid fascia, and then rises up to the skull base. Laterally, the fascia rises up above the level of the zygomatic arch and covers the temporalis muscle. The zygomatic arch is used to subdivide the MS into a suprazygomatic MS (portion above the zygomatic arch) and the nasopharyngeal MS (portion below the level of the zygomatic arch). The contents of the MS include the mandibular division of the fifth cranial nerve, the muscles of mastication, sections of the internal maxillary artery, the pterygoid plexus and the ramus and coronoid of the mandible. Lesions related to the lower alveolus would be related to the most inferior part of the masticator space that is still enclosed by the investing fascia [1, 2].

## Definition of the Paraglottic Space

The paraglottic space (PGS) is not mentioned in the Nomina anatomica [3, 4]. Tucker and Smith [5] and Tucker [6] defined it as the region bounded by the thyroid cartilage anterolaterally, the conus elasticus inferomedially, the laryngeal ventricle and the quadrangular membrane medially, and the mucosal lining of the piriform sinus dorsally. The exact structures have been extensively studied and described by Reidenbach in 1996 [7] and by Maroldi et al. using magnetic resonance imaging for laryngeal cancer [8].

## Extension to Adjacent Sites

In tumours extending to an adjacent site, differentiation between superficial extension and deep extension is necessary. In superficial extension the involvement is limited to the mucosa; in deep extension muscles, bones or other deep structures are invaded.

Superficial extension to adjacent sites is not considered as invasion of adjacent structures.

### Example

A tumour extending from the hypopharynx to the oesophagus and limited to the mucosa (without invasion of muscles, bones or other deep structures) is classified as T3/pT3. If there is invasion of the muscles or other structures of the wall it is classified as T4a/pT4a.

Deep extension to an adjacent site can be the result of vertical invasion of adjacent structures (see above) or the result of horizontal spread not limited to the mucosa but also involving muscles or bones. Such extension is classified as invasion of adjacent structures.

**Example**
An oral cavity carcinoma extending through the skin of cheek is classified as T4a.

Invasion of bone (T4a/pT4a) includes only involvement of spongiosa, not involvement of the cortex.

## Regional Lymph Nodes
The status of the regional lymph nodes in head and neck cancer is of considerable prognostic importance. In addition, it is helpful to subdivide the lymph nodes and possible metastasis into specific anatomic subsites and group these lymph nodes into levels. A consensus guideline from DAHANCA, EORTC, HKNPCSG, NCIC CTG, NCRI, RTOG and TROG has been published and the nodal groups are listed below. However, a number of different classifications exist that use variable level numbers and therefore we recommend the levels be named rather than referred to by number to limit any confusion, although the levels used in the consensus document are given [9]. This proposal is not identical to the classification used by the AJCC [10]. In the consensus classification, the retropharyngeal nodes are classified as level VII, but in the classification used by the AJCC Level VII described the upper mediastinal nodes.

**The lymph node groups are defined as follows (Figures 2.1 to 2.4):**
For information, the level numbers used in the consensus guidelines are given in parentheses. For definitions and descriptions of the anatomical boundaries, refer to the consensus paper [9].

| | |
|---|---|
| Submental nodes | (Ia) |
| Submandibular nodes | (Ib) |
| Upper jugular (deep cervical) nodes | (II) |
| Medial jugular (deep cervical) nodes | (III) |
| Lower/caudal jugular (deep cervical) nodes | (IVa) |
| Medial supraclavicular nodes | (IVb) |
| Upper posterior triangular nodes | (Va) |
| Lower posterior triangular nodes | (Vb) |
| Lateral supraclavicular nodes | (Vc) |
| Anterior jugular nodes | (VIa) |
| Pre-laryngeal, pre-tracheal, paratracheal and recurrent laryngeal nodes | (VIb) |
| Retropharyngeal nodes | (VIIa) |

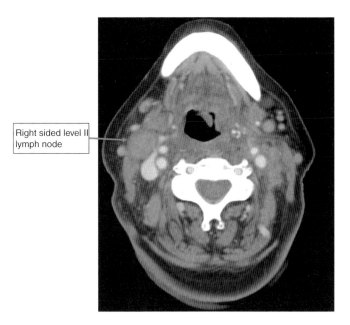

**Figure 2.1** Axial CT scan showing enlarged right upper jugular (deep cervical) level II lymph node measuring 2.5 cm in greatest dimension.

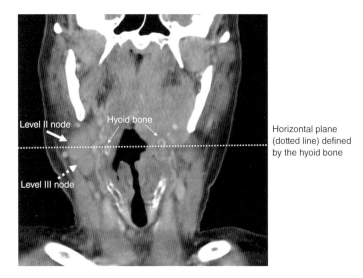

**Figure 2.2** Coronal CT scan showing the same enlarged right upper jugular (deep cervical) level II lymph node measuring 2.5 cm in greatest dimension but also an enlarged right medial jugular (deep cervical) level III lymph node measuring 1.5 cm in greatest dimension. The horizontal plane (dotted line) delineated by the hyoid bone, that defines level II nodes superiorly from level III nodes inferiorly, is marked. This is classified as cN2b: metastasis in multiple ipsilateral lymph nodes, none more than 6 cm in greatest dimension without extranodal extension.

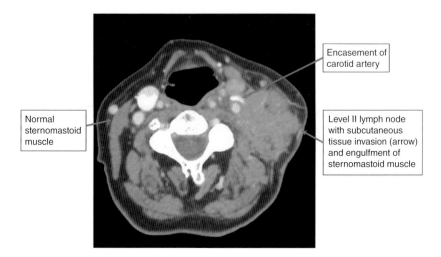

Encasement of carotid artery

Normal sternomastoid muscle

Level II lymph node with subcutaneous tissue invasion (arrow) and engulfment of sternomastoid muscle

**Figure 2.3** Axial CT scan showing clinically fixed right upper jugular (deep cervical) level II lymph node with subcutaneous tissue invasion, engulfment of sternomastoid muscle and encasement of the carotid artery. This is classified as cN3b.

| | |
|---|---|
| Retrostyloid nodes | (VIIb) |
| Parotid nodes | (VIII) |
| Buco-facial nodes | (IX) |
| Retroauricular nodes | (Xa) |
| Occipital nodes | (Xb) |

For the tumour entities listed below a clinical and a pathological N classification have been introduced in the 8th edition of the AJCC [10] and UICC [12] *TNM Classification of Malignant Tumours*:

- Lip and oral cavity
- Oropharynx (p-16-negative or oropharyngeal without p-16-IH performed)
- Hypopharynx
- Pharynx
- Nasal cavity and paranasal sinuses
- Unknown primary – cervical nodes
- Major salivary glands
- Skin carcinoma of head and neck

**Figure 2.4** (*Continued*) sA: subauricular; SAN: spinal accessory nerve; SEJ: superficial external jugular; siP: superficial intraparotid; sMb: submandibular; sMt: submental; sP: subparotid; TCA: transverse cervical artery. (Source: Figure 1, p. 174, Gregoire V, Ang K, Buchach W, et al. Delineation of the neck node levels for head and neck tumors: a 2013 update. DAHANCA, EORTC, HKNPCSG, NCIC CTG, NCRI, RTOG, TROG consensus guidelines. *Radiother Oncol* 2014;110:172–181.)

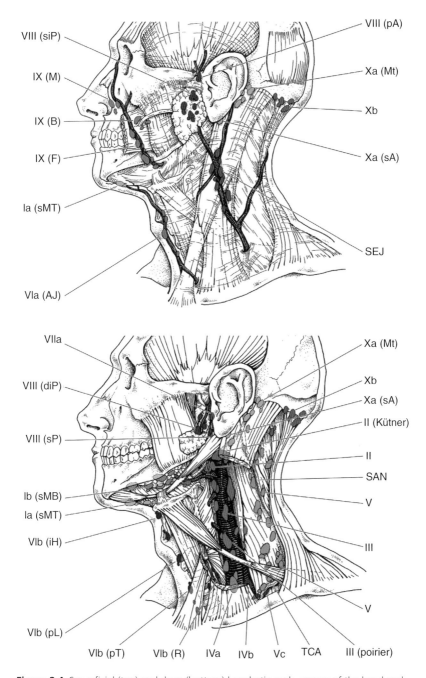

**Figure 2.4** Superficial (top) and deep (bottom) lymphatic node groups of the head and neck. These groups are named according to the node levels modified from Robbins classification (modified from Lengelé B *et al.*, *Radiother Oncol.* 2007 Oct;85(1):146–155). AJ: anterior jugular; B: buccal; diP: deep intraparotid; F: facial; iH: infrahyoid; M: malar; Mt: mastoid; pA: preauricular; pL: pre-laryngeal; pT: pre-tracheal; R: recurrent or paratracheal;

The difference between the clinical (cN) and pathological (pN) classification is obvious in the definition of N2a and pN2a:

| N2a | pN2a |
|---|---|
| Metastasis in a single ipsilateral lymph node, more than 3 cm but not more than 6 cm in greatest dimension without extranodal extension | Metastasis in a single ipsilateral lymph node, 3 cm or less in greatest dimension with extranodal extension, or more than 3 cm but not more than 6 cm in greatest dimension without extranodal extension |

**The following tumour entities have their own N classification:**
- Oropharynx (p16-positive)
- Nasopharynx
- Malignant melanoma of the upper aerodigestive tract
- Thyroid gland

## N Classification

The number of nodes ordinarily examined after surgical resection of most head and neck cancers has been revised so that the histological examination of a selective neck dissection specimen will ordinarily include 10 or more lymph nodes. Histological examination of a radical or modified radical neck dissection specimen will ordinarily include 15 or more lymph nodes [12].

*Size of lymph nodes:* In an advanced lymphatic spread, one often finds perinodal tumour and the confluence of several lymph node metastases into one large tumour conglomerate. In the definition of the N classification, the perinodal component should be included in the size for isolated lymph node metastases; for conglomerates, the overall size of the conglomerate should be considered and not only the size of the individual lymph nodes.

pN classification is based on the size of the metastasis rather than the size of the lymph node(s).

As extranodal extension (ENE) is a major prognostic factor [13] in most head and neck cancers (HPV positive oropharynx and thyroid cancer excepted), an assessment of extranodal status is now incorporated into the N category. Clinical extranodal involvement requires either the presence of skin involvement or soft tissue invasion with deep fixation/tethering to underlying muscle or adjacent structures or clinical signs of nerve involvement and is classified as clinical ENE. ENE is poorly assessed by imaging and is not considered sufficient to classify as ENE if the only evidence is seen on imaging.

ENE is clinically relevant in oral cavity SCC when it has extended more than 1.7 mm beyond the nodal capsule [13]. According to these findings the

AJCC [10] discriminated in histopathological examinations different types of ENE, namely:

ENE-        No extranodal extension
ENE$_{mi}$   Microscopic extranodal extension $\leq 2$ mm
ENE$_{ma}$   ENE > 2 mm or grossly detectable ENE

It is recommended to only use the ENE$_{ma}$ for the histopathological diagnosis of a positive ENE finding in regional lymph node metastasis [10].

## T Classification

Neither in the recent editions of the TNM Classification [14–17] nor in the recent TNM Supplements [18–21] are there any statements concerning the way to measure the pT category, particularly tumour size. However, this should be stated in the pathology report.

The AJCC *Cancer Staging Manual* [10] states that pT is derived from the actual measurement of the unfixed tumour in a surgical specimen. It should be noted that up to 30% shrinkage of soft tissue may occur in a resected specimen after formalin fixation.

There have been reports that size might change from 2.1 cm in an unfixed specimen to 2.0 cm or even less due to fixation resulting in a change from pT2 to pT1.

## Lip and Oral Cavity
### *Lip*
Tumours of the mucosal lip are classified according to the TNM of the 'lip and oral cavity'. It has been proposed that tumours of the lip that affect the vermilion surface and the commissure (ICD-0-3 C00) as well as the skin are assigned to the newly introduced TNM Classification of skin carcinoma of the head and neck. This will be adopted in the 9th edition of TNM.

### Summary – *Lip and Oral Cavity*

| | |
|---|---|
| T1 | Tumour 2 cm or less in greatest dimension and 5 mm or less depth of invasion |
| T2 | Tumour 2 cm or less in greatest dimension and more than 5 mm depth of invasion or tumour more than 2 cm but not more than 4 cm in greatest dimension and depth of invasion no more than 10 mm |
| T3 | Tumour more than 2 cm but not more than 4 cm in greatest dimension and depth of invasion more than 10 mm or tumour more than 4 cm in greatest dimension and not more than 10 mm depth of invasion |

T4a  (*lip*) Tumour invades through the cortical bone, inferior alveolar nerve, floor of the mouth or skin (of the chin or the nose)

T4a  (*oral cavity*) Tumour more than 4 cm in greatest dimension and more than 10 mm depth of invasion or tumour invades through the cortical bone of the mandible or maxilla or involves the maxillary sinus, or invades the skin of the face

T4b  (*lip and oral cavity*) Masticator space, pterygoid plates, skull base, internal carotid artery encasement

## Clinical N

N1  Ipsilateral single ≤ 3 cm (ENE-)
N2  (a) Ipsilateral single > 3 but ≤ 6 cm (ENE-)
     (b) Ipsilateral multiple ≤ 6 cm (ENE-)
     (c) Bilateral or contralateral ≤ 6 cm (ENE-)
N3  (a) > 6 cm (ENE-)
     (b) Any (ENE+)

## Pathological N

N1  Ipsilateral single ≤ 3 cm (ENE-)
N2  (a) Ipsilateral single ≤ 3 cm and ENE+ or ipsilateral single > 3–6 cm (ENE-)
     (b) Ipsilateral multiple ≤ 6 cm (ENE-)
     (c) Bilateral or contralateral ≤ 6 cm (ENE-)
N3  (a) > 6 cm (ENE-)
     (b) Any (ENE+) other than pN2a

## *Oral Cavity*
### *T Classification*

An important modification in the T classification has been the introduction of the depth of invasion (DOI). The depth of invasion has been incorporated into the definition of T category for the floor of the mouth following the assessment of 1792 patients by the International Consortium for Outcomes Research in Head and Neck Cancer and validated by a study combining the MSKCC and University of Toronto surgically managed cases.

The definitions of T3 and T4a given above have been modified from that publication for clarity and to be consistent with the data published by the Consortium [22].

Clinicians experienced in the treatment of head and neck cancer will generally have few problems identifying a less invasive lesion (≤5mm) from those of moderate depth of invasion ($> 5$–$\leq 10$ mm) or deeply invasive carcinomas ($> 10$ mm). When in doubt TNM rule No. 4 should be used, e.g. the less advanced depth. The way depth of invasion should be measured is shown in Plate 2.2.

**Note.**
The lingual tonsil is classified in the oropharynx.

Extrinsic muscle (M. genioglossus, M. hyoglossus, M. palatoglossus, and M. styloglossus) infiltration is no longer a staging criterion for T4 categories because DOI has been shown to be prognostically more important and extrinsic muscle invasion is difficult to assess (clinically and pathologically) [10].

Invasion of the submandibular gland is not classified T4a/b.

Invasion of the sublingual gland by a carcinoma of the floor of mouth does not qualify for T4a/b and is not considered in the T classification.

## Pharynx
The pharynx section has been divided into three separate anatomic regions:

- Oropharynx: HPV-negative and human-papilloma virus-associated (HPV) oropharyngeal cancers
- Nasopharynx
- Hypopharynx

### *Pharynx: Oropharynx*
### Summary – *Oropharynx, p16-negative or Oropharyngeal Cancers*
### *Without p16-immunohistochemistry Performed*

| | |
|---|---|
| T1 | $\leq 2$ cm |
| T2 | $> 2$ but $\leq 4$ cm |
| T3 | $> 4$ cm, or extension lingual surface of epiglottis |
| T4a | Invasion of larynx, deep/extrinsic muscle of the tongue, medial pterygoid, hard palate, mandible |
| T4b | Invasion of lateral pterygoid muscle, pterygoid plates, lateral nasopharynx, skull base, carotid artery |

### Clinical N

| | |
|---|---|
| N1 | Ipsilateral single $\leq 3$ cm (ENE-) |
| N2 | (a) Ipsilateral single $> 3$ but $\leq 6$ cm (ENE-) |
| | (b) Ipsilateral multiple $\leq 6$ cm (ENE-) |
| | (c) Bilateral or contralateral $\leq 6$ cm (ENE-) |
| N3 | (a) $> 6$ cm (ENE-) |
| | (b) Any (ENE+) other than pN2a |

## Pathological N

| | |
|---|---|
| N1 | Ipsilateral single ≤ 3 cm (ENE-) |
| N2 | (a) Ipsilateral single ≤ 3 cm and ENE+ or ipsilateral single > 3–6 cm (ENE-) |
| | (b) Ipsilateral multiple ≤ 6 cm (ENE-) |
| | (c) Bilateral or contralateral ≤ 6 cm (ENE-) |
| N3 | (a) > 6 cm (ENE-) |
| | (b) Any (ENE+) |

### *T Classification*

The intrinsic muscles of the tongue include musculi longitudinalis superior and inferior, transversus linguae and verticalis linguae.

Mucosal extension to the lingual surface of the epiglottis from the primary tumour of the base of the tongue and vallecula does not constitute invasion of the larynx.

A tumour extending from the oropharynx to the nasopharynx or to the hypopharynx or to the oral cavity or larynx and limited to the mucosa (without invasion of muscles, bones or other deep structures) is classified only according to size up to T3.

A tumour invading soft tissue of the neck and paravertebral fascia/muscles is classified as T4b.

*Definition of invasion of the larynx:* invasion of the outer framework (thyroid cartilage, cricoid cartilage, pre-epiglottic space) or internal structures such as arytenoid and epiglottic cartilages.

### Summary – *Oropharynx, p16-positive*

Tumours that have positive p16 immunohistochemistry overexpression.

| | |
|---|---|
| T1 | ≤ 2 cm |
| T2 | > 2 but ≤ 4 cm |
| T3 | > 4 cm or extension to lingual surface of epiglottis |
| T4 | Invasion of larynx, deep/extrinsic muscle of tongue, medial pterygoid, hard palate, mandible, lateral pterygoid muscle, pterygoid plates, lateral nasopharynx, skull base, carotid artery |

### Clinical N

| | |
|---|---|
| N1 | Unilateral metastasis ≤ 6 cm |
| N2 | Contralateral, bilateral ≤ 6 cm |
| N3 | > 6 cm |

## Pathological N

| N1 | 1–4 lymph nodes |
|----|-----------------|
| N2 | 5 or more lymph nodes |

### *T Classification*

Mucosal extension to the lingual surface of epiglottis from the primary tumour of the base of the tongue and vallecula does not constitute invasion of the larynx.

# Nasopharynx
## Summary – *Nasopharynx*

| T1 | Nasopharynx, oropharynx or nasal cavity without parapharyngeal involvement |
|----|---------------------------------------------------------------------------|
| T2 | Parapharyngeal space and/or medial pterygoid, lateral pterygoid and/or prevertebral muscles |
| T3 | Bony structures of skull base, cervical vertebra, pterygoid structures and/or paranasal sinuses |
| T4 | Intracranial extension, cranial nerves, hypopharynx, orbit, parotid gland and/or infiltration beyond the lateral surface of the lateral pterygoid muscle |

## Clinical and Pathological N

| N1 | Unilateral cervical, unilateral or bilateral retropharyngeal lymph nodes $\leq 6$ cm, above the caudal border of cricoid cartilage |
|----|---------------------------------------------------------------------------|
| N2 | Bilateral cervical $\leq 6$ cm, above the caudal border of cricoid cartilage |
| N3 | Cervical $> 6$ cm and/or below the caudal border of cricoid cartilage |

### *T Classification*

Tumours not involving the oropharynx and/or nasal cavity/fossa, but with parapharyngeal extension are classified T2.

The term 'post-nasal space' corresponds to nasopharynx (C11).

### *N Classification*

The previous N classification has been revised: N2 includes nodes above the caudal border of the cricoid, not above the supraclavicular fossa. Similarly, the definition of N3 has been revised to include nodes below the cricoid cartilage. N3 is no longer subdivided into N3a and N3b

N2    Bilateral metastasis in cervical lymph node(s), 6 cm or less in greatest dimension

N3    Metastasis in cervical lymph node(s) greater than 6 cm in dimension and/or extension below the caudal border of cricoid cartilage

## Hypopharynx
### Summary – *Hypopharynx*

| | |
|---|---|
| T1 | ≤2 cm and limited to one subsite |
| T2 | >2 but≤4 cm without hemilarynx fixation or more than one subsite |
| T3 | >4 cm or with hemilarynx fixation or extension to oesophageal mucosa |
| T4a | Invasion of thyroid/cricoid cartilage, hyoid bone, thyroid gland, oesophagus or central compartment of soft tissue |
| T4b | Invasion of prevertebral fascia, carotid artery or mediastinal structures |

### Clinical N

| | |
|---|---|
| N1 | Ipsilateral single≤3 cm (ENE-) |
| N2 | (a) Ipsilateral single>3 but≤6 cm (ENE-) |
| | (b) Ipsilateral multiple≤6 cm (ENE-) |
| | (c) Bilateral or contralateral≤6 cm (ENE-) |
| N3 | (a) >6 cm (ENE-) |
| | (b) Any (ENE+) |

### Pathological N

| | |
|---|---|
| N1 | Ipsilateral single≤3 cm (ENE-) |
| N2 | (a) Ipsilateral single≤3 cm and ENE+ or ipsilateral single>3–6 cm (ENE-) |
| | (b) Ipsilateral multiple≤6 cm (ENE-) |
| | (c) Bilateral or contralateral≤6 cm (ENE-) |
| N3 | (a) >6 cm (ENE-) |
| | (b) Any (ENE+) other than pN2a |

### *T Classification*

Central compartment of soft tissues includes prevertebral strap muscles and subcutaneous fat.

The term 'laryngopharynx' corresponds to hypopharynx (C13.9).

For classification, the hypopharyngeal surface of the aryepiglottic fold (C13.1) belongs to the hypopharynx, while the laryngeal aspect of the aryepiglottic fold (C32.1) is part of the supraglottis.

Fixation of hemilarynx is diagnosed endoscopically by immobility of the arytenoid or vocal cord.

The uncommon tumours limited to one subsite but with vocal cord fixation should be classified as T3.

Involvement of the arytenoid cartilage is T3, not T4a.

A tumour extending from the hypopharynx to the oesophagus and limited to the mucosa (without invasion of muscles, bones or other deeper structures) is classified only according to size up to T3.

## Larynx
### Summary – *Supraglottis*

| | |
|---|---|
| T1 | One subsite, normal mobility |
| T2 | Mucosa of more than one adjacent subsite of supraglottis or glottis or adjacent region outside the supraglottis; without fixation |
| T3 | Limited to larynx with cord fixation and/or invades post-cricoid area, pre-epiglottic space, paraglottic space, thyroid cartilage erosion |
| T4a | Through thyroid cartilage; trachea, soft tissues of neck: deep extrinsic muscle of tongue, strap muscles, thyroid, oesophagus |
| T4b | Prevertebral space, mediastinal structures, carotid artery |

### Summary – *Glottis*

| | |
|---|---|
| T1 | Limited to vocal cord(s), normal mobility |
| | (a) One cord |
| | (b) Two cords |
| T2 | Supraglottis, subglottis, impaired cord mobility |
| T3 | Cord fixation, paraglottic space, thyroid cartilage erosion |
| T4a | Through thyroid cartilage; trachea, soft tissues of neck: deep extrinsic muscle of tongue, strap muscles, thyroid, oesophagus |
| T4b | Prevertebral space, mediastinal structures, carotid artery |

### Summary – *Subglottis*

| | |
|---|---|
| T1 | Limited to subglottis |
| T2 | Extends to vocal cord(s) with normal/impaired mobility |
| T3 | Limited to the larynx with cord fixation |
| T4a | Through cricoid or thyroid cartilage; trachea, soft tissues of neck: deep extrinsic muscle of tongue, strap muscles, thyroid, oesophagus |
| T4b | Prevertebral space, mediastinal structures, carotid artery |

## All Sites

### Clinical N

| | |
|---|---|
| N1 | Ipsilateral single ≤ 3 cm (ENE-) |
| N2 | (a) Ipsilateral single > 3 but ≤ 6 cm (ENE-) |
| | (b) Ipsilateral multiple ≤ 6 cm (ENE-) |
| | (c) Bilateral or contralateral ≤ 6 cm (ENE-) |
| N3 | (a) > 6 cm (ENE-) |
| | (b) Any (ENE+) |

### Pathological N

| | |
|---|---|
| N1 | Ipsilateral single ≤ 3 cm (ENE-) |
| N2 | (a) Ipsilateral single ≤ 3 cm and ENE+ or ipsilateral single > 3 but ≤ 6 cm (ENE-) |
| | (b) Ipsilateral multiple ≤ 6 cm (ENE-) |
| | (c) Bilateral or contralateral ≤ 6 cm (ENE-) |
| N3 | (a) > 6 cm (ENE-) |
| | (b) Any (ENE+) other than pN2a |

## Anatomical Definitions

### Superior and Inferior Boundaries of the Glottis

According to previous editions of AJCC *Cancer Staging Manuals* [23, 24], the inferior boundary of the supraglottis is the horizontal plane passing through the apex of the ventricle. However, the apex of the ventricle is an anatomically variable structure and is difficult to identify during endoscopy. Furthermore, Kleinsasser [25] emphasized embryological and functional reasons for the following definition of the boundary between supraglottis and glottis:

> A plane running horizontally through the opening of the ventricle, posteriorly over the vocal process of the arytenoid cartilage and then rising between the cuneiform and the corniculate cartilage to end over the upper edge of the posterior commissure.

According to the AJCC *Cancer Staging Manual* 2002 and 2009 [23, 24], the lower boundary of the glottis is the horizontal plane 1 cm below the apex of ventricle.

The designation 'apex of ventricle' [23, 24] and 'the opening of the ventricle' [25] are not mentioned in the anatomical international nomenclature. They correspond to the laryngeal saccule (sacculus laryngis, appendix ventriculi laryngis). According to this definition, the variability of the so-called apex and the difficulty of clinical endoscopic assessment have been opposed, and so the following definition is recommended [25]:

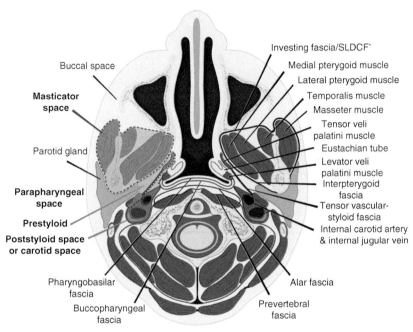

Buccal space

Masticator space

Parotid gland

Parapharyngeal space

Prestyloid

Poststyloid space or carotid space

Pharyngobasilar fascia

Buccopharyngeal fascia

Investing fascia/SLDCF*

Medial pterygoid muscle

Lateral pterygoid muscle

Temporalis muscle

Masseter muscle

Tensor veli palatini muscle

Eustachian tube

Levator veli palatini muscle

Interpterygoid fascia

Tensor vascular-styloid fascia

Internal carotid artery & internal jugular vein

Alar fascia

Prevertebral fascia

*SLDCF: superficial layer of deep cervical fascia

**Plate 2.1** Schematic axial view with colour overlays on left side at the level of the nasopharynx demonstrating the facial boundaries of the masticator (green overlay) and parapharyngeal spaces (blue overlay). Note that the tensor–vascular–styloid fascia subdivides the parapharyngeal space into a pre-styloid and post-styloid (carotid space). (Source: O'Sullivan B, Yu E. Staging of nasopharyngeal carcinoma. In: *Nasopharyngeal Cancer: Multidisciplinary Management. Medical Radiology – Diagnostic Imaging and Radiation Oncology*, Lu JJ, Cooper JS, Lee AWM (eds). New York: Springer; 2010. Reprinted by permission from Springer © 2010.)

*TNM Supplement: A Commentary on Uniform Use*, Fifth Edition.
Edited by Christian Wittekind, James D. Brierley, Anne Lee and Elisabeth van Eycken.
© 2019 UICC. Published 2019 by John Wiley & Sons Ltd.

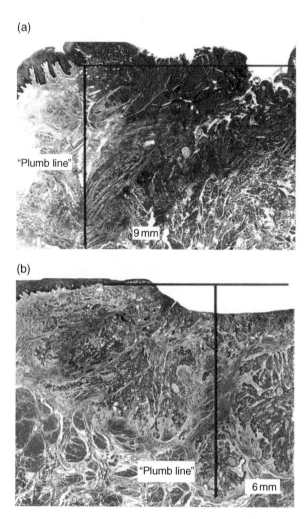

(a)

"Plumb line"

9 mm

(b)

"Plumb line"

6 mm

**Plate 2.2** Measurement of depth of invasion (DOI) in carcinomas of the oral cavity. The horizon is established at the level of the basement membrane relative to the closest intact squamous mucosa. The greatest DOI is measured by dropping a plumb line from the horizon (the reader is referred to Figures 7.6 and 7.7 in the *AJCC Manual*, 8th edition [10]).

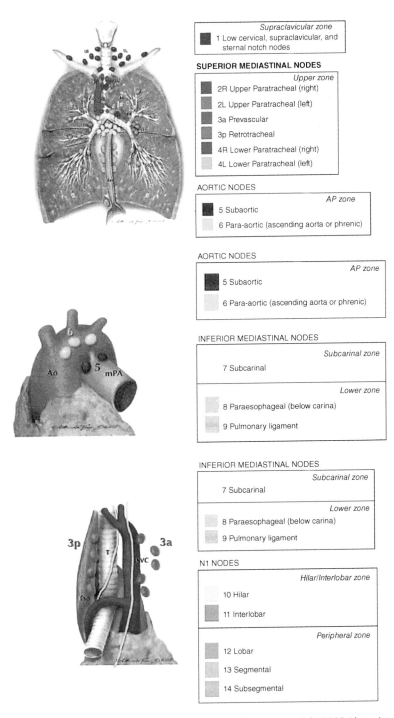

**Plate 2.3** IASLC: Nodal chart with stations and zones. (Source: copyright 2008 Aletta Ann Frazier, MD.)

The inferior boundary of the glottis is a horizontal plane 1 cm inferior to the level of the upper surface of the vocal cords, which is called subglottic space (the reader is referred to Figure 54 [25]).

## Pathological Criteria of Impaired Vocal Cord Mobility or Vocal Cord Fixation

### Impaired Mobility or Fixation

For pathological classification concerning impaired mobility or fixation of vocal cords the information from the clinical T is used for the pathologic T. This is in accordance with TNM rule number 2, where pathological classification 'is based on evidence acquired before treatment, supplemented or modified by additional evidence acquired from surgery and from pathological examination'.

### Associated Carcinoma in Situ

1. For invasive carcinoma, the classification according to horizontal spread is based only on the invasive component.
2. To indicate the presence of associated carcinoma in situ (adjacent or separate) the suffix '(is)' may be added to the respective T category of the invasive carcinoma, e.g. T2(is). The presence of an associated carcinoma in situ influences treatment of the invasive carcinoma and needs identification and separate analysis.

### T Classification

For tumours of the glottis there is a gap of classification between T3 with thyroid cartilage erosion and T4a through thyroid cartilage: tumours with an invasion of the thyroid cartilage corpus should be classified as T3/pT3.

## Nasal Cavity and Paranasal Sinuses

### Summary – *Maxillary Sinus, Nasal Cavity and Ethmoid Sinus*

| Maxillary Sinus | |
|---|---|
| T1 | Mucosa |
| T2 | Bone erosion/destruction, hard palate, middle nasal meatus |
| T3 | Posterior bony wall maxillary sinus, subcutaneous tissues, floor/medial wall of orbit, pterygoid fossa, ethmoid sinus |
| T4a | Anterior orbit, skin of cheek, pterygoid plates, infratemporal fossa, cribriform plate, sphenoid/frontal sinus |
| T4b | Orbital apex, dura, brain, middle cranial fossa, cranial nerves other than V2, nasopharynx, clivus |

## Nasal Cavity and Ethmoid Sinus

| | |
|---|---|
| T1 | One subsite |
| T2 | Two subsites or adjacent nasoethmoidal site |
| T3 | Medial wall/floor orbit, maxillary sinus, palate, cribriform plate |
| T4a | Anterior orbit, skin of nose/cheek, anterior cranial fossa (minimal), pterygoid plates, sphenoid/frontal sinuses |
| T4b | Orbital apex, dura, brain, middle cranial fossa, cranial nerves other than V2, nasopharynx, clivus |

## All Sites

### Clinical N

| | |
|---|---|
| N1 | Ipsilateral single ≤ 3 cm (ENE-) |
| N2 | (a) Ipsilateral single > 3 but ≤ 6 cm (ENE-) |
| | (b) Ipsilateral multiple ≤ 6 cm (ENE-) |
| | (c) Bilateral or contralateral ≤ 6 cm (ENE-) |
| N3 | (a) > 6 cm (ENE-) |
| | (b) Any (ENE+) |

### Pathological N

| | |
|---|---|
| N1 | Ipsilateral single ≤ 3 cm (ENE-) |
| N2 | (a) Ipsilateral single ≤ 3 cm and ENE+ or ipsilateral single > 3 but ≤ 6 cm (ENE-) |
| | (b) Ipsilateral multiple ≤ 6 cm (ENE-) |
| | (c) Bilateral or contralateral ≤ 6 cm (ENE-) |
| N3 | (a) > 6 cm (ENE-) |
| | (b) Any (ENE+) other than pN2a |

## Unknown Primary – Cervical Lymph Nodes

There should be histological confirmation of squamous cell carcinoma with lymph node metastasis but without an identified primary carcinoma. Histological (immunohistochemical) methods should be used to identify EBV and HPV/p16-related tumours. If there is evidence of EBV, the TNM Classification of tumours of the nasopharynx is applied (see page 45). If there is evidence of HPV and positive immunohistochemistry p16 overexpression, the p16-positive oropharyngeal classification should be applied.

### Summary – *Unknown Primary with Cervical Lymph Node Metastasis*

| | |
|---|---|
| T0 | No evidence of primary tumour |

## *N Classification*

### Clinical N

| | |
|---|---|
| N1 | Ipsilateral single ≤ 3 cm (ENE-) |
| N2 | (a) Ipsilateral single > 3 but ≤ 6 cm (ENE-) |
| | (b) Ipsilateral multiple ≤ 6 cm (ENE-) |
| | (c) Bilateral ≤ 6 cm (ENE-) |
| N3 | (a) > 6 cm (ENE-) |
| | (b) Any (ENE+) |

### Pathological N

| | |
|---|---|
| N1 | Ipsilateral single ≤ 3 cm (ENE-) |
| N2 | (a) Ipsilateral single ≤ 3 cm and ENE+ or ipsilateral single > 3 but ≤ 6 cm (ENE-) |
| | (b) Ipsilateral multiple ≤ 6 cm (ENE-) |
| | (c) Bilateral ≤ 6 cm (ENE-) |
| N3 | (a) > 6 cm (ENE-) |
| | (b) Any (ENE+) other than pN2a |

### Stage

| | | | |
|---|---|---|---|
| Stage III | T0 | N1 | M0 |
| Stage IVA | T0 | N2 | M0 |
| Stage IVB | T0 | N3 | M0 |
| Stage IVC | T0 | N1, N2, N3 | M1 |

# Malignant Melanoma of the Upper Aerodigestive Tract

ICD-O-3 Topography codes: C00-06, C09.0, C9.1, C9.9, C10–14, C30–32

The classification applies to mucosal melanomas of the head and neck region, i.e. of the upper aerodigestive tract.

A grading is not applicable.

There is no stage classification of other mucosal melanoma. However, it has been suggested that this classification could be used for other mucosal melanomas such as the anal canal; this proposal is described in Chapter 4.

### Summary – *Melanoma: Upper Aerodigestive Tract*

| | |
|---|---|
| T3 | Epithelium/submucosa (mucosal disease) |
| T4a | Deep soft tissue, cartilage, bone or overlying skin |
| T4b | Brain, dura, skull base, lower cranial nerves, masticator space, carotid artery, prevertebral space, mediastinal structures |
| N0 | No regional lymph node metastasis |
| N1 | Regional lymph node metastasis |

## Salivary Glands
### Summary – *Salivary Glands*

| | |
|---|---|
| T1 | ≤2 cm, without extraparenchymal extension |
| T2 | >2 to 4 cm, without extraparenchymal extension |
| T3 | >4 cm and/or extraparenchymal extension |
| T4a | Skin, mandible, ear canal, facial nerve |
| T4b | Skull, pterygoid plates, carotid artery |

### Clinical N

| | |
|---|---|
| N1 | Ipsilateral single ≤3 cm (ENE-) |
| N2 | (a) Ipsilateral single >3 but ≤6 cm (ENE-) |
| | (b) Ipsilateral multiple ≤6 cm (ENE-) |
| | (c) Bilateral or contralateral ≤6 cm (ENE-) |
| N3 | (a) >6 cm (ENE-) |
| | (b) Any (ENE+) |

### Pathological N

| | |
|---|---|
| N1 | Ipsilateral single ≤3 cm (ENE-) |
| N2 | (a) Ipsilateral single ≤3 cm and ENE+ or ipsilateral single >3 but ≤6 cm (ENE-) |
| | (b) Ipsilateral multiple ≤6 cm (ENE-) |
| | (c) Bilateral or contralateral ≤6 cm (ENE-) |
| N3 | (a) >6 cm (ENE-) |
| | (b) Any (ENE+) other than pN2a |

### *T Classification*
Tumours arising in minor salivary glands localized to the mucus membrane of the upper aerodigestive tract are classified according to the rules for tumours of the oral cavity or pharynx.

Classification by histological type should be done to permit separation of squamous mucosal tumours from minor salivary gland tumours.

## Thyroid
### Summary – *Thyroid*

| | |
|---|---|
| T1 | ≤2 cm, limited to the thyroid |
| | T1a ≤1 cm, limited to the thyroid |
| | T1b >1 cm to 2 cm, limited to the thyroid |
| T2 | >2 but ≤4 cm, limited to the thyroid |
| T3 | >4 cm or minimal thyroid extension |
| | T3a >4 cm, limited to the thyroid |

| | | |
|---|---|---|
| | T3b | Any size, gross extrathyroidal extension: strap muscles (sternohyoid, sternothyroid, omohyoid) |
| T4a | | Subcutaneous soft tissues, larynx, trachea, oesophagus, recurrent laryngeal nerve |
| T4b | | Prevertebral fascia, mediastinal vessels, carotid artery |
| N1a | | Level VI |
| N1b | | Other unilateral, bilateral, contralateral cervical (Levels I, II, III, IV, V) or retropharyngeal (VIIa) |

The classification applies to differentiated thyroid carcinoma (papillary and follicular including Hürthle cell) and to poorly differentiated, medullary and anaplastic (undifferentiated) carcinomas.

### T Classification

Minor extrathyroidal extension was removed from the definition of T3 disease. As a result, minor extrathyroidal extension does not affect either the T category or overall stage.

The T3 category has been divided into T3a and T3b with T3a being a tumour > 4 cm limited to the thyroid and T3b being defined as a tumour of any size with gross extrathyroidal extension (ETE). This separation does not consider a possible prognostic importance of a minimal extrathyroidal extension because the thyroid capsule is incomplete and the capsule and the gland contain varying proportions of muscle, fibrous and adipose tissue; the criteria for defining minimal (pT3) ETE are subjective and problematic. However, a ramification of the T categories is proposed in Chapter 5 (see page 210), taking into consideration cases without or with extrathyroidal extension.

All anaplastic/undifferentiated carcinomas are considered to be T4.

### N Classification

The definition of central neck (N1a) lymph nodes was expanded to include both level VI and upper mediastinal lymph node compartments. In the previous TNM classification [16, 17], upper mediastinal lymph nodes were classified as lateral neck lymph nodes (N1b).

### Stage

Separate stages are recommended for differentiated (papillary and follicular including the Hürthle cell carcinomas) and poorly differentiated carcinomas, medullary carcinomas and anaplastic (undifferentiated) carcinomas.

As there is increasing evidence that 45 years of age is too young a cutoff point for change in prognosis, worse prognosis being associated with a higher age, the age at diagnosis cutoff used for staging was increased from 45 to 55 years [26].

### Stage – Papillary and Follicular, Hürthle cell, under 55 years, poorly differentiated

| | | | |
|---|---|---|---|
| Stage I | Any T | Any N | M0 |
| Stage II | Any T | Any N | M1 |

### Stage – Papillary and Follicular, Hürthle cell, 55 years and older

| | | | |
|---|---|---|---|
| Stage I | T1a, T1b, T2 | N0 | M0 |
| Stage II | T3 | N0 | M0 |
| | T1, T2, T3 | N1 | M0 |
| Stage III | T4a | Any N | M0 |
| Stage IVA | T4b | Any N | M0 |
| Stage IVB | Any T | Any N | M1 |

### Stage – Medullary

| | | | |
|---|---|---|---|
| Stage I | T1a, T1b | N0 | M0 |
| Stage II | T2, T3 | N0 | M0 |
| Stage III | T1, T2, T3 | N1a | M0 |
| Stage IVA | T1, T2, T3 | N1b | M0 |
| | T4a | Any N | M0 |
| Stage IVB | T4b | Any N | M0 |
| Stage IVC | Any T | Any N | M1 |

### Stage – Anaplastic

| | | | |
|---|---|---|---|
| Stage IVA | T1, T2, T3a | N0 | M0 |
| Stage IVB | T1, T2, T3a | N1 | M0 |
| | T3b, T4a, T4b | N0, N1 | M0 |
| Stage IVC | Any T | Any N | M1 |

## Digestive System Tumours

### Rules for Classification

The classification applies to all types of carcinoma. Differentiated neuroendo-crine tumours (G1 and G2) have their own classifications, which are shown at the end of Digestive System Tumours section (page 80). Gastrointestinal stromal tumours are treated within the Tumours of Bones and Soft Tissues section in Chapter 3 (page 157).

## Oesophagus
### Summary – *Oesophagus (includes Oesophagogastric Junction)*

| | |
|---|---|
| T1 | Lamina propria, muscularis mucosae (T1a), submucosa (T1b) |
| T2 | Muscularis propria |
| T3 | Adventitia |
| T4a | Pleura, pericardium, azygos vein, diaphragm, peritoneum |
| T4b | Aorta, vertebral body, trachea |
| N1 | 1–2 regional |
| N2 | 3–6 regional |
| N3 | 7 or more regional |

A tumour whose epicentre is in the stomach within 2 cm of the oesophagogastric junction and also extends into the oesophagus is classified and staged using the oesophageal scheme.

Cancers involving the oesophagogastric junction (OGJ) whose epicentre is within the proximal 2 cm of the cardia (Siewert types I/II) are to be staged as oesophageal carcinomas.

There is a proposal to divide carcinomas of the oesophagogastric junction into three entities [27–29]:

- Adenocarcinoma of the distal oesophagus (AEG I, so-called Barrett carcinoma)
- 'Real' carcinoma of the cardia (AEG II)
- Subcardial carcinoma of the stomach, infiltrating the distal oesophagus (AEG III)

These proposals give some indication of the epidemiology and biology of the tumours. By sampling worldwide data on oesophageal and oesophagogastric junction cancers it has been shown that patients with Siewert's type I/II carcinoma have a similar poor prognosis as patients with oesophageal cancer [28, 29]. Therefore, those types are classified according to tumours of the oesophagus.

Cancers whose epicenter is more than 2 cm distal from the OGJ will be staged using the stomach Cancer TNM and stage, even if the OGJ is involved [30].

### T Classification
The presence of additional synchronous primary carcinomas that are only histologically demonstrable is classified as multifocality and is not considered in the TNM classification. For the separation of these multifocal carcinomas from skip metastasis (intramural metastasis), the configuration of tumour cells as well as the presence of intraepithelial neoplasia are considered. In contrast to multifocality, multiplicity, i.e. the presence of additional macroscopically detectable synchronous primary carcinomas, is indicated in brackets, e.g. T2(m) or pT2(3).

So-called skip metastasis (intramural metastasis) are tumour foci (orally or aborally) separate from the primary carcinoma in the wall of the oesophagus or stomach, particularly in the submucosa. Such skip metastasis can be found in 10–15% in an oesophageal tumour resection specimen. They are considered to be the result of lymphatic spread in the oesophageal wall. These 'skip metastasis' are not considered in the TNM/pTNM classification and are not considered as metastasis.

Invasion of adventitia (cT3/pT3) corresponds to invasion of perioesophageal soft tissue. This is not considered to be invasion of the mediastinum or invasion of adjacent structures and is not classified as T4a/pT4a.

Invasion of pleura, pericardium, azygos vein, peritoneum or diaphragm (structures that are usually considered resectable) are classified as T4a/pT4a.

A carcinoma of the oesophagus that has invaded the stomach and shows a perforation there is classified as T4a/pT4a (equivalent to tumours of the stomach).

Invasion of bronchi, lung, heart, aorta, vena cava, and invasion of recurrent nerve(s) or phrenic or sympathetic nerves (structures that are usually considered unresectable) are classified as T4b.

Invasion in fistulas between the oesophagus and trachea or the oesophagus and bronchus or compression of vena cava is classified as T4b.

### N Classification

The definition of the regional lymph nodes of the oesophagus has been simplified in the 7th edition [17]:

The regional lymph nodes, irrespective of the site of the primary tumour, are those in the oesophageal drainage area, including coeliac axis nodes and paraoesophageal nodes in the neck but not the supraclavicular lymph nodes.

Paraoesophageal lymph nodes within the neck are considered regional. All other involved lymph nodes above the clavicles (supraclavicular) are classified as distant metastasis.

In the AJCC *Cancer Staging Manual* 2017 [10] the regional lymph nodes are listed in detail.

## Regional Lymph Nodes

| Number | Designation | Site |
| --- | --- | --- |
| 1R | Right lower cervical, | Between the supraclavicular space paratracheal nodes and the apex of the lung |
| 1L | Left lower cervical Paratracheal nodes | Between the supraclavicular space and the apex of the lung |

| | | |
|---|---|---|
| 2R | Right upper paratracheal nodes | Between the intersection of the caudal margin of the brachiocephalic artery with the trachea and the apex of the lung |
| 2L | Left upper paratracheal nodes | Between the top of the aortic arch and the apex of the lung |
| 4R | Right lower paratracheal nodes | Between the intersection of the caudal margin of the brachiocephalic artery with the trachea and cephalic border of the azygos vein |
| 4L | Left lower paratracheal nodes | Between the top of the aortic arch and the carina |
| 7 | Subcarinal nodes | Caudal to the carina of the trachea |
| 8U | Upper thoracic paraoesophageal nodes | From the apex of the lung to the tracheal bifurcation |
| 8M | Middle thoracic paraoesophageal nodes | From the tracheal bifurcation to the caudal margin of the inferior pulmonary vein |
| 8Lo | Lower thoracic paraoesophageal nodes | From the caudal margin of the inferior pulmonary vein to the oesophagogastric junction |
| 9R | Pulmonary ligament nodes | Within the right inferior pulmonary ligament |
| 9L | Pulmonary ligament nodes | Within the left inferior pulmonary ligament |
| 15 | Diaphragmatic nodes | On the dome of the diaphragm and adjacent to or behind its crura |
| 16 | Paracardial nodes | Adjacent to the oesophagogastric junction |
| 17 | Left gastric nodes | Along the course of the left gastric artery |
| 18 | Common hepatic nodes | On the proximal common hepatic artery |
| 19 | Splenic nodes | On the proximal splenic artery |
| 20 | Coeliac nodes | On the base of the coeliac artery |

In the 7th edition of the TNM *Classification of Malignant Tumours* of UICC and AJCC there has been a difference in classification of supraclavicular lymph nodes in that they have been classified as distant metastasis in the UICC system [17] and as regional in the AJCC Manual [24].

To correct this problem, the following sentence was placed in AJCC 8th edition [10], page 189:

> The nomenclature for cervical regional nodes follows that of head and neck chapters (see Chapter 6) and are located in periesophageal levels VI and VII. Lymph nodes in continuity with the esophagus would be considered regional.

On page 59 of the 8th edition of the *AJCC Cancer Staging Manual*, Figure 5.1 and Table 5.1 clarify this definition. Supraclavicular lymph nodes are in boundary levels IV and VB. Since they are not in levels VI and VII (which are perioesophageal) they are not regional lymph nodes for the oesophagus. They are distant metastases. In other words, supraclavicular nodes that are perioesophageal are regional but all other supraclavicular nodes are considered to be distant metastases.

Another problem arises by a rule of the TNM System (see page 8). If a tumour involves more than one site or subsite, e.g. contiguous extension to another site or subsite, the regional lymph nodes include those of all involved sites and subsites. According to this rule all nodes regional for the stomach have to be considered as regional for tumours of the oesophagus and also of the oesophagogastric junction. However, in the AJCC list the following stations are missing: perigastric/lesser curvature, perigastric/greater curvature, suprapyloric, infrapyloric, at the splenic hilum.

## Stages and Prognostic Groups

The T, N and M categories used by the UICC and the AJCC are identical. The UICC presents two options for stages and prognostic groups:

1. A purely anatomic approach: T-, N-, M-categories that apply to all histological types, and a separate clinical and pathological stage for squamous cell carcinoma as well as for adenocarcinoma.
2. A prognostic approach – similar to the AJCC approach – that has two separate classifications for squamous cell and adenocarcinoma, with the former taking the histological grade and subsite into consideration and the latter including the histological grade only. The definitions of the prognostic groups for squamous cell and adenocarcinoma of UICC and AJCC are identical. The AJCC Manual has only the prognostic scheme; it is called AJCC Prognostic Stage Groups.

In the 8th edition [12] a clinical (cTNM) as well as a pathological (pTNM) TNM stage have been newly introduced for both squamous cell and adenocarcinomas of the oesophagus. Clinical stages are based on clinically determined T-, N- and M- categories.

## Clinical Stage – Squamous Cell Carcinomas – Pathological Stage

| | | | | | | | |
|---|---|---|---|---|---|---|---|
| Stage 0 | Tis | N0 | M0 | | pTis | pN0 | M0 |
| Stage I | T1 | N0, N1 | M0 | IA | pT1a | pN0 | M0 |
| | | | | IB | pT1b | pN0 | M0 |
| | | | | | pT2 | pN0 | M0 |
| Stage II | T2 | N0, N1 | M0 | IIA | pT2 | pN0 | M0 |
| | T3 | N0 | M0 | IIB | pT1 | pN1 | M0 |
| | | | | | pT3 | pN0 | M0 |
| Stage III | T1, T2 | N2 | M0 | IIIA | pT1 | pN2 | M0 |
| | | | | | pT2 | pN1 | M0 |
| | T3 | N1, N2 | M0 | IIIB | pT2 | pN2 | M0 |
| | | | | | pT3 | pN1, pN2 | M0 |
| | | | | | pT4a | pN0, pN1 | M0 |
| Stage IVA | T4a, T4b | N0, N1, N2 | M0 | IVA | pT4a | pN2 | M0 |
| | | | | | pT4b | Any pN | M0 |
| | | | | | Any pT | pN3 | M0 |
| | Any T | N3 | M0 | IVB | Any pT | Any pN | M1 |
| Stage IVB | Any T | Any N | M1 | | | | |

## Pathological Prognostic Group – Squamous Cell Carcinoma

| Group | T | N | M | Grade | Location* |
|---|---|---|---|---|---|
| 0 | Tis | 0 | 0 | 1 | Any |
| IA | 1 | 0 | 0 | 1, X | Any |
| IB | 1 | 0 | 0 | 2, 3 | Any |
| | 2, 3 | 0 | 0 | 1, X | Lower, X |
| IIA | 2, 3 | 0 | 0 | 1, X | Upper, middle |
| | 2, 3 | 0 | 0 | 2, 3 | Lower, X |
| IIB | 2, 3 | 0 | 0 | 2, 3 | Upper, middle |
| | 1, 2 | 1 | 0 | Any | Any |
| IIIA | 1, 2 | 2 | 0 | Any | Any |
| | 3 | 1 | 0 | Any | Any |
| | 4a | 0 | 0 | Any | Any |
| IIIB | 3 | 2 | 0 | Any | Any |
| Stage IVA | 4a | 2 | 0 | Any | Any |
| | 4b | Any | 0 | Any | Any |
| | Any | 3 | 0 | Any | Any |
| Stage IVB | Any | Any | 1 | Any | Any |

*Lower, middle and upper correspond to the intrathoracic third of the oesophagus.

## Clinical Stage – Adenocarcinoma – Pathological Stage

| | | | | | | | |
|---|---|---|---|---|---|---|---|
| Stage 0 | Tis | N0 | M0 | | pTis | pN0 | M0 |
| Stage I | T1 | N0, N1 | M0 | IA | pT1a | pN0 | M0 |
| | | | | IB | pT1b | pN0 | M0 |
| Stage IIA | T1 | N1 | M0 | IIA | pT2 | pN0 | M0 |
| Stage IIB | T2 | N0 | M0 | IIB | pT1 | pN1 | M0 |
| | | | | | pT3 | pN0 | M0 |
| Stage III | T2 | N1 | M0 | IIIA | pT1 | pN2 | M0 |
| | | | | | pT2 | pN1 | M0 |
| | T3, T4a | N0, N1 | M0 | IIIB | pT2 | pN2 | M0 |
| | | | | | pT3 | pN1, pN2 | M0 |
| | | | | | pT4a | pN0, pN1 | M0 |
| Stage IVA | T1-T4a | Any N | M0 | IVA | pT4a | pN2 | M0 |
| | T4b | N0, N1, N2 | M0 | | pT4b | Any pN | M0 |
| | Any T | N3 | M0 | | Any pT | pN3 | M0 |
| Stage IVB | Any T | N3 | M1 | IVB | Any pT | Any pN | M1 |

In addition, the Pathological Prognostic Groups were kept in the same way as in the 7th edition.

## Pathological Prognostic Group – Adenocarcinoma

| Group | T | N | M | Grade |
|---|---|---|---|---|
| 0 | Tis | 0 | 0 | N/A |
| IA | 1a | 0 | 0 | 1, X |
| IB | 1a | 0 | 0 | 2 |
| | 1b | 0 | 0 | 1, 2 |
| | 1b | 0 | 0 | X |
| IC | 1a, 1b | 0 | 0 | 3 |
| | 2 | 0 | 0 | 1, 2 |
| IIA | 2 | 0 | 0 | 3 |
| | 2 | 0 | 0 | X |
| IIB | 3 | 0 | 0 | Any |
| | 1, 2 | 1 | 0 | Any |
| IIIA | 1 | 2 | 0 | Any |
| | 2 | 1 | 0 | Any |
| IIIB | 2 | 2 | 0 | Any |
| | 3 | 1, 2 | 0 | Any |
| | 4a | 0, 1 | 0 | Any |

| IVA | 4a | 2 | 0 | Any |
|-----|-----|-----|-----|-----|
|  | 4b | Any | 0 | Any |
|  | Any | 3 | 0 | Any |
| IVB | Any | Any | 1 | Any |

Barbour et al. [31] have emphasized that the current staging system (UICC/AJCC) for oesophageal cancer is inadequate for patients who receive neoadjuvant chemoradiotherapy.

The AJCC offers in the 8th edition an additional stage after post-neoadjuvant therapy of patients with squamous cell carcinoma [10] based on WECC data [32–34]. The UICC did not include this in the TNM Classification since it is a measure of response to treatment and may differ depending on the preoperative treatment given and the time interval to surgery.

| yStage I | T0, T1, T2 | N0 | M0 |
|-----|-----|-----|-----|
| yStage II | T3 | N0 | M0 |
| yStage IIIA | T0, T1, T2 | N1 | M0 |
| yStage IIIB | T3 | N1 | M0 |
|  | T0, T1, T2, T3 | N2 | M0 |
|  | T4a | N0 | M0 |
| yStage IVA | T4a | N1, N2 | M0 |
|  | T4a | NX | M0 |
|  | T4b | N0, N1, N2 | M0 |
|  | Any T | N3 | M0 |
| yStage IVB | Any T | Any N | M1 |

The AJCC also offers an additional stage after post-neoadjuvant therapy for patients with adenocarcinoma and adenocarcinoma of the oesophagogastric junction [10] based on WECC data [32–36].

| yStage I | T0, T1, T2 | N0 | M0 |
|-----|-----|-----|-----|
| yStage II | T3 | N0 | M0 |
| yStage IIIA | T0, T1, T2 | N1 | M0 |
| yStage IIIB | T3 | N1 | M0 |
|  | T0, T1, T2, T3 | N2 | M0 |
|  | T4a | N0 | M0 |
| yStage IVA | T4a | N1, N2 | M0 |
|  | T4a | NX | M0 |
|  | T4b | N0, N1, N2 | M0 |
|  | Any T | N3 | M0 |
| yStage IVB | Any T | Any N | M1 |

## Stomach

### Anatomy

Adenocarcinomas that straddle the junction of the oesophagus and stomach are considered tumours of the oesophagogastric (OG) junction. This definition includes many tumours formerly called cancers of the gastric cardia. The convention regarding how to classify such tumours is discussed in the oesophagus section of this chapter (see page 55).

In the presence of Barrett oesophagus, an adenocarcinoma in both the cardia and lower oesophagus (within 2 cm from the oesophagogastric junction) is most likely oesophageal (as is a squamous cell carcinoma). In the absence of Barrett oesophagus such an adenocarcinoma is most likely to be gastric. These biological considerations have no influence on TNM Classification, which classifies these tumours as oesophageal.

## Anatomical Definitions of Lymph Node Stations [37–39]

The regional lymph nodes of the stomach are in groups 1–12:

| | |
|---|---|
| 1 | Right paracardial LNs, including those along the first branch of the ascending limb of the left gastric artery |
| 2 | Left paracardial LNs, including those along the oesophagogastric branch of the left subphrenic artery |
| 3a | Lesser curvature LNs along the branches of the left gastric artery |
| 3b | Lesser curvature LNs along the second branch and distal part of the right gastric artery |
| 4sa | Left greater curvature LNs along the short gastric arteries (perigastric area) |
| 4sb | Left greater curvature LNs along the left gastroepiploic artery (perigastric area) |
| 4d | Right greater curvature LNs along the second branch and distal part of the right gastroepiploic artery |
| 5 | Suprapyloric LNs along the first branch and proximal part of the right gastric artery |
| 6 | Infrapyloric LNs along the first branch and proximal part of the right gastroepiploic artery down to the confluence of the right gastroepiploic vein and the anterior superior pancreatoduodenal vein |
| 7 | LNs along the left gastric artery between its root and the origin of its ascending branch |
| 8a | Anteriosuperior LNs along the common hepatic artery |
| 8b | Posterior LNs along the common hepatic artery |
| 9 | Coeliac artery LNs |

| 10 | Splenic hilar LNs including those adjacent to the splenic artery distal to the pancreatic tail, those on the roots of the short gastric arteries and those along the left gastroepiploic artery proximal to its first gastric branch |
|---|---|
| 11p | Proximal splenic artery LNs from its origin to halfway between its origin and the pancreatic tail end |
| 11d | Distal splenic artery LNs from halfway between its origin and the pancreatic tail end to the end of the pancreatic tail |
| 12a | Hepatoduodenal ligament LNs along the proper hepatic artery, in the caudal half between the confluence of the right and left hepatic ducts and the upper border of the pancreas |
| 12b | Hepatoduodenal ligament LNs along the bile duct, in the caudal half between the confluence of the right and left hepatic ducts and the upper border of the pancreas |
| 12p | Hepatoduodenal ligament LNs along the portal vein in the caudal half between the confluence of the right and left hepatic ducts and the upper border of the pancreas |
| 13 | LNs on the posterior surface of the pancreatic head cranial to the duodenal papilla |
| 14v | LNs along the superior mesenteric vein |
| 15 | LNs along the middle colic vessels |
| 16a1 | Para-aortic LNs in the diaphragmatic aortic hiatus |
| 16a2 | Para-aortic LNs between the upper margin of the origin of the coeliac artery and the lower border of the left renal vein |
| 16b1 | Para-aortic LNs between the lower border of the left renal vein and the upper border of the origin of the inferior mesenteric artery |
| 16b2 | Para-aortic LNs between the upper border of the origin of the inferior mesenteric artery and the aortic bifurcation |
| 17 | LNs on the anterior surface of the pancreatic head beneath the pancreatic sheath |
| 18 | LNs along the inferior border of the pancreatic body |
| 19 | Infradiaphragmatic LNs predominantly along the subphrenic artery |
| 20 | Paraoesophageal LNs in the diaphragmatic oesophageal hiatus |
| 110 | Paraoesophageal LNs in the lower thorax |
| 111 | Supradiaphragmatic LNs separate from the oesophagus |
| 112 | Posterior mediastinal LNs separate from the oesophagus and the oesophageal hiatus |

**Note.**

The numerical order corresponds to the proposals of the Japanese Gastric Cancer Association [37].

Stations 7, 8, 9 and 11 ('along the ... ', 'around the ...') include only lymph nodes along the main trunk of the mentioned arteries. Lymph nodes along the ramifications of the left gastric artery are classified as perigastric nodes.

In the case of gastric stump carcinoma (following previous distal gastrectomy and localized at the anastomosis) lymph nodes in the mesentery of the intestinal loop used for anastomosis are classified as gastric regional nodes.

In the case of gastric carcinoma, the epicentre of which is more than 2 cm from the oesophagogastric junction, with invasion of the oesophagus the infradiaphragmatic lymph nodes (No. 19) and the lymph nodes of the oesophageal hiatus (No. 20) are considered as additional regional lymph nodes [39, 40].

### Summary – *Stomach*

| | |
|---|---|
| T1 | Lamina propria, muscularis mucosae (T1a), submucosa (T1b) |
| T2 | Muscularis propria |
| T3 | Subserosa |
| T4a | Perforates serosa |
| T4b | Adjacent structures |
| N1 | 1–2 regional |
| N2 | 3–6 regional |
| N3a | 7–15 regional |
| N3b | 16 or more regional |

### *T Classification*

Invasion of the transverse mesocolon is considered analogous to invasion of the gastrocolic ligament and is therefore classified as T3/pT3 if the covering visceral peritoneum is not perforated. The same applies to direct invasion of the greater omentum.

The adjacent structures of the stomach include the spleen, transverse colon, liver diaphragm, pancreas, abdominal wall, adrenal gland, kidney, small intestine and retroperitoneum.

Intramural extension to the duodenum or oesophagus is classified by the depth of invasion in any of these sites, including the stomach.

Tumour nodules in the greater omentum that are separate from the primary tumour are classified as distant (peritoneal) metastasis (M1 PER).

### *N Classification*

For pN0 histological examination of a regional lymphadenectomy specimen will ordinarily include 16 or more lymph nodes.

Metastasis in lymph nodes other than those defined above are classified as distant metastasis, e.g. signet ring cell carcinoma of the gastric antrum with submucosal invasion and with 34 regional lymph nodes without metastasis but one lymph node metastasis in a retropancreatic lymph nodes is classified as pT1bpN0(0/34)pM1 LYM.

Extracapsular spread in regional lymph nodes has been described as an independent prognostic factor and can be recorded separately to obtain further data [41].

The presence of isolated tumour cells (ITC) in the regional lymph nodes did not affect the prognosis of patients with stomach carcinoma who underwent gastrectomy with D2 lymph node dissection [42–44].

### *M Classification*

So-called omental deposits of stomach carcinoma distant from the primary tumour are classified as M1/pM1.

### *Stages*

Based on the data of the ICGA staging project [30] in the 8th edition [10, 12] a clinical stage as well as a pathological stage were introduced.

### Clinical Stage

| Stage 0 | Tis | N0 | M0 |
|---|---|---|---|
| Stage I | T1, T2 | N0 | M0 |
| Stage IIA | T1, T2 | N1, N2, N3 | M0 |
| Stage IIB | T3, T4a | N0 | M0 |
| Stage III | T3, T4a | N1, N2, N3 | M0 |
| Stage IVA | T4b | Any N | M0 |
| Stage IVB | Any T | Any N | M1 |

### Pathological Stage

| Stage 0 | Tis | N0 | M0 |
|---|---|---|---|
| Stage IA | T1 | N0 | M0 |
| Stage IB | T1 | N1 | M0 |
| | T2 | N0 | M0 |
| Stage IIA | T1 | N2 | M0 |
| | T2 | N1 | M0 |
| | T3 | N1 | M0 |
| | T4a | N0 | M0 |
| Stage IIB | T1 | N3a | M0 |
| | T2 | N2 | M0 |
| | T1 | N1 | M0 |
| Stage IIIA | T2 | N3a | M0 |
| | T3 | N1 | M0 |
| | T4a | N1, N2 | M0 |
| | T4b | N0 | M0 |

| Stage IIIB | T1, T2 | N3b | M0 |
|---|---|---|---|
| | T3, T4a | N3a | M0 |
| | T4b | N1, N2 | M0 |
| Stage IIIC | T3, T4a | N3b | M0 |
| | T4b | N3a, N3b | M0 |
| Stage IV | Any T | Any N | M1 |

The AJCC published prognostic groups for use after neoadjuvant therapy (categories with the prefix 'y') [44, 45].

It will have to be evaluated whether these new stages after neoadjuvant therapy will be helpful for clinical purposes. Comparisons of outcome results among different sort of stages should be performed.

## Small Intestine

### Summary – *Small Intestine*

| | |
|---|---|
| T1 | Lamina propria or muscularis mucosae (T1a), submucosa (T1b) |
| T2 | Muscularis propria |
| T3 | Subserosa, non-peritonealized perimuscular tissues (mesentery, retroperitoneum), without perforation of the serosa |
| T4 | Perforates visceral peritoneum or invades other organs/structures including small bowel loops, mesentery, retroperitoneum, abdominal wall (via serosa) |
| | Duodenum only: invasion of pancreas |
| N1 | 1–2 regional |
| N2 | ≥3 regional |

### *T Classification*

The very uncommon carcinoma in a Meckel diverticulum may be classified according to the classification for small intestine carcinoma, although supporting data are not available.

Intramural extension of an ileal carcinoma directly into the caecum (not by way of the serosa) does not affect the T classification, and in particular does not qualify for T4. The T should reflect the deepest invasion in either site.

### *N Classification*

For pN0 histological examination of a regional lymphadenectomy the specimen will ordinarily include 6 or more lymph nodes.

In rare cases, tumour deposits (satellites) can be observed in carcinomas of the small bowel. These findings should be documented. Presently, these findings are not classified in the N classification in the same manner as for carcinomas of the appendix or colon/rectum.

## Appendix

The classification applies to adenocarcinomas of the appendix. Neuroendocrine tumours are classified separately (see page 80). There should be histological confirmation of the disease and separation of carcinomas into mucinous and non-mucinous adenocarcinomas.

Goblet cell carcinoids are classified according to the carcinoma scheme.

Grading is of particular importance for mucinous carcinomas.

### Summary – *Appendix Carcinoma*

| | |
|---|---|
| Tis | Carcinoma in situ: intraepithelial or invasion of lamina propria |
| Tis (LAMN) | LAMN confined to appendix |
| T1 | Submucosa |
| T2 | Muscularis propria |
| T3 | Subserosa or mesoappendix |
| T4 | Perforates visceral peritoneum, including mucinous peritoneal tumour or acellular mucin on the serosa of the appendix/mesoappendix, and/or directly invades other organs/structures |
| | T4a Perforates visceral peritoneum, including mucinous peritoneal tumour or acellular mucin on the serosa of the appendix/mesoappendix |
| | T4b Invasion of other organs or structures |
| N1 | 1–3 regional |
| | N1a Metastasis in 1 regional lymph node |
| | N1b Metastasis in 2–3 regional lymph nodes |
| | N1c Tumour deposits (satellites) in the subserosa or in non-peritonealized pericolic or perirectal soft tissues without regional lymph nodes |
| N2 | 4 or more regional |
| M1 | Distant |
| | M1a Intraperitoneal acellular mucin only |
| | M1b Intraperitoneal metastasis only including mucinous epithelium |
| | M1c Non-peritoneal |

### *T Classification*

Tis/pTis includes cancer cells confined within the glandular basement membrane (intraepithelial) or lamina propria (intramucosal) with no extension through muscularis mucosae into the submucosa.

Low-grade appendiceal mucinous neoplasm (LAMN) confined to the appendix (defined as involvement by acellular mucin or mucinous epithelium that may extend into muscularis propria) is classified Tis/pTis.

LAMN with involvement of the subserosa or the serosal surface (visceral peritoneum) should be classified as T3 or T4a, respectively.

Direct invasion in T4 includes invasion of other intestinal segments by way of the serosa, e.g. invasion of the ileum.

Tumour that is adherent to other organs or structures, macroscopically, is classified T4b. However, if no tumour is present in the adhesion, microscopically, the classification should be pT1, pT2 or pT3.

### N Classification

Tumour deposits (satellites) are discrete macroscopic or microscopic nodules of cancer in the adipose tissue's lymph drainage area of a primary carcinoma that are discontinuous from the primary and without histological evidence of a residual lymph node or identifiable vascular or neural structures. If a vessel wall is identifiable on H&E, elastic or other stains, it should be classified as venous invasion (V1/V2) or lymphatic invasion (L1). Similarly, if neural structures are identifiable, the lesion should be classified as perineural invasion (Pn1).

### M Classification

Distant metastases were newly subdivided [11, 12]:

| M1 | Distant metastasis |
| | M1a | Intraperitoneal acellular mucin only |
| | M1b | Intraperitoneal metastasis only including mucinous epithelium |
| | M1c | Non-peritoneal metastasis |

### Stage – Appendix Carcinoma

Stage 0 has been newly introduced in the 8th edition [10, 12] and Stage IV was subdivided in Stages IVA-IVC.

| Stage 0 | Tis | N0 | M0 | |
| Stage 0 | Tis(LAMN) | N0 | M0 | |
| Stage I | T1, T2 | N0 | M0 | |
| Stage IIA | T3 | N0 | M0 | |
| Stage IIB | T4a | N0 | M0 | |
| Stage IIC | T4b | N0 | M0 | |
| Stage IIIA | T1, T2 | N1 | M0 | |
| Stage IIIB | T3, T4 | N1 | M0 | |
| Stage IIIC | Any T | N2 | M0 | |
| Stage IVA | Any T | Any N | M1a | Any G |
| | Any T | Any N | M1b | G1 |
| Stage IVB | Any T | Any N | M1b | G2, G3, GX |
| Stage IVC | Any T | Any N | M1c | Any G |

### G – Histopathological Grading

Determination of the histologic grade has prognostic significance and is needed to define Stage IVA tumours as either IVA or IVB.

Appendiceal mucinous adenocarcinomas (those with > 50% of the tumour mass consisting of extracellular mucin) that spread into the peritoneum have a better prognosis than non-mucinous tumours.

| | | |
|---|---|---|
| GX | Grade of differentiation cannot be assessed | |
| G1 | Well differentiated | Mucinous low grade |
| G2 | Moderately differentiated | Mucinous high grade |
| G3 | Poorly differentiated | Mucinous high grade |
| G4 | Undifferentiated | |

## Colon and Rectum

### Anatomical Sites and Subsites

1. A tumour located at the border between two subsites is registered as a tumour of the subsite that is more involved.

   **Example**
   A carcinoma with a longitudinal diameter of 6 cm, 2 cm in the caecum and 4 cm in the ascending colon is classified as a carcinoma of the ascending colon (C 18.2).

   If two subsites are involved to the same extent, the lesion is classified as an overlapping lesion.

   **Example**
   If the carcinoma involves 2 cm of the caecum and 2 cm of the ascending colon, the code C 18.8 (overlapping lesion of the colon) is used.

2. The rectum is defined as the distal large intestine commencing opposite the sacral promontory and ending at the upper border of the anal canal. When measured from below with a rigid sigmoidoscope, it extends 16 cm from the anal verge. A tumour is classified as rectal if its lower margin lies 16 cm or less from the anal verge [46, 47]. A tumour is considered rectal if any is located at least within the supply of the superior rectal artery. Tumours are classified as rectosigmoid when differentiation between the rectum and sigmoid according to the above rules is not possible.

   According to the recommendations of the International Documentation System [46] and its actualized version [47] a tumour is classified as rectal if its lower margin lies 16 cm or less from the anal verge, when measured from below with a rigid sigmoidoscope. In Europe, most authors follow this rule, while others use 15 cm as the boundary. However, in the US, generally only tumours with a lower margin of 12 cm or less from the anal margin are classified as rectal. Because of these differences, the definition of rectal carcinoma used should be stated in relevant publications.

Owing to differences in treatment and prognosis, the rectum may be subdivided into three parts according to the distance of the lower margin of the tumour from the anal verge (assessed by rigid sigmoidoscopy) [47]:

| | |
|---|---|
| Upper third/upper rectum | 12–16 cm |
| Middle third/middle rectum | 6–< 12 cm |
| Lower third/lower rectum | < 6 cm |

For tumours of the colon, frequently only the colonoscopic measurement of the distance between the tumour and anal verge is available. In this case, the site can be coded according to the recommendations of the SEER Program [48].

### Local Recurrence

A local recurrence after previous colon resection should be classified with the prefix 'r' (for recurrence). The recurrent tumour is topographically assigned to the proximal segment of the anastomosis.

### Regional Lymph Nodes

Metastasis in the external iliac or common iliac nodes is classified as distant metastasis (M1a/pM1a) as metastasis in lymph nodes along the superior mesenteric artery, provided this is the only site of metastasis.

In case of direct invasion of the small intestine, lymph nodes in the mesentery of the invaded intestinal loop are considered as regional lymph nodes.

### Summary – Colon and Rectum

| | |
|---|---|
| Tis | Carcinoma in situ (lamina propria) |
| T1 | Submucosa |
| T2 | Muscularis propria |
| T3 | Subserosa, non-peritonealized pericolic/perirectal tissues |
| T4a | Perforates visceral peritoneum |
| T4b | Invades other organs or structures |
| N1a | 1 regional |
| N1b | 2–3 regional |
| N1c | Satellite(s) without regional lymph nodes |
| N2a | 4–6 regional |
| N2b | 7 or more regional |
| M1 | Distant metastasis |
| | M1a One organ (liver, lung, ovary, non-regional lymph node(s), without peritoneal metastasis |
| | M1b >one organ |
| | M1c Peritoneum, with or without other organs |

## T Classification

Tis includes cancer cells confined within the mucosal lamina propria (intramucosal) with no extension through the muscularis mucosae in the submucosa. High-grade intraepithelial neoplasia (dysplasia) should not be assigned to the category 'Tis/pTis' any longer because these lesions lack potential for invasive cancer spread (no invasion through the basement membrane).

T3/pT3: The perirectal tissue includes the mesorectum (paraproctium).

Tumour extension into the peritoneal cavity is classified as T4a. Perforation of the visceral peritoneum at the microscopic level requires identification of the tumour directly extending to and growing on the peritoneal surface and/or positive cytology on specimens obtained by scraping the serosa overlying the primary tumour [49].

Intramural direct extension from one subsite (segment) of the colon to an adjacent one is not considered in the T classification. The same applies to intramural direct extension from the rectum to the sigmoid colon and vice versa and from the rectum to the anal canal.

Intramural extension of a caecal carcinoma directly into the ileum (not by way of serosa) does not affect the T classification, in particular it does not qualify for T4b. In contrast, direct extension via serosa or via mesocolon is classified T4b, e.g. extension of a sigmoid colon carcinoma to caecum.

Perforation of the bowel does not justify pT4a unless the tumour itself is at the perforation.

Vaginal involvement by rectal adenocarcinoma can be classified T4b/pT4b if there is invasion of the vaginal wall.

Tumour cells in lymphatics or veins do not affect the pT classification. The V and L classifications can be used to record such spread.

### Example

Carcinoma with continuous local spread into the submucosa, tumour cells in a small vein within the muscularis propria - pT1, V1 (muscularis propria).

Perineural invasion is considered part of the T classification, but can also be recorded as Pn1.

### Example

Carcinoma with continuous local spread into the submucosa, tumour cells in perineural structures in the pericolorectal adipous tissue – pT3, Pn1.

Direct invasion of the Musculus sphincter ani internus and/or externus and/or levator ani should be classified as T4b/pT4b.

A tumour nodule in the soft tissues beneath a perineal surgical skin scar after abdominoperineal resection for rectal carcinoma after a disease-free interval is classified as rT(+) not M1.

A rectal tumour extending into the presacral fascia is considered T4b/pT4b.

An omental deposit that is not a tumour deposit or satellite is considered to be a peritoneal metastases and staged as cM1c/pM1c.

### N/pN Classification and Tumour Deposits (Satellites)

Macroscopic or microscopic detectable nodules of cancer found in the pericolic or perirectal adipous tissue in the lymph drainage area of a primary carcinoma that are discontinuous from the primary tumour and without histological evidence of residual lymph node or identifiable vascular (venous) or neural structures are considered to be tumour deposits (TDs) or satellite nodules.

If a vessel is identifiable on H&E, elastic or other stains, it should be classified as venous invasion (V1/V2) or lymphatic invasion (L1). Similarly, if neural structures are identifiable, the lesion should be classified as perineural invasion (Pn1).

The presence of tumour deposits does not change the primary tumour T/pT categories, but change the node status (N) to pN1c, if all examined regional lymph nodes are negative on pathological examination.

There is no size criterion for TD. This proposal was modelled after the N2/3 satellite category of skin melanoma where no size is given.

There is no consensus on how far the TD is from the bowel wall, but it must be discontinuous extension.

If TDs are recorded after neoadjuvant radiation therapy or neoadjuvant chemotherapy, or a combination of both, where tumour regression and isolated clusters of cells are common, it is vital to document the neoadjuvant treatment to separate these cases from those receiving surgery without pre-operative neoadjuvant therapy. The pathologic classification after neoadjuvant therapy must use the 'y' prefix, ypTNM, to further distinguish these cases.

### Example

Carcinoma with continuous local spread into the muscularis propria, 3 satellites in the subserosal soft tissue, no regional lymph node metastasis in 18 lymph nodes and no distant metastasis is classified as pT2pN1c(0/18)(3TDs)cM0.

### Example

Carcinoma with continuous local spread into the muscularis propria, 3 satellites in the subserosal soft tissue and an additional 3 lymph node metastasis in 24 examined regional lymph nodes and no distant metastasis is classified as pT2pN1b(3/24)(3TDs)cM0.

Involvement of the apical lymph node(s) does not influence the N/pN classification.

## M Classification

Tumour nodule(s) in an abdominal scar after removal of an intra-abdominal tumour (with a disease-free interval) should be classified as M1c/pM1c, e.g. rcT0cN0pM1c.

A tumour deposit that is discontinuous from the primary tumour and perforates the serosa with access to the peritoneal cavity should be classified as M1c/pM1c.

# Anal Canal and Perianal Skin

The anal canal extends from the rectum to the perianal skin (to the junction with hair-bearing skin). It is lined by the mucous membrane overlying the internal sphincter, including the transitional epithelium and dentate line.

Tumours of the anal margin and perianal skin defined as within 5 cm of the anal margin (ICD-O C44.5) are now classified with carcinomas of the anal canal.

It should be emphasized that three different types of carcinomas are included in this TNM classification: tumours of the anal canal, tumours of the anal margin and tumours of perianal skin. The latter two have a different lymphatic drainage leading only to inguinal and not to intrapelvic lymph nodes.

The classification applies to all types of carcinoma including those arising within an anorectal fistula as well as squamous cell (cloacogenic) carcinoma.

## Regional Lymph Nodes

The regional lymph nodes are differently defined by the UICC and AJCC.

| UICC [12] | AJCC [10] |
| --- | --- |
| Perirectal lymph nodes | Mesorectal lymph nodes |
| Internal iliac lymph nodes | Internal iliac lymph nodes (hypogastric) |
| External iliac lymph nodes | External iliac lymph nodes |
| Inguinal lymph nodes | Inguinal lymph nodes (superficial, deep) |
| | Superior rectal (haemorrhoidal) |

## Summary – *Anal Canal*

| | |
| --- | --- |
| T1 | ≤2 cm |
| T2 | >2 – 5 cm |
| T3 | >5 cm |
| T4 | Adjacent organ(s) |
| N1 | Metastasis in regional lymph node(s) |
| | N1a  Inguinal, and/or internal iliac |
| | N1b  External iliac |
| | N1c  External iliac and inguinal, and/or internal iliac |

### T Classification

The tumour is classified by size (T1-T3) except when there is invasion of adjacent organ(s) such as the vagina, urethra, bladder (T4/pT4). Direct invasion of the rectal wall, perianal skin, subcutaneous tissue or the sphincter muscle(s) alone is not classified as T4/pT4 but according to the size of the tumour (T1–T3).

### N Classification

In previous editions the regional nodes were defined as perirectal, internal iliac and inguinal not external iliac. There is lack of evidence on the prognostic significance of the different lymph node regions and no evidence that external iliac node involvement should be classified as metastatic. Tumours below the dentate line may spread to the inguinal and external iliac nodes, while tumours above the dentate line spread to the pararectal and internal iliac nodes. To facilitate collection of data of the prognostic significance of nodal disease the N category was revised.

N1a    Metastases in inguinal, mesorectal and/or internal iliac lymph nodes
N1b    Metastases in external iliac lymph nodes
N1c    Metastases in external iliac and in inguinal, mesorectal and/or internal iliac lymph nodes

## Liver – Hepatocellular Carcinoma

The classification applies only to hepatocellular carcinoma.

Fibrolamellar carcinoma, previously known as fibrolamellar variant of HCC, lacks a specific staging system. Thus, the current HCC staging system should be used.

### Summary – *Hepatocellular Carcinoma*

| | |
|---|---|
| T1a | Solitary, ≤ 2 cm, with or without vascular invasion |
| T1b | Solitary, > 2 cm without vascular invasion |
| T2 | Solitary with vascular invasion, > 2 cm or multiple ≤ 5 cm |
| T3 | Multiple > 5 cm |
| T4 | Invades major branch of portal or hepatic vein, or invasion of adjacent organs (including diaphragm) other than the gallbladder, perforates visceral peritoneum |
| N1 | Regional |

### T Classification

'Multiplicity' includes multiple nodules representing multiple, independent primary tumours and intrahepatic metastasis from a single primary hepatic carcinoma.

'Vascular invasion' is diagnosed clinically by imaging procedures. In the pathological classification it includes macroscopic as well as microscopic involvement of vessels.

Major vascular invasion is defined as invasion of the branches of the main portal vein (right or left portal vein, excluding the sectoral and segmental branches), one or more of the three hepatic veins (right, middle or left) or the main branches of the proper hepatic artery (right or left hepatic artery) [10, 50].

Multiple tumours include satellitosis, multifocal tumours and intrahepatic metastasis.

T4: 'major branches of the portal or hepatic veins' are the right and left branches of the portal vein and the corresponding hepatic veins (not segmental or subsegmental branches).

Involvement of the right, left and (not always existent) intermediate branches of the hepatic artery is also classified as T4.

Invasion of the hepatic ducts or common bile duct or the hepatoduodenal ligament is recommended to be classified as T4/pT4.

Although the presence of cirrhosis is an independent prognostic factor it does not affect the TNM classification, being an independent prognostic variable.

## Liver – Intrahepatic Bile Ducts

The staging system applies to intrahepatic cholangiocarcinoma (cholangiocellular carcinoma) and combined hepatocellular-cholangiocarcinoma (mixed hepato-cholangiocarcinoma). It also applies to intrahepatic biliary cystadenocarcinoma.

The AJCC [10] indicates that primary neuroendocrine tumours of the liver should be classified according to this system.

### Summary – *Intrahepatic Bile Ducts*

| | |
|---|---|
| T1a | Solitary, ≤ 5 cm, without vascular invasion |
| T1b | Solitary, > 5 cm, without vascular invasion |
| T2 | Solitary, with intrahepatic vascular invasion or multiple with/without vascular invasion |
| T3 | Perforation of the visceral peritoneum |
| T4 | Adjacent extrahepatic structures (direct hepatic invasion) |
| N1 | Regional |

### *T/pT Classification*

Lesions classified as carcinoma in situ should meet histologic criteria for biliary intraepithelial neoplasia grade 3 (BilIN-3) or for high-grade dysplasia in an intraductal papillary lesion or mucinous cystic lesion.

Intrahepatic cholangiocarcinoma directly invading the gallbladder wall should be classified as T3/pT3.

Invasion of the hepatic ducts or common bile duct or the hepatoduodenal ligament (hilar fat) is recommended to be classified as T4/pT4, as well as invasion of the retrohepatic vena cava and visceral structures (e.g. duodenum, colon).

'Periductal invasion' characterizes a rare (about 10%) tumour type of intrahepatic cholangiocarcinoma with primarily growth along the intrahepatic large and small bile ducts, usually without mass formation. Patients with this type have been shown to have a very poor prognosis. This growth pattern was eliminated from staging in the 8th edition [10, 12] but is still recommended for data collection.

## Gallbladder

The staging system applies to gallbladder carcinoma (ICD-O-3 C23.9) and to carcinoma of the cystic duct (ICD-O C24.0). The latter ICD-O Code is identical to tumours of the extrahepatic bile ducts (perihilar and distal).

### Summary – *Gallbladder and Cystic Duct*

| | |
|---|---|
| T1 | Lamina propria or muscular layer |
| T1a | Lamina propria |
| T1b | Muscularis propria |
| T2 | Perimuscular connective tissue, no extension beyond serosa or into liver |
| | T2a Perimuscular connective tissue on the peritoneal side (no extension to serosa) |
| | T2b Perimuscular connective tissue on the hepatic side (no extension into liver) |
| T3 | Perforates serosa (visceral peritoneum), and/or liver, and/or invades one organ/structure |
| T4 | Main portal vein or hepatic artery or invades two or more extrahepatic organs/structures |
| N1 | 1–3 regional |
| N2 | 4 or more regional |

### T Classification

T2/pT2 tumours are now subdivided into two groups: T2a/pT2a tumours are on the peritoneal side and T2b/pT2b tumours are on the hepatic side. It has been shown that patients with a hepatic side tumour have a worse prognosis [51].

Adjacent organs or structures are: stomach, duodenum, colon, pancreas, omentum, extrahepatic bile ducts.

Invasion of the hepatoduodenal ligament (hilar fat) is classified as T4/pT4.

### N Classification

The definitions of the N categories changed from location-based definitions to number-based definitions. N categories have been revised to define N1/pN1 as one to three positive lymph nodes and N2/pN2 as four or more positive lymph nodes.

The recommendation that six or more regional lymph nodes should be removed and examined has been added (in contrast to three regional lymph nodes in the 7th edition [10, 12]).

## Extrahepatic Bile Ducts
In TNM-8 [10, 12] there are two classifications for extrahepatic bile ducts:

1) The perihilar extrahepatic bile ducts (so-called Klatskin tumour) and
2) Extrahepatic bile ducts distal to the insertion of the cystic duct.

Carcinoma of the cystic duct and carcinoma in a choledochal cyst are classified as gallbladder carcinoma.

### Anatomical Sites
If a tumour site is designated 'bile duct' or 'extrahepatic bile duct' the classification should follow that of the distal bile duct.

In cases in which the gallbladder including the cystic duct has been removed the surgical clip should be used to separate perihilar and distal sites.

## 1) Perihilar Extrahepatic Bile Ducts
The classification applies to carcinomas of the extrahepatic bile ducts of perihilar localization (Klatskin tumour). Included are the right, left and the common hepatic ducts. The tumours are located in the extrahepatic biliary tree proximal to the origin of the cystic duct.

### Summary – *Perihilar Bile Ducts*

| | |
|---|---|
| T1 | Confined to the bile duct, with extension up to the muscle layer or fibrous tissue |
| T2a | Invades beyond the wall of the bile duct to surrounding adipose tissue |
| T2b | Invades adjacent hepatic parenchyma |
| T3 | Tumour invades unilateral branches of the portal vein or hepatic artery |
| T4 | Invades main portal vein or its branches bilaterally, common hepatic artery or the second-order biliary radicals bilaterally; or unilateral second-order biliary radicals with contralateral portal vein or hepatic artery involvement |
| N1 | 1–3 regional |
| N2 | 4 or more regional |

### T Classification

The definition of Tis/pTis has been expanded to include high-grade biliary intraepithelial neoplasia (BilIn-3). High-grade dysplasia (BilIn-3), a non-invasive neoplastic process, is synonymous with carcinoma in situ at this site.

According to the anatomical nomenclature the terms 'confined to the bile ducts' and invasion 'beyond the wall of the bile duct' are defined as follows:

T1/pT1 (confined to the bile duct) includes tumours confined to the subepithelial connective tissue (tunica mucosa) or the fibromuscular layer (tunica muscularis) only.

T2/pT2 (beyond the wall of the bile duct) includes tumours with invasion of the perifibromuscular connective tissue.

The T3/pT3 hepatic artery corresponds to the common hepatic artery.

Tumours directly invading the pancreas (per continuitatem) are classified as T3/pT3.

Bilateral second-order biliary radical invasion (Bismuth–Corlette type IV) has been removed from the T4/pT4 category.

This classification does not apply to carcinomas of the ampulla of Vater.

### N Classification

N categories have been revised to define N1/pN1 as one to three positive lymph nodes and N2/pN2 as four or more positive lymph nodes.

## 2) Distal Extrahepatic Bile Ducts

### Summary – *Distal Extrahepatic Bile Ducts*

| | |
|---|---|
| T1 | Confined to the bile duct wall < 5 mm |
| T2 | Confined to the bile duct wall 5–≤ 12 mm |
| T3 | Confined to the bile duct wall > 12 mm |
| T4 | Invades coeliac axis, superior mesenteric artery and/or common hepatic artery |
| N1 | 1–3 regional |
| N2 | 4 or more regional |

### T Classification

The definition of Tis/pTis has been expanded to include high-grade biliary intraepithelial neoplasia (BilIn-3). High-grade dysplasia (BilIn-3), a noninvasive neoplastic process, is synonymous with carcinoma in situ at this site.

Definitions of T1/pT1, T2/pT2 and T3/pT3 have been revised based on the measured depth of invasion. The descriptive extent of invasion should also be recorded. Depth of invasion is better than the descriptive extent of tumour invasion in predicting patient outcomes [15, 52].

## Ampulla of Vater

This staging system applies to all primary carcinomas that arise in the ampulla or on the duodenal papilla. This system does not apply to well-differentiated neuroendocrine tumours (G1 and G2) but does apply to high-grade neuroendocrine carcinomas, such as small cell carcinomas and large cell neuroendocrine carcinomas.

### Regional lymph nodes

The definition of regional lymph nodes has changed and is now the same as that of the pancreas.

### Summary – *Ampulla of Vater*

| | |
|---|---|
| T1a | Ampulla or sphincter of Oddi |
| T1b | Beyond sphincter of Oddi and/or duodenal submucosa |
| T2 | Muscularis propria of duodenum |
| T3 | Pancreas or peripancreatic tissue |
| | T3a ≤0.5 cm in pancreas |
| | T3b >0.5 cm, extends into peripancreatic tissue, duodenal serosa |
| T4 | Involvement of superior mesenteric artery, coeliac axis, common hepatic artery |
| N1 | 1–3 regional |
| N2 | 4 or more regional |

### T Classification

An invasive adenocarcinoma arising in an intraampullary papillary neoplasm, extensively infiltrating the duodenum and periduodenal/peripancreatic soft tissue with focal minimal infiltration of the pancreas without duodenal serosal involvement, should be classified as pT3b [12].

## Pancreas

The classification applies to carcinomas of the exocrine pancreas and/or high-grade pancreatic neuroendocrine carcinomas.

## Summary – *Pancreas*

T1  ≤2 cm
    T1a  ≤0.5 cm
    T1b  >0.5–1 cm
    T1c  >1–2 cm
T2  >2 cm–≤4 cm
T3  >4 cm
T4  Coeliac axis, superior mesenteric artery and/or common hepatic artery
N1  1–3 regional
N2  4 or more regional

### *T Classification*

T1–T3 categories are based on the size of the tumour.

Invasion of peripancreatic soft tissue is no longer a criterion for T3. This is because the peripancreatic soft tissue is poorly defined and invasion does not appear to be discriminatory in determining prognosis [53].

Invasion of the coeliac axis, superior mesenteric artery and/or common hepatic artery is classified as T4. Invasion of the coeliac axis comprises invasion of the vessels belonging to the coeliac trunk.

Invasion of the caval vein is classified as T4.

The coeliac axis comprises the anatomical plane surrounding the origin of the coeliac artery from the anterior aorta. This plane is defined by imaging studies or the inability to create a plane between the tumour and the arterial wall at the time of operative resection.

Tumour extension in the mesocolon, omentum, extrapancreatic biliary tract, duodenum and the ampulla of Vater for pancreatic head tumours does not affect the T category. Tumour extension in the stomach, spleen, left adrenal gland and peritoneum for the pancreatic body or tail tumours does not affect the T category any more.

## Neuroendocrine Tumours

The classification system applies to well-differentiated neoplasms, i.e. neuroendocrine tumours G1 and G2 – formerly called carcinoid and atypical carcinoid tumours – of the gastrointestinal tract. Pancreatic well-differentiated neoplasms, i.e. neuroendocrine tumours, are graded G1, G2 and G3 [54, 55]. It is intended that the UICC, AJCC and ENETS classifications of neuroendocrine tumours will all be aligned.

Neuroendocrine neoplasms of the lung should be classified according to the criteria of the WHO Classification 2015 [56] and appropriate TNM.

Merkel cell carcinoma of the skin has a separate TNM classification.

Poorly differentiated (high-grade) neuroendocrine neoplasms (i.e. neuroendocrine carcinomas) are excluded and should be classified according to the criteria applied to conventional carcinomas at the respective site.

## Histopathological Grading

The following histopathological grading scheme is in use for gastrointestinal and pancreatic well-differentiated neuroendocrine neoplasms, i.e. neuroendocrine tumours.

| Grade | Mitotic count (per 10 HPF)[a] | Ki-67 index (%)[b] |
|-------|-------------------------------|--------------------|
| G1    | <2                            | ≤2 (< 3)[c]        |
| G2    | 2–20                          | 3–20               |
| G3    | >20                           | >20                |

[a] 10 HPF (high power field)=2 mm², at least 40 fields (at 40× magnification) evaluated in areas of highest mitotic density.
[b] Ki-67-MIB1 antibody: % of 500–2000 tumour cells in areas of highest nuclear labelling (hot spot).
[c] Applies only to pancreatic neuroendocrine neoplasms.

### Regional Lymph Nodes

The regional lymph nodes correspond to those listed under the appropriate sites for conventional carcinomas.

## Neuroendocrine Neoplasms of the Stomach

This classification applies to well-differentiated tumours (G1 and G2) of the stomach. The classification of the poorly differentiated (high grade) neoplasms (i.e. neuroendocrine carcinomas) follows the criteria for classifying conventional adenocarcinoma.

### Summary – Gastric Neuroendocrine Tumours

| | |
|--|--|
| T1 | Mucosa or submucosa, ≤ 1 mm in size |
| T2 | Invades muscularis propria or > 1 cm |
| T3 | Invades subserosa |
| T4 | Perforates visceral peritoneum (serosa) or invades adjacent organs and structures |
| N1 | Regional |
| M1 | Distant metastasis |
| | M1a  Hepatic only |
| | M1b  Extrahepatic only |
| | M1c  Hepatic and extrahepatic |

**Note.**
For any T, add (m) for multiple tumours.

## Neuroendocrine Neoplasms of the Duodenum and Ampulla of Vater

This classification applies to well-differentiated tumours (G1 and G2) of the duodenum and ampulla of Vater. The classification of the poorly differentiated (high grade) neoplasms (i.e. neuroendocrine carcinomas) follows the criteria for classifying conventional adenocarcinoma.

### Summary – *Duodenal/Ampullary Neuroendocrine Tumours*

T1  Duodenal: Mucosa or submucosa, $\leq 1$ cm
    Ampullary: Confined within sphincter of Oddi, $\leq 1$ cm
T2  Duodenal: Muscularis propria or > 1 cm
    Ampullary: Through sphincter into duodenal submucosa or muscularis propria or > 1 cm
T3  Pancreas or peripancreatic adipose tissue
T4  Perforates visceral peritoneum (serosa) or invades adjacent organs or structures
N1  Regional lymph node metastasis
M1  Distant metastasis
    M1a  Hepatic only
    M1b  Extrahepatic only
    M1c  Hepatic and extrahepatic

**Note.**
For any T, add (m) for multiple tumours.

## Neuroendocrine Neoplasms of the Jejunum and Ileum

This classification applies to well-differentiated tumours (G1 and G2) of the jejunum and ileum. The classification of the poorly differentiated (high grade) neoplasms (i.e. neuroendocrine carcinomas) follows the criteria for classifying conventional adenocarcinoma.

### Summary – *Jejunal/Ileal Neuroendocrine Tumours*

T1  Mucosa or submucosa, $\leq 1$ cm
T2  Muscularis propria or > 1 cm
T3  Subserosa without penetration of overlying serosa (jejunal or ileal)
T4  Perforates visceral peritoneum (serosa) or invades adjacent organs or structures
N1  < 12 regional lymph node metastasis without mesenteric mass(es) > 2 cm

N2   $\geq 12$ regional lymph nodes and/or mesenteric mass(es)$>2$ cm
M1   Distant metastasis
    M1a   Hepatic only
    M1b   Extrahepatic only
    M1c   Hepatic and extrahepatic

**Note.**
For any T, add (m) for multiple tumours.

## Neuroendocrine Neoplasms of the Appendix

This classification applies to well-differentiated tumours (G1 and G2) of the appendix. The classification of the poorly differentiated (high grade) neoplasms (i.e. neuroendocrine carcinomas) and goblet cell carcinoids follows the criteria for classifying conventional adenocarcinoma.

### Summary – *Appendiceal Neuroendocrine Tumours*

T1   $\leq 2$ cm
T2   $>2$ cm to 4 cm or with extension to the cecum
T3   $>4$ cm or with subserosal invasion or involvement mesoappendix
T4   Perforation of peritoneum, or invades other adjacent organs or structures, e.g. abdominal wall and skeletal muscle
N1   Regional lymph node metastasis
M1   Distant metastasis
    M1a   Hepatic only
    M1b   Extrahepatic only
    M1c   Hepatic and extrahepatic

### T Classification

High-grade neuroendocrine carcinomas, mixed adenoneuroendocrine carcinomas and so-called goblet-cell carcinoids are excluded and should be classified according to criteria for classifying carcinoma.

Tumour that is adherent to other organs or structures, macroscopically, is classified as cT4. However, if no tumour is present in the adhesion, microscopically, this should be classified as pT1–pT3.

## Neuroendocrine Neoplasms of the Colon and Rectum

This chapter applies to well differentiated (G1 and G2) neuroendocrine tumours of the colon and rectum. The classification of the poorly differentiated (high grade) neoplasms (i.e. neuroendocrine carcinomas) follows the criteria for classifying conventional adenocarcinoma.

## Summary – *Colon and Rectal Neuroendocrine Tumours*

T1    Mucosa or submucosa, $\leq$ 2 cm

    T1a   < 1 cm

    T1b   1 to 2 cm

T2    Muscularis propria or > 2 cm

T3    Subserosa, non-peritonealized pericolic/perirectal tissues

T4    Perforates visceral peritoneum (serosa) or invades other organs

N1    Regional lymph node metastasis

M1    Distant metastasis

    M1a   Hepatic only

    M1b   Extrahepatic only

    M1c   Hepatic and extrahepatic

## Neuroendocrine Neoplasms of the Pancreas

The classification system applies to well-differentiated neuroendocrine neoplasms (i.e. neuroendocrine tumours) as well as to G3 neuroendocrine tumours of the pancreas. The classification of the poorly differentiated (high grade) neoplasms (i.e. neuroendocrine carcinomas) follows the criteria for classifying ductal adenocarcinoma.

### Summary – *Pancreatic Neuroendocrine Tumours*

T1    Limited to pancreas, $\leq$ 2 cm

T2    Limited to pancreas, > 2 and $\leq$ 4 cm

T3    Limited to pancreas, > 4 cm, or invasion of duodenum or bile duct

T4    Invasion of adjacent organs (stomach, spleen, colon, adrenal gland) or wall of large vessels (coeliac axis, superior mesenteric artery)

N1    Regional lymph node metastasis

M1    Distant metastasis

    M1a   Hepatic metastasis only

    M1b   Extrahepatic metastasis only

    M1c   Hepatic and extrahepatic metastases

**Note.**

For T1, T2 and T3, this includes invasion of peripancreatic adipose tissue, but excludes invasion of adjacent organs. For any T, add (m) for multiple tumours.

### *T Classification*

The Tis/pTis distinction was eliminated.

T1–T3: Invasion of adjacent peripancreatic adipose tissue is accepted within the respective T category but invasion of adjacent organs is excluded and should be classified as T4.

# Lung, Pleural and Thymic Tumours

The classification applies to carcinomas of the lung including non-small cell carcinomas, small cell carcinomas and bronchopulmonary carcinoid tumours (typical and atypical carcinoids), malignant mesothelioma of pleura and thymic tumours.

## Lung

The classification applies to carcinomas of the lung including non-small cell carcinomas, small cell carcinomas and bronchopulmonary carcinoid tumours (typical and atypical carcinoids).

It does not apply to sarcomas and other rare tumours.

**Changes to the 7th edition are based upon recommendations from the International Association for the Study of Lung Cancer (IASLC) Lung Cancer Staging Project [57–69].**

### Regional Lymph Nodes

The regional lymph nodes extend from the supraclavicular region to the diaphragm (see pages 90–91). Direct extension of the primary tumour into lymph nodes is classified as lymph node metastasis.

### Summary – *Lung*

Tis  Carcinoma in situ[1]
     Tis(AIS) adenocarcinoma in situ, Tis(SCIS) squamous cell carcinoma in situ
T1   ≤ 3 cm, surrounded by lung or visceral pleura, without bronchoscopic evidence of invasion more proximal than the lobar bronchus[2]
     T1mi  Minimal invasive adenocarcinoma[3]
     T1a   ≤ 1 cm
     T1b   > 1–2 cm
     T1c   > 2–3 cm
T2   > 3–5 cm or tumour with any of the following features[4]
     – Main bronchus, without involvement of the carina
     – Invades visceral pleura
     – Atelectasis (or obstructive pneumonitis) extending into the hilar region (part of or entire lung)
     T2a   > 3–4cm
     T2b   > 4–5 cm
T3   > 5–7 cm or invasion of any of the following:
     parietal pleura, chest wall, phrenic nerve, parietal pericardium or separate tumour nodule(s) in the same lobe

T4  > 7 cm or any size with invasion of any of the following:
diaphragm, mediastinum, heart, great vessels, trachea, recurrent laryngeal
nerve, oesophagus, vertebral body, carina, separate tumour nodule(s) in a
different ipsilateral lobe

N1  Ipsilateral peribronchial and/or ipsilateral hilar, ipsilateral intrapulmonary

N2  Ipsilateral mediastinal and/or subcarinal

N3  Contralateral mediastinal or hilar, scalene or supraclavicular

M1  Distant metastasis

M1a  Separate tumour nodule(s) in a contralateral lobe; tumour with
pleural or pericardial nodules or malignant pleural or pericardial
effusion[5]

M1b  Single extrathoracic in a single organ[6]

M1c  Multiple extrathoracic in a single or multiple organs

**Notes**

[1] Tis includes adenocarcinoma in situ and squamous cell carcinoma in situ.

[2] The uncommon superficial spreading tumour of any size with its invasive component
limited to the bronchial wall, which may extend proximal to the main bronchus, is also
classified as T1a.

[3] Solitary adenocarcinoma (not more than 3 cm in greatest dimension), with a predominantly
lepidic pattern and not more than 5 mm invasion in greatest dimension, in any one focus.

[4] T2 tumours with these features are classified as T2a if 4 cm or less, or if size cannot be
determined, and T2b if greater than 4 cm but not larger than 5 cm.

[5] Most pleural (pericardial) effusions with lung cancer are due to a tumour. In a few
patients, however, multiple microscopical examinations of pleural (pericardial) fluid are
negative for the tumour and the fluid is non-bloody and is not an exudate. Where these
elements and clinical judgement dictate that the effusion is not related to the tumour,
the effusion should be excluded as a staging descriptor.

[6] This includes involvement of a single non-regional node.

### Clinical and Pathological Classification

Clinical classification (pre-treatment clinical classification), designated TNM (or
cTNM), is essential to select and evaluate therapy. This is based on evidence
acquired before treatment. Such evidence arises from physical examination,
imaging (e.g. computed tomography and positron emission tomography),
endoscopy (bronchoscopy or oesophagoscopy, with/without ultrasound directed
biopsies (EBUS, EUS)), biopsy (including mediastinoscopy, mediastinotomy, thora-
cocentesis and video-assisted thoracoscopy), as well as surgical exploration and
other relevant examinations such as pleural/pericardial aspiration for cytology.

Pathological classification (post-surgical histopathological classification),
designated pTNM, provides the most precise data to estimate prognosis and
calculate end results. This is based on the evidence acquired before treatment,
supplemented or modified by the additional evidence acquired from surgery and
from pathological examination. The pathological assessment of the primary

tumour (pT) entails a resection of the primary tumour or biopsy adequate to evaluate the highest pT category. Removal of nodes adequate to validate the absence of regional lymph node metastasis is required for pN0. The pathological assessment of distant metastasis (pM) entails microscopic examination.

Pathologic staging depends on the proven anatomic extent of disease, whether or not the primary lesion has been completely removed. If a biopsied primary tumour technically cannot be removed, or when it is unreasonable to remove it, the criteria for pathologic classification and staging are satisfied without total removal of the primary cancer if:

(a) Biopsy has confirmed a pT category and there is microscopical confirmation of nodal disease at any level (pN1-3).
(b) There is microscopical confirmation of the highest N category (pN3), or
(c) There is microscopical confirmation of pM1.

General Rule No. 3 states that clinical and pathological data may be combined when only partial information is available in either the pathological classification or the clinical classification, e.g. the classification of a case designated as cT1pN2cM1 or pT2cN0cM1 would be considered a clinical classification while in a case designated pT2pN2cM1, cT2pN3cM0 or cT2cN0pM1 it would be appropriate to designate a pathological classification.

### *T Classification*

Invasion of visceral pleura (T2) is defined as 'invasion beyond the elastic layer including invasion to the visceral pleural surface'. The use of elastic stains is recommended when this feature is not clear on routine histology [70].

A tumour with direct invasion of an adjacent lobe, across the fissure or by direct extension at a point where the fissure is deficient, should be classified as T2a/pT2a unless other criteria assign a higher T category.

Invasion of the phrenic nerve is classified as T3. Note that invasion of the mediastinal pleura is no longer considered as a T descriptor.

Vocal cord paralysis (resulting from involvement of the recurrent branch of the vagus nerve), superior vena cava obstruction or compression of the trachea or oesophagus may be related to direct extension of the primary tumour or to lymph node involvement. If associated with direct extension of the primary tumour a classification of T4/pT4 is recommended. If the primary tumour is peripheral, vocal cord paralysis is usually related to the presence of N2 disease and should be classified as such.

T4: the 'great vessels' are:

- Aorta
- Superior vena cava
- Inferior vena cava

- Main pulmonary artery (pulmonary trunk)
- Intrapericardial portions of the right and left pulmonary artery
- Intrapericardial portions of the superior and inferior right and left pulmonary veins

Invasion of more distal branches does not qualify for classification as T4.

The designation of a 'Pancoast' tumour relates to the symptom complex or syndrome caused by a tumour arising in the superior sulcus of the lung that involves the inferior branches of the brachial plexus (C8 and/or T1) and, in some cases, the stellate ganglion. Some superior sulcus tumours are more anteriorly located and cause fewer neurological symptoms but encase the subclavian vessels. The extent of disease varies in these tumours and they should be classified according to the established rules. If there is evidence of invasion of the vertebral body or spinal canal, encasement of the subclavian vessels or unequivocal involvement of the superior branches of the brachial plexus (C8 or above), the tumour is then classified as T4/pT4. If no criteria for T4/pT4 disease are present, the tumour is classified as T3/pT3.

Direct extension to parietal pericardium is classified as T3/pT3 and to visceral pericardium, T4/pT4.

A tumour extending to rib is classified as T3/pT3.

The uncommon superficial spreading tumour of any size with its invasive component limited to the bronchial wall, which may extend proximal to the main bronchus, is classified as T1a.

The classification of additional tumour nodules in lung cancer depends on their histological appearances.

(a) In most situations in which additional tumour nodules are found in association with a lung primary, these are metastatic nodules with identical histological appearances to that of the primary tumour. If limited to the lobe of the primary tumour such tumours are classified as T3/pT3, when found in other ipsilateral lobes are designated as T4/pT4 and if found in the contralateral lung are designated M1a/pM1a.

(b) Multiple tumours may be considered to be synchronous primaries if they are of different histological cell types. Multiple tumours of similar histological appearance should only be considered to be synchronous primary tumours if in the opinion of the pathologist, based on differences in morphology, immunohistochemistry and/or molecular studies, or, in the case of squamous cancers, are associated with carcinoma in situ, they represent differing subtypes of the same histopathological cell type. Such cases should also have no evidence of mediastinal nodal metastases or of nodal metastases within a common nodal drainage. These circumstances are most commonly encountered when dealing with either bronchioloalveolar carcinomas or adenocarcinoma of mixed subtype with a bronchioloalveolar component.

Multiple synchronous primary tumours should be staged separately. The highest T category and stage of disease should be assigned and the multiplicity or the number of tumours should be indicated in parenthesis, e.g. T2(m) or T2(5). This distinction may require histopathological confirmation of cell type from more than one tumour nodule, where clinically appropriate.

**Note.**
In the above classification lung differs from other sites in the application of General Rule No. 5 as the classification of additional tumour nodules applies not only to grossly recognizable tumours but also those that are microscopic or otherwise only discovered on pathological examination, a not unusual finding in lung cancer.

Invasion into mediastinal fat is T4/pT4. However, if such an invasion is clearly limited to fat within the hilum, classification as T2a/pT2a or T2b/pT2b is appropriate, depending on size, unless other features dictate a higher T category.

### N Classification
The regional lymph nodes are the intrathoracic, scalene and supraclavicular nodes.

The internal mammary lymph nodes are not defined as 'loco-regional lymph nodes' and are not in the IASLC lymph node map. Therefore, they cannot be considered in the N classification. Metastasis in the lymph nodes should be classified as M1. Because these nodes are outside the parietal pleural (they are extrathoracic), they should be classified as M1b if single or M1c if multiple.

The International Association for the Study of Lung Cancer (IASLC) lymph node definitions are now the recommended means of describing regional lymph node involvement for lung cancers [71] (see Plate 2.3 and Table 2.1). In this nomenclature ipsilateral or contralateral node involvement in #1 would be classified as N3/pN3. Involvement of mediastinal nodes, if limited to the midline stations or ipsilateral stations (#2–9), would be classified as N2/pN2. Involvement of #10–14 if ipsilateral would be classified as N1/pN1. Contralateral involvement of #2, 4, 5, 6, 8, 9, 10–14 would be classified as N3/pN3.

The IASLC nodal chart has been adopted as the new international chart for the documentation of nodal stations at clinical or pathological staging where a detailed assessment of lymph nodes has been made, usually by invasive techniques or at thoracotomy. The concept of the nodal zone was suggested in the 7th edition of the TNM classification of lung cancer [17, 24] as a simpler, more

**Table 2.1** IASLC Nodal definitions [71]

| Nodal station | Description | Definition |
|---|---|---|
| #1 (Left/Right) | Low cervical, supraclavicular and sternal notch nodes | Upper border: lower margin of cricoid cartilage<br>Lower border: clavicles bilaterally and, in the midline, the upper border of the manubrium<br>**#L1 and #R1 are limited by the midline of the trachea.** |
| #2 (Left/Right) | Upper paratracheal nodes | 2R: Upper border: apex of lung and pleural space and, in the midline, the upper border of the manubrium<br>Lower border: intersection of caudal margin of innominate vein with the trachea<br>2L: Upper border: apex of the lung and pleural space and, in the midline, the upper border of the manubrium<br>Lower border: superior border of the aortic arch<br>**As for #4, in #2 the oncologic midline is along the left lateral border of the trachea.** |
| #3 | Pre-vascular and retrotracheal nodes | 3a: Pre-vascular<br>**On the right**<br>Upper border: apex of chest<br>Lower border: level of carina<br>Anterior border: posterior aspect of sternum<br>Posterior border: anterior border of superior vena cava<br>**On the left**<br>Upper border: apex of chest<br>Lower border: level of carina<br>Anterior border: posterior aspect of sternum<br>Posterior border: left carotid artery<br>3p: Retrotracheal<br>Upper border: apex of chest<br>Lower border: carina |
| #4 (Left/Right) | Lower paratracheal nodes | 4R: includes right paratracheal nodes and pretracheal nodes extending to the left lateral border of trachea<br>Upper border: intersection of caudal margin of innominate vein with the trachea<br>Lower border: lower border of azygos vein<br>4L: includes nodes to the left of the left lateral border of the trachea, medial to the ligamentum arteriosum |

| | | |
|---|---|---|
| | | Upper border: upper margin of the aortic arch |
| | | Lower border: upper rim of the left main pulmonary artery |
| #5 | Subaortic nodes (aortopulmonary window) | Subaortic lymph nodes lateral to the ligamentum arteriosum Upper border: lower border of the aortic arch Lower border: upper rim of the left main pulmonary artery |
| #6 | Para-aortic nodes (ascending aorta or phrenic) | Lymph nodes anterior and lateral to the ascending aorta and aortic arch Upper border: a line tangential to the upper border of the aortic arch Lower border: the lower border of the aortic arch |
| #7 | Subcarinal nodes | Upper border: the carina of the trachea Lower border: the upper border of the lower lobe bronchus on the left; the lower border of the bronchus intermedius on the right |
| #8 (Left/Right) | Paraoesophageal nodes | Nodes lying adjacent to the wall of the oesophagus (below and to the right or left of the midline, excluding the carina and subcarinal nodes) Upper border: the upper border of the lower lobe bronchus on the left; the lower border of the bronchus intermedius on the right Lower border: the diaphragm |
| #9 (Left/Right) | Pulmonary ligament nodes | Nodes lying within the pulmonary ligament Upper border: the inferior pulmonary vein Lower border: the diaphragm |
| #10 (Left/Right) | Hilar nodes | Includes nodes immediately adjacent to the mainstem bronchus and hilar vessels including the proximal portions of the pulmonary veins and main pulmonary artery Upper border: the lower rim of the azygos vein on the right; upper rim of the pulmonary artery on the left Lower border: interlobar region bilaterally |
| #11 | Interlobar nodes | Between the origin of the lobar bronchi are optional subcategories: #11s: between the upper lobe bronchus and bronchus intermedius on the right #11i: between the middle and lower lobe bronchi on the right |
| #12 | Lobar nodes | Adjacent to the lobar bronchi |
| #13 | Segmental nodes | Adjacent to the segmental bronchi |
| #14 | Subsegmental nodes | Adjacent to the subsegmental bronchi |

utilitarian system for clinical staging where surgical exploration of lymph nodes has not been performed. An exploratory analysis suggested that the nodal extent could be grouped into three categories with different prognoses:

i) Involvement of a single N1 zone, designated as N1a.
ii) Involvement of more than one N1 zone, designated as N1b, or a single N2 zone, designated as N2a, and
iii) Involvement of more than one N2 zone, designated as N2b.

It was suggested that radiologists, clinicians and oncologists use the classification prospectively, where more detailed data on nodal status is not available, to assess the utility of such a classification for future revision.

**Note [71].**
For the 8th edition, quantification of regional lymph node involvement has been based on the number of nodal stations involved. The survival analyses performed on patients whose tumours were resected and had an adequate intraoperative nodal evaluation revealed four categories with different prognosis:
i) Involvement of a single N1 station,
ii) involvement of more than one N1 station, designated as N1b, or involvement of one N2 station without N1 involvement (skip metastasis), designated as N2a1,
iii) involvement of one N2 station with N1 metastasis, designated as N2a2, and
iv) involvement of more than one N2 station, designated as N2b.

From the analyses of nodal zones and stations, it is evident that the amount of nodal disease has a prognostic impact. It is suggested that quantification of nodal disease be made with the available methods at clinical staging and with systematic nodal dissection at the time of lung resection, either open or video-assisted. Quantifying nodal disease assists physicians in refining prognosis and in planning therapy and follow-up.

The UICC [12] recommends that at least 6 lymph nodes/stations be removed/sampled and confirmed on histology to be free of disease to confer pN0 status. Three of these nodes/stations should be mediastinal, including the subcarinal nodes (#7) and three from N1 nodes/stations.

If all resected/sampled lymph nodes are negative, but the number recommended is not met, classify as pN0. If resection has been performed and otherwise fulfils the requirements for complete resection, it should be classified as R0.

### M Classification
Pleural/pericardial effusions are classified as M1a. Most pleural (pericardial) effusions with lung cancer are due to tumour. In a few patients, however, multiple microscopical examinations of pleural (pericardial) fluid are negative for tumour,

and the fluid is non-bloody and is not an exudate. Where these elements and clinical judgement dictate that the effusion is not related to the tumour, the effusion should be excluded as a staging element and the patient should be classified as cM0.

Tumour foci in the ipsilateral parietal and visceral pleura that are discontinuous from direct pleural invasion by the primary tumour are classified M1a.

Pericardial effusion/pericardial nodules are classified as M1a, the same as pleural effusion/nodules.

Separate tumour nodules of similar histological appearance are classified as M1a if in the contralateral lung (vide supra regarding synchronous primaries).

Distant metastases are classified as M1b/pM1b if single and M1c/pM1c if multiple in one or several organs.

Discontinuous tumours outside the parietal pleura in the chest wall or in the diaphragm are classified as M1b/pM1b or M1c/pM1c depending on the number of lesions.

In cases classified as M1b/pM1b or M1c/pM1c due to distant metastases it is important to document all of the sites of metastatic disease, whether the sites are solitary or multiple and in addition if the metastases at each site are solitary or multiple.

## Stage – Lung Carcinoma

| | | | |
|---|---|---|---|
| Occult carcinoma | TX | N0 | M0 |
| Stage 0 | Tis | N0 | M0 |
| Stage IA | T1 | N0 | M0 |
| Stage IA1 | T1mi | N0 | M0 |
| | T1a | N0 | M0 |
| Stage IA2 | T1b | N0 | M0 |
| Stage IA3 | T1c | N0 | M0 |
| Stage IB | T2a | N0 | M0 |
| Stage IIA | T2b | N0 | M0 |
| Stage IIB | T1a–c, T2a, T2b | N1 | M0 |
| | T3 | N0 | M0 |
| Stage IIIA | T1a–c, T2a, T2b | N2 | M0 |
| | T3 | N1 | M0 |
| | T4 | N0, N1 | M0 |
| Stage IIIB | T1a–c, T2a, T2b | N3 | M0 |
| | T3, T4 | N2 | M0 |
| Stage IIIC | T3, T4 | N3 | M0 |
| Stage IV | Any T | Any N | M1 |
| Stage IVA | Any T | Any N | M1a, M1b |
| Stage IVB | Any T | Any N | M1c |

### V Classification

In the lung, arterioles are frequently invaded by cancers. For this reason, the V classification is applicable to indicate vascular invasion, whether venous or arteriolar.

### Small Cell Carcinoma

The TNM classification and stage grouping should be applied to small cell lung cancer (SCLC). TNM is of significance for prognosis of small cell carcinoma [62] and has the advantage of providing a uniform detailed classification of tumour spread. TNM should be used when undertaking trials in SCLC. The former categories 'limited' and 'extensive' for small cell carcinoma have been inconsistently defined and used.

### Bronchopulmonary Carcinoid Tumours

The TNM classification and stages should be applied to carcinoid tumours, typical and atypical variants [72, 73].

### Isolated Tumour Cells (ITC)

Isolated tumour cells (ITC) are single tumour cells or small clusters of cells not more than 0.2 mm in greatest dimension, which are detected by routine histological stains, immunohistochemistry or molecular methods. Cases with ITC cells in lymph nodes or at distant sites should be classified as cN0 or cM0, respectively. The same applies to cases with findings suggestive of tumour cells or their components by non-morphologic techniques such as flow cytometry or DNA analysis.

The following classification may be used:

| | |
|---|---|
| (p)N0 | No regional lymph node metastasis histologically, no examination for isolated tumour cells (ITC) |
| (p)N0(i–) | No regional lymph node metastasis histologically, negative morphological findings for ITC |
| (p)N0(i+) | No regional lymph node metastasis histologically, positive morphological findings for ITC |
| (p)N0(mol-) | No regional lymph node metastasis histologically, negative non-morphological findings for ITC |
| (p)N0(mol+) | No regional lymph node metastasis histologically, positive non-morphological findings for ITC |

**Note.**
This approach is consistent with TNM General Rule No. 4.

### Involvement of Visceral Pleura

A standardized definition of visceral pleural invasion (VPI) has been incorporated into the 7th edition of TNM and recommendations included on the use of elastic stains in the determination of VPI [70]. It is important that data be collected using this definition so that the utility of this pT2 descriptor can be assessed more accurately in future revisions. A subclassification has been proposed [70] based upon a system published by the Japan Lung Cancer Society [74] and by Hammar [75]. It is proposed that the PL category be used to describe the pathological extent of pleural invasion:

| | |
|---|---|
| PL0 | Tumour is within the subpleural lung parenchyma or invades superficially into the pleural connective tissue beneath the elastic layer |
| PL1 | Tumour invades beyond the elastic layer |
| PL2 | Tumour invades to the pleural surface |
| PL3 | Tumour invades into any component of the parietal pleura. |

**Note.**
In the TNM 7th edition PL0 is not regarded as a T descriptor and the T category should be assigned to other features. PL1 or PL2 indicate 'visceral pleural invasion', i.e. T2a/pT2a. PL3 indicates invasion of the parietal pleura, i.e. T3/pT3.

It is recommended that pathologists prospectively collect data based upon these subcategories to facilitate future revisions of TNM.

### Chest Wall Invasion

There are suggestions that the depth of chest wall invasion may influence prognosis following a resection of lung cancer. A subclassification has been proposed, based upon the histopathological findings of the resection specimen, dividing such pT3 tumours into pT3a if invasion is limited to the parietal pleura (PL 3), pT3b if invasion involves the endothoracic fascia and pT3c if invasion involves the rib or soft tissue.

   Pathologists are encouraged to collect this information prospectively to facilitate analysis and future revisions.

### Classification of Lung Cancers with Multiple Sites of Involvement

To avoid ambiguity and to facilitate the homogeneous classification of lung cancer with multiple sites of disease, an ad hoc subcommittee of the IASLC Staging and Prognostic Factors Committee developed the following recommendations based on the analyses of the IASLC database where data were available, the review of published reports and a wide multidisciplinary and international consensus [71]. The following recommendations apply to grossly recognizable tumours and to those identified at microscopic examination, and differ depending on the pattern of disease [64–67].

- **Synchronous and metachronous primary lung cancers**
  Regardless of tumour location, a separate TNM is defined for each tumour. The clinical and pathological criteria to differentiate second primary from related tumours are defined as follows:

  *Clinical Criteria* (note that a comprehensive histological assessment is not included in clinical staging, as it requires that the entire specimen has been resected)

  **Tumours may be considered separate primary tumours if:**
  They are clearly of a different histological type (e.g. squamous carcinoma and adenocarcinoma) by biopsy

  **Tumours may be considered to be arising from a single tumour source if:**
  Exactly matching breakpoints are identified by comparative genomic hybridization

  **Relative arguments that favour separate tumours:**

  - Different radiographic appearance or metabolic uptake
  - Different biomarker pattern (driver gene mutations)
  - Different rates of growth (if previous imaging is available)
  - Absence of nodal or systemic metastases

  **Relative arguments that favour a single tumour source:**

  - Same radiographic appearance
  - Similar growth patterns (if previous imaging is available)
  - Significant nodal or systemic metastases
  - Same biomarker pattern (and same histotype)

  *Pathologic Criteria (i.e. after resection)* (pathologic information should be supplemented with any clinical information that is available)

  **Tumours may be considered separate primary tumours if:**

  - They are clearly of a different histological type (e.g. squamous carcinoma and adenocarcinoma)
  - They are clearly different by a comprehensive histological assessment
  - They are squamous carcinomas that have arisen from carcinoma in situ

  **Tumours may be considered to be arising from a single tumour source if:**

  - Exactly matching breakpoints are identified by comparative genomic hybridization

**Relative arguments that favour separate tumours:**

– Different pattern of biomarkers
– Absence of nodal or systemic metastases

**Relative arguments that favour a single tumour source (to be considered together with clinical factors):**

– Matching appearance on comprehensive histological assessment
– Same biomarker pattern
– Significant nodal or systemic metastasis

- **Separate tumour nodules with similar histopathologic features (intrapulmonary metastases)**
  Classification depends on the location of the separate tumour nodule(s): T3, if the separate tumour nodule(s) is (are) in the same lobe of the primary tumour; T4, if located in a different ipsilateral lobe; M1a, if located in the contralateral lung. If there are additional extrathoracic metastases, the tumour will be classified as M1b or M1c depending on the number of metastatic sites. The clinical and pathological criteria to categorize separate tumour nodules (intrathoracic metastasis) are defined as follows:

  There is a separate tumour nodule(s) of cancer in the lung with a similar histologic appearance to a primary lung cancer and provided that the lesions are not judged to be synchronous primary lung cancers and the lesions are not multiple foci of LPA, MIA, AIS.

*Clinical Criteria*
**Tumours should be considered to have a separate tumour nodule(s) if:**
There are a solid lung cancer and a separate tumour nodule(s) with similar solid appearance and with (presumed) matching histologic appearance.

- This applies whether or not a biopsy has been performed on the lesions, provided that there are strong suspicions that the lesions are histologically identical.
- This applies whether or not there are sites of extrathoracic metastases and provided that the lesions are NOT judged to be synchronous primary lung cancers.

The lesions are not multifocal GG/L lung cancer/multiple nodules (with ground glass/lepidic features) or a pneumonic type of lung cancer.

*Pathologic Criteria*

**Tumours should be considered to have a separate tumour nodule(s) (intrapulmonary metastasis) if:**

There is a separate tumour nodule(s) of cancer in the lung with a similar histologic appearance to a primary lung cancer and provided that the lesions are not judged to be synchronous primary lung cancer and provided that:

The lesions are not judged to be synchronous primary lung cancers.
The lesions are not multiple foci of LPA, MIA, AIS.

**Note.**

A radiographically solid appearance and the specific histological subtype of solid adenocarcinoma denote different things.

   AIS, adenocarcinoma in situ: GG/L, ground glass/lepidic; LPA, lepidic predominant adenocarcinoma; MIA, minimally invasive adenocarcinoma.

- **Multifocal pulmonary adenocarcinoma with ground glass/lepidic features:**
  Regardless of the location of the tumours, the rule of the highest T with the number (#) or (m) for multiple in parentheses, and an N and an M for all the multiple tumours collectively applies for these tumours.

*Clinical Criteria*

Tumours should be considered multifocal GG/L lung adenocarcinoma if:

   There are multiple subsolid nodules (either pure ground glass or part-solid), with at least one suspected (or proven) to be cancerous.

- This applies whether or not a biopsy has been performed on the nodules.
- This applies if the other nodule(s) are found on biopsy to be AIS, MIA or LPA.
- This applies if a nodule has become > 50% solid but is judged to have arisen from a GGN, provided there are other subsolid nodules.
- GGN lesions < 5 mm or lesions to be suspected to be AAH are not counted.

*Pathologic Criteria*

There are multiple foci of LPA, MIA or AIS:

- This applies whether a detailed histologic assessment (i.e. proportion of subtypes, etc.) shows a matching or different appearance.
- This applies if one lesion(s) is LPA, MIA or AIS and there are other subsolid nodules on which a biopsy has not been performed.

- This applies whether the nodule(s) is/are identified pre-operatively or only on pathologic examination.
- Foci of AAH are not counted.

### Diffuse pneumonic-type lung adenocarcinoma:

(A) Single focus of disease. The general TNM classification is applied, with the T category defined by tumour size.
(B) Multiple foci of disease. Tumour classification is based on the location of the involved areas (including miliary involvement): T3, if located in one lobe; T4, if located in other ipsilateral lobes; M1a, if the contralateral lung is involved, with the T category defined by the largest tumour.
(C) If tumour size is difficult to determine. T4 applies if there is evidence of involvement of another ipsilateral lobe. In all circumstances, the N category should apply to all pulmonary sites and the appropriate M category should be applied depending on the number and location of metastases.

### *Clinical Criteria*
### Tumours should be considered as a pneumonic-type of adenocarcinoma if:

The cancer manifests in a regional distribution, similar to a pneumonic infiltrate or consolidation.

- This applies whether there is one confluent area or multiple regions of disease. The region(s) may be confined to one lobe, in multiple lobes, or bilateral, but should involve a regional pattern of distribution.
- The involved areas may appear to be ground glass, solid consolidation, or a combination thereof.
- This can be applied when there is compelling suspicion of malignancy whether or not a biopsy has been performed on the area(s).
- This should not be applied to discrete nodules (i.e. GG/L nodules).
- This should not be applied to tumours causing bronchial obstruction with resultant obstructive pneumonia or atelectasis.

### *Pathologic Criteria*
There is a diffuse distribution of adenocarcinoma throughout a region(s) of the lung as opposed to a single well-demarcated mass or multiple discrete well-demarcated nodules.

- This typically involves an invasive mucinous adenocarcinoma, although a mixed mucinous and non-mucinous pattern may occur.
- The tumour may show a heterogeneous mixture of acinar, papillary and micropapillary growth patterns, although it is usually lepidic predominant.

## Expansion of the R Classification
**RX Presence of residual tumour cannot be assessed**
**R0 Complete Resection**

All of the following are satisfied:

(a) Resection margins confirmed to be clear on microscopy.
(b) Six nodes/nodal stations removed/sampled for histological examination.

These should include three nodes/stations from the mediastinum, one of which should be subcarinal node #7, and three nodes/stations from the hilum or other N1 locations.

**Note.**
If all resected/sampled lymph nodes are negative, but the number ordinarily included in a lymphadenectomy specimen is not met, classify as pN0. If resection has been performed, and otherwise fulfils the requirements for complete resection, it should be classified as R0.

### R1(cy+)
The requirements for R0 have been met, but pleural lavage cytology (PLC) is positive for malignant cells (see pages 15–19).

A recent meta-analysis [76] has confirmed that PLC, undertaken immediately on thoracotomy and shown to be positive for cancer cells, has an adverse and independent prognostic impact following complete resection. Such patients may be candidates for an adjuvant chemotherapy. Surgeons and pathologists are encouraged to undertake this simple addition to intraoperative staging and collect data on PLC +ve cases. Where the resection fulfils all of the requirements for classification as a complete resection, R0, but PLC has been performed and is positive, the resection should be classified as R1(cy+).

### R1(is)
The requirements for R0 have been met, but in situ carcinoma is found at the bronchial resection margin (see pages 15–19).

### R1 Microscopic Incomplete Resection
Microscopic evidence of residual disease found at any of the following sites:

(a) Resection margins
(b) Extracapsular extension at margins of resected nodes
(c) Positive cytology of pleural/pericardial effusions (R1(cy+))

### R2 Macroscopic Incomplete Resection
Macroscopic evidence of residual disease found at any of the following sites:

(a) Resection margins
(b) Extracapsular extension at margins of resected nodes

(c) Positive nodes not resected at surgery

(d) Pleural/pericardial nodules

A new category, '**R0(un)**', is proposed to document those other features that fall within the proposed category of '**uncertain resection**', i.e. no macroscopic or microscopic evidence of residual disease but any of the following reservations applies:

i)  Nodal assessment has been based on less than the number of nodes/stations recommended for complete resection.

ii) The highest mediastinal node removed/sampled is positive.

This extension of the R classification for lung cancers has been confirmed recently [77].

## Pleural Mesothelioma

There has been no substantial change in the classification of malignant pleural mesotheliomas from the 7th TNM edition [17, 24].

The staging system applies only to malignant pleural mesothelioma [78, 79].

### Regional Lymph Nodes

The regional lymph nodes are the intrathoracic, internal mammary, scalene and supraclavicular lymph nodes.

**The IASLC definition is as follows:** The regional lymph nodes extend from the supraclavicular region to the diaphragm. Direct extension of the primary tumour into lymph nodes is classified as lymph node metastasis.

### Summary – *Pleural Mesothelioma*

---

T1    Ipsilateral parietal pleura with/without visceral, mediastinal or diaphragmatic pleura

T2    Ipsilateral parietal or visceral pleura with at least one of the following:
- Diaphragmatic muscle
- Lung parenchyma

T3    Ipsilateral parietal or visceral pleura with at least one of the following:
- Endothoracic fascia
- Mediastinal fat
- Solitary focus of tumour invading soft tissue of the chest wall
- Non-transmural pericardium

T4    Ipsilateral parietal or visceral pleura with at least one of the following:
- Chest wall with/without rib destruction (diffuse/multifocal)

- Peritoneum (via direct transdiaphragmatic extension)
- Contralateral pleura
- Mediastinal organs (oesophagus, trachea, heart, great vessels)
- Vertebra, neuroforamen, spinal cord
- Internal surface of the pericardium (transmural invasion with/without pericardial effusion)

N1 Ipsilateral intrathoracic (ipsilateral bronchopulmonary, hilar, subcarinal, paratracheal, aortopulmonary, paraoesophageal, peridiaphragmatic, pericardial fat pad, intercostal, internal mammary nodes)

N2 Contralateral intrathoracic
Ipsilateral or contralateral supraclavicular

### T Classification

T3 describes locally advanced but potentially resectable tumour [71].
T4 describes advanced technically unresectable tumour [71].

### N Classification

In the 8th edition [10, 12, 71] changes in the definitions of the regional lymph nodes have been introduced, basically with a simplification.

### Stage – Pleural Mesothelioma

| Stage IA | T1 | N0 | M0 |
|---|---|---|---|
| Stage IB | T2, T3 | N0 | M0 |
| Stage II | T1, T2 | N1 | M0 |
| Stage IIIA | T3 | N1 | M0 |
| Stage IIIB | T1, T2, T3 | N2 | M0 |
| | T4 | Any N | M0 |
| Stage IV | Any T | Any N | M1 |

## Thymic Tumours

The classification applies to epithelial tumours of the thymus, including thymomas, thymic carcinomas and neuroendocrine tumours of the thymus.

It does not apply to sarcomas, malignant lymphomas and other rare tumours.

This classification is new to the 8th edition and is based upon recommendations from the International Association for the Study of Lung Cancer (IASLC) Staging Project and the International Thymic Malignancies Interest Group (ITMIG) [80–82].

### Regional Lymph Nodes

The regional lymph nodes are the anterior (perithymic) lymph nodes, the deep intrathoracic lymph nodes and the cervical lymph nodes.

### Summary – *Thymus Tumours*

| | |
|---|---|
| T1 | Encapsulated or extending into mediastinal fat, may involve mediastinal pleura |
| | T1a   No mediastinal pleura |
| | T1b   Direct invasion of mediastinal pleura |
| T2 | Direct involvement of pericardium |
| T3 | Direct invasion of any of the following: lung, brachiocephalic vein, superior vena cava, phrenic nerve, chest wall, extrapericardial pulmonary artery or vein |
| T4 | Invasion of any of the following: aorta (ascending arch or descending) arch vessels, intrapericardial pulmonary artery, myocardium, trachea, oesophagus |
| N1 | Anterior (perithymic) lymph modes |
| N2 | Deep intrathoracic or cervical lymph nodes |
| M1 | Distant metastasis |
| | M1a   Separate pleural or pericardial |
| | M1b   Distant beyond pleura or pericardium |

### T Classification

The presence or absence of a capsular invasion or invasion beyond is not a descriptor in the T classification [81]. The IASLC – Thymic Malignancy Interest Group (IASLC-ITMIG) analysis of a large global dataset demonstrated that these descriptors have no impact on outcomes, as have been shown by others [83].

While it is recommended that tumour size is recorded, it does not affect the T classification. In the IALSC-ITMIG global database the largest dimension of tumour size had no impact.

### N Classification

Direct extension of the primary tumour into lymph nodes is classified as lymph node metastasis.

### Stage – Thymic Tumours

| | | | |
|---|---|---|---|
| Stage I | T1 | N0 | M0 |
| Stage II | T2 | N0 | M0 |
| Stage IIIA | T3 | N0 | M0 |
| Stage IIIB | T4 | N0 | M0 |

| Stage IVA | Any T | N1 | M0 |
|-----------|-------|--------|---------|
| | Any T | N0, N1 | M1a |
| Stage IVB | Any T | N2 | M0, M1a |
| | Any T | Any N | M1b |

## Bone Tumours

The classification applies to all primary malignant bone tumours except malignant lymphoma, multiple myeloma, surface/juxtacortical osteosarcoma and juxtacortical chondrosarcoma.

For different tumour entities we refer to the *WHO Classification of Tumours of Bone and of Tissues*, 2013 [84].

In the 8th edition [10, 12] different TNM definitions for different sites of bone tumours have been introduced with different definitions of T categories:

- Appendicular skeleton, trunk, skull and facial bones
- Spine
- Pelvis

### Summary – *Bone Tumours*

#### Appendicular skeleton, trunk, skull and facial bones
| | |
|------|------|
| T1 | ≤8 cm |
| T2 | >8 cm |
| T3 | Discontinuous tumours in primary site |

#### Spine
| | |
|------|------|
| T1 | Single vertebral segment or two adjacent segments |
| T2 | Three adjacent vertebral segments |
| T3 | Four adjacent vertebral segments |
| T4a | Spinal canal |
| T4b | Adjacent vessels or tumour thrombosis within adjacent vessels |

#### Pelvis
| | |
|------|------|
| T1a | ≤8 cm, confined to single pelvic segment, no extraosseous extension |
| T1b | >8 cm, confined to single pelvic segment, no extraosseous extension |
| T2a | ≤8 cm, confined to single pelvic segment, with extraosseous extension *or* two adjacent pelvic segments without extraosseous extension |
| T2b | >8 cm, confined to single pelvic segment, with extraosseous extension *or* two adjacent pelvic segments without extraosseous extension |
| T3a | ≤8 cm, confined to two pelvic segments, with extraosseous extension |

| T3b | >8 cm, confined to two pelvic segments, with extraosseous extension |
|---|---|
| T4a | Three adjacent pelvic segments *or* crossing the sacroiliac joint to the sacral neuroforamen |
| T4b | Encasing external iliac vessels *or* gross tumour thrombus in major pelvic vessels |
| N1 | Regional |
| M1 | Distant metastasis |
| M1a | Lung |
| M1b | Other distant sites |

### *T Classification*

Figures 2.5 and 2.6 show important definitions of the T categories.

Skip metastasis in the same bone as the primary are classified as T3. Metastasis in another bone is classified as distant metastasis.

### G Histopathological Grading

The grading of bone sarcomas is based on a three-tiered grade classification. In this classification, grade 1 is considered 'low grade' and grades 2 and 3 'high grade.

### Stage – Bone Sarcoma – Appendicular Skeleton, Trunk, Skull and Facial Bones

| Stage IA | T1 | N0 | M0 | G1, GX (Low grade) |
|---|---|---|---|---|
| Stage IB | T2, T3 | N0 | M0 | G1, GX (Low grade) |
| Stage IIA | T1 | N0 | M0 | G2, G3 (High grade) |
| Stage IIB | T2 | N0 | M0 | G2, G3 (High grade) |
| Stage III | T3 | N0 | M0 | G2, G3 (High grade) |
| Stage IVA | Any T | N0 | M1a | Any G |
| Stage IVB | Any T | N1 | Any M | Any G |
| | Any T | Any N | M1b | Any G |

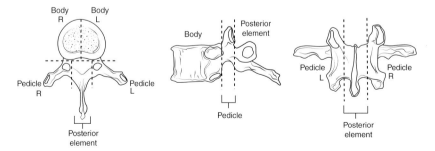

**Figure 2.5** Spine segment for staging. (Source: Figure 38.1 in the AJCC *Cancer Staging Manual* 2017 [10].)

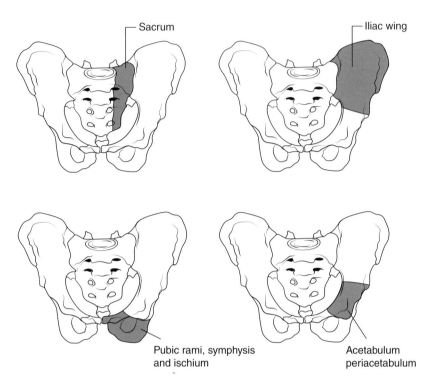

**Figure 2.6** Pelvic segments for staging. (Source: Figure 38.2 in the AJCC *Cancer Staging Manual* 2017 [10].)

### Stage – Bone Sarcoma – Spine and Pelvis
There is no stage for bone sarcomas of the spine and pelvis.

## Soft Tissue Tumours

### Histological Types of Tumours
The following histological types are not included:

- Kaposi sarcoma
- Dermatofibrosarcoma (protuberans)
- Fibromatosis (desmoid tumour)
- Sarcoma arising from the dura mater or brain
- Angiosarcoma, an aggressive sarcoma, is excluded because its natural history is not consistent with the classification

**Note.**
Cystosarcoma phyllodes of the breast is staged as a soft tissue sarcoma of the superficial trunk.

In the AJCC *Cancer Staging Manual*, 8th edition [10], the Kaposi sarcoma, fibromatosis (desmoid tumour) and sarcoma arising from the dura mater or brain, are not included.

Angiosarcoma (deep) is included in the AJCC classification. In the UICC classification, angiosarcoma is excluded because its natural history is not consistent with the classification.

A TNM classification and stages of the Kaposi sarcoma are not provided. The prognosis of the Kaposi sarcoma associated with AIDS is determined by AIDS.

In the 8th edition [10, 12] different TNM definitions for different sites of soft tissue tumours have been introduced with different definitions of T categories:

- Extremity and superficial trunk
- Retroperitoneum
- Head and neck
- Thoracic and abdominal viscera

### Summary – *Soft Tissue Tumours*

#### Extremity and Superficial Trunk, Retroperitoneum

| | |
|---|---|
| T1 | ≤5 cm |
| T2 | >5–10 cm |
| T3 | >10–15 cm |
| T4 | >15 cm |

#### Head and Neck

| | |
|---|---|
| T1 | ≤2 cm |
| T2 | >2–4 cm |
| T3 | >4 cm |
| T4a | Orbit, skull base or dura, central compartment viscera, facial skeleton and/or pterygoid muscles |
| T4b | Brain parenchyma, carotid artery, prevertebral muscle *or* central nervous system by perineural spread |

#### Thoracic and Abdominal Viscera

| | |
|---|---|
| T1 | Single organ |
| T2a | Serosa or visceral peritoneum |
| T2b | Microscopic extension beyond the serosa |
| T3 | Another organ or macroscopic extension beyond the serosa |
| T4a | Multifocal involving no more than 2 sites in one organ |
| T4b | Multifocal involving more than 2 sites but not more than 5 |
| T4c | Multifocal involving more than 5 |
| N1 | Regional |

## G Histopathological Grading

The grading of soft tissue sarcomas is based on a three-tiered grade classification. In this classification, grade 1 is considered 'low grade' and grades 2 and 3 'high grade'.

### Stage – Soft Tissue Sarcomas – Extremity, Superficial Trunk, Retroperitoneum

| Stage IA | T1 | N0 | M0 | G1, GX (Low grade) |
|---|---|---|---|---|
| Stage IB | T2, T3, T4 | N0 | M0 | G1, GX (Low grade) |
| Stage II | T1 | N0 | M0 | G2, G3 (High grade) |
| Stage IIIA | T2 | N0 | M0 | G2, G3 (High grade) |
| Stage IIIB | T3, T4 | N0 | M0 | G2, G3 (High grade) |
| | Any T | N1* | M0 | Any G |
| Stage IV | Any T | Any N | M1 | Any G |

**\*Note.**
AJCC classifies N1 as Stage IV for sarcomas of extremities and superficial trunk.

### Stage – Soft Tissue Sarcoma – Head and Neck, Thoracic and Abdominal Viscera

There is no stage for soft tissue sarcomas of the head and neck and thoracic and abdominal viscera.

## Gastrointestinal Stromal Tumour (GIST)

It is recommended to stage all GISTs by TNM even if they might be benign. It is very rare for a pathologist to diagnose a GIST as benign since GISTs can be unpredictable.

The classification applies to gastrointestinal stromal tumours of the following sites and subsites:

- Oesophagus (C15)
- Stomach (C16)
- Small intestine (C17)
  1. Duodenum (C17.0)
  2. Jejunum (C17.1)
  3. Ileum (C17.2)
- Colon (C18-C19)
- Rectum (C20)
- Omentum (C48.1)
- Mesentery (C48.1)

## Summary – *Gastrointestinal Stromal Tumour*

| | |
|---|---|
| T1 | ≤2 cm |
| T2 | >2–5 cm |
| T3 | >5–10 cm |
| T4 | >10 cm |
| N1 | Regional |

### Note.

Regional lymph node involvement is rare for GISTs, so that cases in which the nodal status is not assessed clinically or pathologically could be recorded as N0 instead of NX or pNX.

### G Histopathological Grading

Grading for GIST is dependent on the mitotic rate.

Low mitotic rate: 5 or fewer per 50 hpf

High mitotic rate: over 5 per 50 hpf

### Note.

The mitotic rate of GIST is best expressed as the number of mitoses per 50 high power fields (hpf) using the 40× objective (total area of 5 mm$^2$ in 50 fields).

### Stage

Staging criteria for gastric tumours can be applied in primary, solitary omental GISTs. Staging criteria for small intestinal tumours can be applied to GISTs in less common sites such as the oesophagus, colon, rectum and mesentery.

### Stage Grouping – Gastric GIST

| | | | | Mitotic rate |
|---|---|---|---|---|
| Stage IA | T1, T2 | N0 | M0 | Low |
| Stage IB | T3 | N0 | M0 | Low |
| Stage II | T1, T2 | N0 | M0 | High |
| | T4 | N0 | M0 | Low |
| Stage IIIA | T3 | N0 | M0 | High |
| Stage IIIB | T4 | N0 | M0 | High |
| Stage IV | Any T | N1 | M0 | Any rate |
| | Any T | Any N | M1 | Any rate |

### Stage Grouping – Small Intestinal GIST

| | | | | |
|---|---|---|---|---|
| Stage I | T1, T2 | N0 | M0 | Low |
| Stage II | T3 | N0 | M0 | Low |
| Stage IIIA | T1 | N0 | M0 | High |
| | T4 | N0 | M0 | Low |

| | | | | |
|---|---|---|---|---|
| Stage IIIB | T2, T3, T4 | N0 | M0 | High |
| Stage IV | Any T | N1 | M0 | Any rate |
| | Any T | Any N | M1 | Any rate |

## Skin Tumours

The classification applies to

- Carcinoma of the skin (excluding the eyelid and skin carcinoma of the head and neck)
- Skin carcinoma of the head and neck (excluding the eyelid)
- Carcinoma of the skin of the eyelid

**The classification does not apply to**

- Carcinoma of the perianal skin
- Carcinoma of the skin of the vulva
- Carcinoma of the skin of the penis

*Anatomical Sites*
The following sites are identified by ICD-O-3 topography rubrics:

- Lip (C44.0) excluding the vermilion surface (C00)
- Eyelid (C44.1)
- External ear (C44.2)
- Other and unspecified parts of the face (C44.3)
- Scalp and neck (C44.4)
- Trunk (excluding the anal margin and perianal skin) (C44.5)
- Upper limb and shoulder (C44.6)
- Lower limb and hip (C44.7)
- Scrotum (C63.2)

**Malignant Melanoma of Skin:** ICD-O C44, C51.0, C60.9, C63.2
In addition, the AJCC Manual [10] lists:

| | |
|---|---|
| C51.1 | Labium minus |
| C51.2 | Clitoris |
| C51.8 | Overlapping lesions |
| C51.9 | Vulva, NOS |
| C60.0 | Prepuce |
| C60.1 | Glans penis |
| C60.2 | Body of penis |
| C60.8 | Overlapping lesions of penis |
| C60.9 | Penis, NOS |

**Merkel Cell Carcinoma of Skin:** ICD-O C44.0-9, C63.2

In addition, the AJCC Manual [10] lists:

| | |
|---|---|
| C51.0 | Labium majus |
| C51.1 | Labium minus |
| C51.2 | Clitoris |
| C51.8 | Overlapping lesions |
| C51.9 | Vulva, NOS |
| C60.0 | Prepuce |
| C60.1 | Glans penis |
| C60.2 | Body of penis |
| C60.8 | Overlapping lesions of penis |
| C60.9 | Penis, NOS |

**Carcinoma of Skin (excluding eyelid, head and neck, perianal, vulva and penis)**

The classification applies to carcinomas of the skin (AJCC [10]: Cutaneous squamous cell carcinoma and other cutaneous carcinomas, e.g. basal cell carcinoma and carcinomas of skin appendages).

There should be histological confirmation of the disease and division of cases by histological type.

An entirely new classification was introduced for Merkel cell carcinoma in the 7th edition [17, 24] (see page 117), which therefore is no longer included in the TNM classification of carcinomas of the skin.

Grading is not applicable to basal cell carcinomas.

**Summary – *Skin Carcinoma***

| | |
|---|---|
| T1 | ≤2 cm |
| T2 | >2 cm–≤4 cm |
| T3 | > 4 cm or minor bone erosion or perineural invasion or deep invasion* |
| T4a | Gross cortical bone/marrow invasion |
| T4b | Axial skeleton invasion including foraminal involvement and/or vertebral foramen involvement to the epidural space |
| N1 | Single, ≤ 3 cm |
| N2 | Single, > 3–6 cm |
| | Multiple ipsilateral, < 6 cm |
| N3 | >6 cm |

**Note.**

* Deep invasion is defined as invasion beyond the subcutaneous or >6 mm (as measured from the granular layer of adjacent normal epidermis to the base of the tumour); perineural invasion for T3 classification is defined as clinical or radiographic involvement of named nerves without foramen or skull base invasion or transgression.

In the case of multiple simultaneous tumours, the tumour with the highest T category is classified and the number of separate tumours is indicated in parentheses, e.g. T2(5).

# ▮ Skin Carcinoma of Head and Neck

## Summary – *Skin Carcinoma of Head and Neck*

| | |
|---|---|
| T1 | ≤2 cm |
| T2 | >2 cm and ≤4 cm |
| T3 | >4 cm or minor bone erosion or perineural invasion or deep invasion |
| T4a | Gross cortical bone/marrow invasion |
| T4b | Skull base or axial skeleton invasion with foraminal involvement and/or vertebral foramen involvement to the epidural space |

### Note.

Deep invasion for T3 classification is defined as invasion beyond the subcutaneous fat or >6 mm (as measured from the granular layer of adjacent normal epidermis to the base of the tumour); perineural invasion for T3 classification is defined as clinical or radiographic involvement of named nerves without foramen or skull base invasion or transgression.

## Clinical N

| | |
|---|---|
| N1 | Ipsilateral single ≤3 cm (ENE-) |
| N2 | (a) Ipsilateral single >3–6 cm (ENE-) |
| | (b) Ipsilateral multiple ≤6 cm (ENE-) |
| | (c) Bilateral or contralateral ≤6 cm (ENE-) |
| N3 | (a) >6 cm (ENE-) |
| | (b) Any (ENE+) |

## Pathological N

| | |
|---|---|
| N1 | Ipsilateral single ≤3 cm (ENE-) |
| N2 | (a) Ipsilateral single ≤3 cm and ENE+ or ipsilateral single >3–6 cm (ENE-) |
| | (b) Ipsilateral multiple ≤6 cm (ENE-) |
| | (c) Bilateral or contralateral ≤6 cm (ENE-) |
| N3 | (a) >6 cm (ENE-) |
| | (b) Any (ENE+) other than pN2a |

## *T Classification*

Some consider verrucous carcinoma to be an in situ lesion (giant condyloma of Buschke-Löwenstein) whereas others consider it a malignant (invasive) tumour. In the WHO Classification, Buschke-Löwenstein is used as a synonym for verrucous squamous cell carcinoma (ICD-C M 8051/3) [85].

In the case of multiple simultaneous tumours, the tumour with the highest T category is classified and the number of separate tumours is indicated in parentheses, e.g. T2(5).

## *N Classification*

For carcinomas of the skin of the head and neck a clinical as well as a pathological N classification have been introduced in the 8th edition [10, 12].

The presence of skin involvement or soft tissue invasion with deep fixation/ tethering to underlying muscle or adjacent structures or clinical signs of nerve involvement is classified as clinical extranodal extension.

## Eyelid Carcinoma

There should be histological confirmation of the disease and division of cases by histological type, e.g. basal cell, squamous cell, sebaceous carcinoma.

Malignant melanoma of the eyelid is classified with the TNM for melanoma skin tumours (see page 114).

Although not stated in the *TNM Classification*, 8th edition, Merkel cell carcinoma of the eyelid should be classified using the criteria in this section rather than the criteria for Merkel cell carcinoma at other skin sites, owing to size considerations.

### Summary – *Carcinoma of the Skin of Eyelid*

| | | |
|---|---|---|
| T1 | ≤ 10 mm | |
| | T1a | Not invading the tarsal plate or eyelid margin |
| | T1b | Tarsal plate or eyelid margin |
| | T1c | Full thickness of eyelid |
| T2 | > 10–20 mm | |
| | T2a | Not invading the tarsal plate or eyelid margin |
| | T2b | Tarsal plate or eyelid margin |
| | T2c | Full thickness of eyelid |
| T3 | > 20 mm | |
| | T3a | Not invading the tarsal plate or eyelid margin |
| | T3b | Tarsal plate or eyelid margin |
| | T3c | Full thickness of eyelid |
| T4 | Adjacent ocular, orbital, facial structures | |
| | T4a | Ocular or intraorbital structures |
| | T4b | Invades (or erodes through) bony walls of orbit, extends to paranasal sinuses or invades the lacrimal sac/nasolacrimal duct or brain |
| N1 | Single ipsilateral, ≤ 3 cm | |
| N2 | Single ipsilateral, > 3 cm *or* bilateral *or* contralateral | |

## Malignant Melanoma of Skin

Melanoma thickness continues to be used in defining the T categories that can only be determined after excision (pT classification).

The number of involved lymph nodes and the differentiation between clinically occult (microscopic) and clinically apparent (macroscopic) metastases are used in the M category.

The site of distant metastases and the presence of elevated serum lactic dehydrogenase (LDH) are used in the M category.

The classification applies to malignant melanoma of skin of all sites, including the eyelid, vulva, penis and scrotum.

This classification does not apply to melanomas arising in mucous membranes (oral cavity, nasopharynx, vagina, urethra, anal canal) or to melanomas of the conjunctiva and uvea. The last two sites have separate classifications.

There is no classification for melanoma of the visceral sites, except mucosal melanomas of the upper aerodigestive tract.

## Summary – *Skin Malignant Melanoma*

| | |
|---|---|
| pT1a | < 0.8 mm, no ulceration |
| pT1b | < 0.8 mm + ulceration or ≥ 0.8–1.0 mm, +/- ulceration |
| pT2a | > 1–2 mm in thickness, no ulceration |
| pT2b | > 1–2 mm in thickness, ulceration |
| pT3a | > 2–4 mm in thickness, no ulceration |
| pT3b | > 2–4 mm in thickness, ulceration |
| pT4a | > 4 mm, no ulceration |
| pT4b | > 4 mm, ulceration |
| | |
| N1 | 1 lymph node *or* intralymphatic regional without nodal metastasis |
| | N1a Microscopic (clinically occult) |
| | N1b Macroscopic (clinically apparent) |
| | N1c Satellite or in-transit metastasis without regional node metastasis |
| N2 | 2–3 lymph nodes or satellites/in-transit *or* intralymphatic regional with nodal metastasis |
| | N2a Microscopic |
| | N2b Macroscopic |
| | N2c Satellite or in-transit metastasis with 1 regional node metastasis |
| N3 | ≥ 4 lymph nodes; matted; satellite(s); in transit with 2 or more regional lymph nodes |
| | N3a Microscopic |
| | N3b Macroscopic |
| | N3c Satellite(s) or in-transit metastasis with two or more regional nodes |
| M1 | Distant metastasis |
| | M1a Skin, subcutaneous tissues, lymph node(s) beyond the regional |
| | M1b Lung |
| | M1c Other non-central nervous system sites |
| | M1d Central nervous system |

**Notes.**
Suffixes for the M category:
(0) Lactic dehydrogenase (LDH) – not elevated
(1) LDH – elevated
Thus M1a(1) is metastasis in skin, subcutaneous tissue or lymph node(s) beyond the regional lymph nodes with elevated LDH.
No suffix is used if LDH is not recorded or unspecified.

## pT Classification

Maximum thickness of the tumour is measured with an ocular micrometer after embedding in paraffin at right angles to the adjacent normal skin. The upper reference point is the top of the granular cell layer of the epidermis of the overlying skin or the base of the ulcer if the tumour is ulcerated. The lower reference point is usually the deepest point of invasion. It may be the invading edge of a single tumour mass or an isolated cell or group of cells deep in the main mass. Melanoma cells within the epithelium of structures such as hair follicles and sebaceous glands of the skin are not taken into consideration.

Ulceration is defined as the absence of an intact epidermis overlying a major portion of the primary melanoma based on microscopic examination of the histologic section [10].

## Synchronous primary malignant melanomas

If two primary malignant melanomas occur in the same anatomical region as defined by ICD-O, such as two distinct tumours arising on the trunk, one on one side and the other on the contralateral side, these two lesions are counted only once and the most advanced is coded, e.g. pT4a(2)N0M0.

## N Classification

Classification based solely on sentinel node biopsy without subsequent axillary lymph node dissection is designated (sn) for sentinel node, e.g. pN1(sn) (see page 10).

Positive sentinel nodes should be classified as pN1(sn) as mentioned on page 7 of the 8th TNM edition. It is not recommended to use the subcategories of N1a, N1b, etc., because the findings of 1 or 2 sentinel lymph nodes can be less reliable for a more detailed pN classification.

Regarding positive sentinel lymph nodes for melanoma, (mi) should be used if a metastasis is no larger than 0.2 cm, e.g. pN1(sn)(mi). It allows further analysis on prognosis for these patients when compared to patients with metastasis larger than 2 mm.

In contrast to other tumours, ITCs in a lymph node of a malignant melanoma are classified as (p)N1 (and not as pN0(i+)).

## Clinical Stage – Malignant Melanoma of Skin

| | | | |
|---|---|---|---|
| Stage 0 | pTis | N0 | M0 |
| Stage IA | pT1a | N0 | M0 |
| Stage IB | pT1b | N0 | M0 |
| | pT2a | N0 | M0 |
| Stage IIA | pT2b | N0 | M0 |
| | pT3a | N0 | M0 |
| Stage IIB | pT3b | N0 | M0 |
| | pT4a | N0 | M0 |
| Stage IIC | pT4b | N0 | M0 |
| Stage III | Any pT | N1, N2, N3 | M0 |
| Stage IV | Any pT | Any N | M1 |

## Pathological Stage

| | | | |
|---|---|---|---|
| Stage 0 | pTis | N0 | M0 |
| Stage I | pT1 | N0 | M0 |
| Stage IA | pT1a | N0 | M0 |
| | pT1b | N0 | M0 |
| Stage IB | pT2a | N0 | M0 |
| Stage IIA | pT2b | N0 | M0 |
| | pT3a | N0 | M0 |
| Stage IIB | pT3b | N0 | M0 |
| | pT4a | N0 | M0 |
| Stage IIC | pT4b | N0 | M0 |
| Stage III | Any pT | N1, N2, N3 | M0 |
| Stage IIIA | pT1a, pT1b, pT2a | N1a, N2a | M0 |
| Stage IIIB | pT1a, pT1b, pT2a | N1b, N1c, N2b | M0 |
| | pT2b, pT3a | N1, N2a, N2b | M0 |
| Stage IIIC | pT1a-b, pT2a-b, pT3a | N2c, N3 | M0 |
| | pT3b, pT4a | N1, N2, N3 | M0 |
| | pT4b | N1, N2 | M0 |
| Stage IIID | pT4b | N3 | M0 |
| Stage IV | Any T | Any N | M1 |

## Note.

If lymph node(s) are identified with no apparent primary, the stage is:

| | | | |
|---|---|---|---|
| Stage IIIB | pT0 | N1b, N1c | M0 |
| Stage IIIC | pT0 | N2b, N2c, N3b, N3c | M0 |

## Merkel Cell Carcinoma of Skin

Merkel cell carcinoma of the eyelid is classified according to the eyelid carcinoma scheme (see page 113).

Histopathological grading is not applicable.

### Summary – *Merkel Cell Carcinoma*

| | |
|---|---|
| T1 | ≤2 cm |
| T2 | >2–5 cm |
| T3 | >5 cm |
| T4 | Deep extradermal structures (cartilage, skeletal muscle, fascia, bone) |
| N1 | Regional |
| N2 | In-transit metastasis without lymph node metastasis |
| N3 | In-transit metastasis with lymph node metastasis |
| pN1 | Regional |
| | pN1a(sn)  Microscopic metastasis on sentinel lymph node biopsy |
| | pN1a     Microscopic on lymph node dissection |
| | pN1b     Macroscopic (clinically apparent) |
| pN2 | In-transit metastasis without lymph node metastasis |
| pN3 | In-transit metastasis with lymph node metastasis |
| M1 | Distant metastasis |
| | M1a      Skin, subcutaneous tissues *or* non-regional lymph node(s) |
| | M1b      Lung |
| | M1c      Other site(s) |

**Note.**

In transit metastasis: a discontinuous tumour distinct from the primary lesion and located between the primary lesion and the draining regional lymph nodes or distal to the primary lesion.

### Stage – Merkel Cell Carcinoma of Skin

**Clinical Stage**

| | | | |
|---|---|---|---|
| Stage 0 | Tis | N0 | M0 |
| Stage I | T1 | N0 | M0 |
| Stage IIA | T2, T3 | N0 | M0 |
| Stage IIB | T4 | N0 | M0 |
| Stage III | Any T | N1, N2, N3 | M0 |
| Stage IV | Any T | Any N | M1 |

**Pathological Stage**

| | | | |
|---|---|---|---|
| Stage 0 | Tis | N0 | M0 |
| Stage I | T1 | N0 | M0 |

| Stage IIA | T2, T3 | N0 | M0 |
| Stage IIB | T4 | N0 | M0 |
| Stage IIIA | T0 | N1b | M0 |
| | T1, T2, T3, T4 | N1a, N1a(sn) | M0 |
| Stage IIIB | T1, T2, T3, T4 | N1b, N2, N3 | M0 |
| Stage IV | Any T | Any N | M1 |

## Breast Tumours

The basic strategy and criteria for assigning the T category have not changed in the 8th edition [10, 12].

The pathologic tumour size remains a function of the size of the invasive component. In cases of multifocal or multicentric carcinoma, the largest tumour is used to designate the T category. The size of multiple tumours is not added.

H & E preparations remain the main tool in determining the N category, but immunohistochemistry and polymerase chain reaction (PCR) have been considered in the detection of tumour cells in the 6th edition [16]. The designation of sentinel node involvement is discussed in Chapter 1 (page 11).

Since the involvement of supraclavicular and infraclavicular lymph nodes has a better prognosis than distant dissemination of the tumour, use of the N3 category is still assigned to these sites.

The pN3a category metastasis has undergone a clarification:

pN3a    Metastasis in 10 or more ipsilateral axillary lymph nodes (at least one larger than 2 mm) or metastasis in infraclavicular lymph nodes/level III lymph nodes.

### Summary – *Breast Tumours*

| Tis | Carcinoma in situ |
| Tis (DCIS) | Ductal carcinoma in situ |
| Tis (LCIS) | Lobular carcinoma in situ |
| Tis (Paget) | Paget disease of the nipple[a] |
| T1 | ≤2 cm |
| | T1mi ≤0.1 cm[b] |
| | T1a >0.1– 0.5 cm[c] |
| | T1b >0.5 cm–1.0 cm |
| | T1c >1.0–2.0 cm |
| T2 | >2–5 cm |
| T3 | >5 cm |

| | | | |
|---|---|---|---|
| T4 | Chest wall/skin ulceration, skin nodules, inflammatory | | |
| | T4a | Chest wall | |
| | T4b | Skin ulceration, satellite skin nodules, skin oedema | |
| | T4c | Both T4a and T4b | |
| | T4d | Inflammatory carcinoma | |

| | | | |
|---|---|---|---|
| N1 | Movable axillary level I/II | pN1 | Micrometastasis, 1–3 axillary nodes |
| | | pN1mi | Micrometastasis > 0.2–2 mm |
| | | pN1a | 1–3 axillary nodes (at least one > 2 mm) |
| | | pN1b | Internal mammary nodes |
| | | pN1c | 1–3 axillary nodes and internal |
| N2a | Axillary, fixed or matted | pN2a | 4–9 axillary nodes (at least one > 2 mm) |
| N2b | Internal mammary nodes, clinically detected,[d] without axillary nodes | pN2b | Internal mammary nodes, clinically detected, without axillary nodes |
| N3a | Axillary level III, infraclavicular | pN3a | Axillary ipsilateral ≥ 10 (at least one > 2 mm), Infraclavicular, level III lymph nodes |
| N3b | Axillary and internal mammary | pN3b | Internal mammary nodes and axillary nodes, > 3 axillary nodes and in internal mammary nodes with microscopic or macroscopic metastasis detected by sentinel node biopsy but not clinically detected |
| N3c | Supraclavicular lymph nodes | pN3c | Ipsilateral supraclavicular lymph nodes |

**Notes.**

[a] Paget disease of the nipple is not associated with invasive carcinoma and/or carcinoma in situ (DCIS and/or LCIS) in the underlying breast parenchyma.

Carcinomas in the breast parenchyma associated with Paget disease are categorized based on the size and characteristics of the parenchymal disease, although the presence of Paget disease should still be noted.

[b] Microinvasion is the extension of cancer cells beyond the basement membrane into the adjacent tissues with no focus more than 0.1 cm in greatest dimension. When there are multiple foci of microinvasion, the size of only the largest focus is used to classify the microinvasion. (Do not use the sum of all individual foci.) The presence of multiple foci of microinvasion should be noted, as it is with multiple larger invasive carcinomas.

ᶜ When classifying pT the tumour size is a measurement of the invasive component. If there is a large in situ component (e.g. 4 cm) and a small invasive component (e.g. 0.5 cm), the tumour is coded pT1a.

ᵈ Clinically detected is defined as detected by clinical examination or by imaging studies (excluding lymphoscintigraphy) and having characteristics highly suspicious for malignancy or a presumed pathological macrometastasis based on fine needle aspiration biopsy with cytologic examination. Confirmation of clinically detected metastatic disease by fine needle aspiration without excision biopsy is designated with an (f) suffix, e.g. cN3a(f).

Excisional biopsy of a lymph node or biopsy of a sentinel node, in the absence of assignment of a pT, is classified as a clinical N, e.g. cN1. Pathologic classification (pN) is used for excision or sentinel lymph node biopsy only in conjunction with a pathologic T assignment.

Pathological classification (pN) is used for excision or sentinel lymph node biopsy only in conjunction with a pathological T assignment (pT).

### T Classification

The classification applies to carcinomas of the male as well as of the female breast.

The rules for multiple simultaneous primary cancers in one breast (General Rule No. 5, page 5) do not apply to a single grossly detected tumour associated with multiple separate microscopic foci (satellites).

The clinical estimation of tumour size by physical examination and mammography frequently give different results [86]. Accuracy can be improved by using the following formula:

Size for classification $= 0.5 \times$ physical examination size $+ 0.5 \times$ mammographic size [86].

Only clinically/grossly detected satellite skin nodules are classified as T4b (histologically detected foci are not considered).

T4: direct invasion to 'chest wall' includes ribs, intercostal muscles and serratus anterior muscle but not the pectoral muscle.

Dimpling of the skin, nipple retraction, nipple involvement or other skin changes, except those in T4b and T4d, may occur in T1, T2 or T3 without affecting the classification. This also applies to microscopic invasion of the skin (dermis): invasion of the dermis alone does not qualify as T4.

On mastectomy specimens oedema of the skin (T4b) may be inapparent at the time of pathological examination. Therefore, the surgeon should inform the pathologist of such a clinical finding to guarantee its consideration and to prevent pathological understaging.

Invasion of lymphatic vessels is not considered in the T/pT category.

If there is a clinical picture of inflammatory carcinoma (cT4d), but a biopsy of the skin is negative for tumour and a measurable breast cancer is present, the pT category is based on the size of the tumour (pT1, 2 or 3).

Microscopic involvement of dermal lymphatic vessels by a tumour without the clinical picture of inflammatory carcinoma is classified by the size of the tumour.

For T classification the size of a tumour in a biopsy should be added to the size of a tumour in the definitive resection specimen if the biopsy specimen has a positive margin.

The post-neoadjuvant therapy pathological T category (ypT) must be based on the largest continuous focus of residual invasive cancer (if present). Treatment-related fibrosis adjacent to a residual tumour or between foci of a residual tumour should not be taken into account to classify ypT. Multiple foci of residual cancer should be classified accordingly with the 'm' symbol.

### N/pN Classification

Not clinically detected = not detected by clinical examination or by imaging studies (excluding lymphoscintigraphy).

Clinically detected = detected by clinical examination or by imaging studies (excluding lymphoscintigraphy) or grossly visible pathologically.

Invasion of lymph vessels in the axillary fatty tissue is not considered in the N classification. It can be classified in the L – Lymphatic invasion classification (page 10, TNM 8th edition [12]).

Intramammary lymph nodes are coded as axillary lymph nodes level I.

Infraclavicular (subclavicular) (ipsilateral) lymph nodes are listed separately in the list of regional lymph nodes (page 152, TNM 8th edition [12]) while they are included in level III axillary nodes in the 8th edition of the AJCC staging manual [10]. Level III and infraclavicular lymph nodes are considered as (p)N3.

Isolated tumour cell clusters (ITC) are single tumour cells or small clusters of cells not more than 0.2 mm in greatest extent and can be detected by routine H&E stains or immunohistochemistry. An additional criterion has been proposed to include a cluster of fewer than 200 cells in a single histological cross-section. Nodes containing only ITCs are excluded from the positive node count for purposes of N classification and should be included in the total number of nodes evaluated (see page 13, TNM 7th edition [17]).

It is recommended to avoid the cNX category as physical and/or imaging examination are sufficient to use the cN0 category. Only when the nodes in the relevant node basin have been removed, and therefore cannot be examined, should a cNX category be used.

For sentinel lymph nodes see page 8, TNM 8th edition [12].

### Post-treatment ypN

The post-neoadjuvant therapy pathological N category (ypN) must be based on the largest continuous focus of residual cancer in the lymph nodes. Treatment-related fibrosis is not included in the ypN classification.

ypNX will be used if no yp post-treatment SN or axillary dissection was performed.

### Prognostic stage group

The AJCC [10] also publish a prognostic stage group for breast tumours.

We refer to the publication of prognostic stage groups in the AJCC [86] and to the revised breast cancer chapter, available after registration with an email address, https://cancerstaging.us10.list-manage.com/subscribe?u=e4fcf2de02a fbcaa9a2820fea&id=08450ea96e.

## Gynaecological Tumours

### Vulva

The definitions of TNM and stage grouping have changed in the 7th edition and reflect new staging adopted by the International Federation of Gynaecology and Obstetrics (FIGO) 2009 [87, 88].

Changes to the staging classification reflect a belief that tumour size independent of other factors (spread to adjacent structures, nodal metastasis) is less important in predicting survival. The current revision of N classification adopted reflects a recognition that the number and size of lymph node metastasis more accurately reflect prognosis than the previous criteria.

**Summary – *Vulva***

| TNM | Vulva | FIGO |
|---|---|---|
| T1[a] | Confined to vulva/perineum | I |
| | T1a ≤ 2 cm with stromal invasion ≤ 1.0 mm | IA |
| | T1b > 2 cm or stromal invasion > 1.0 mm | IB |
| T2 | Lower urethra/vagina/anus | II |
| T3[b] | Upper urethra/vagina, bladder, rectal/mucosa, fixed to pelvic bone | IVA |
| N1a | One or two nodes < 5 mm | IIIA |
| N1b | One node ≥ 5 mm | IIIA |
| N2a | 3 or more nodes < 5 mm | IIIB |
| N2b | 2 or more nodes ≥ 5 mm | IIIB |
| N2c | Extracapsular spread | IIIC |
| N3 | Fixed, ulcerated | IVA |
| M1 | Distant | IVB |

**Notes.**

[a] The depth of invasion is defined as the measurement of the tumour from the epithelial–stromal junction of the adjacent most superficial dermal papilla to the deepest point of invasion.

[b] T3 is not used by FIGO. They label it IV.

### *T Classification*

Invasion of the mucosa: Lower urethra    T2

Invasion of the mucosa: Upper urethra    T3

   Upper urethra corresponds to the proximal half, lower urethra to the distal half.

## Vagina

The definitions of TNM and stage grouping for this tumour have not changed from the 7th edition [17, 24].

   FIGO recommended that a vaginal carcinoma occurring 5 years after successful treatment (complete resection) of a carcinoma of the cervix is considered a primary vaginal carcinoma.

   A tumour involving the vulva is classified as carcinoma of the vulva.

   There should be histological confirmation of the disease.

### Summary – *Vagina*

| TNM | Vagina | FIGO |
|-----|--------|------|
| T1 | Vaginal wall | I |
| T2 | Paravaginal tissue | II |
| T3 | Pelvic wall | III |
| T4 | Mucosa of bladder/rectum, beyond pelvis | IVA |
| N1 | Regional | |
| M1 | Distant metastasis | IVB |

### *T Classification*

'Frozen pelvis' is a clinical term, which means that tumour extends to the pelvic wall(s). It is classified as T3.

   Invasion of the rectal wall or bladder wall (not mucosa) is classified as T2. Mucosal involvement is T4.

   A tumour of the upper two thirds of the vagina with inguinal lymph node metastasis is classified as M1 (Stage IVB).

   A tumour of the lower third of the vagina with pelvic lymph node metastasis is classified as M1 (Stage IVB).

## Cervix Uteri

The definitions of TNM and the Stages Grouping reflect the staging adopted by the International Federation of Gynaecology and Obstetrics [87, 88].

**Summary – *Cervix Uteri***

| TNM | Cervix uteri | | FIGO |
|---|---|---|---|
| T1 | Confined to cervix | | I |
| | T1a | Diagnosed only by microscopy | IA |
| | T1a1 | Depth $\leq 3$ mm, horizontal spread $\leq 7$ mm | IA1 |
| | T1a2 | Depth $> 3 - 5$ mm, horizontal spread $< 7$ mm | IA2 |
| | T1b | Clinically visible or microscopic lesion greater than T1a2 | IB |
| | T1b1 | $\leq 4$ cm | IB1 |
| | T1b2 | $> 4$ cm | IB2 |
| T2 | Beyond uterus but not pelvic wall or lower third vagina | | II |
| | T2a | No parametrium | IIA |
| | T2a1 | $\leq 4$ cm | IIA1 |
| | T2a2 | $> 4$ cm | IIA2 |
| | T2b | Parametrium | IIB |
| T3 | Lower third vagina/pelvic wall/ hydronephrosis/non-functioning kidney | | III |
| | T3a | Lower third vagina | IIIA |
| | T3b | Pelvic wall/hydronephrosis/non-functioning kidney | IIIB |
| T4 | Mucosa of bladder or rectum; beyond true pelvis | | IVA |
| N1 | Regional | | |
| M1 | Distant metastasis (includes inguinal lymph nodes and intraperitoneal disease). It excludes metastasis to vagina, pelvic serosa and adnexa | | IVB |

*T Classification*

The FIGO stages are based on clinical staging. TNM stages are based on clinical and/or pathological classification.

A description of cervical tumour size is important, especially for T1–T3 carcinomas (Stages II–III) where tumour size shows prognostic utility. The 2009 FIGO classification [87, 88] has adopted T subclassification based on tumour size $\leq 4$ cm (T2a1) and $> 4$ cm (T2a2) for cervical carcinoma spreading beyond the cervix but not to the pelvic side wall or lower 1/3 of the vagina (T2 lesions).

In the rare multifocal T1a tumours for horizontal spread FIGO [87, 88] classifies by the largest focus. This is in accordance with TNM rule number 5.

The presence of tumour cells in lymphatics (lymph vessels) or veins of the parametrium does not qualify for T2b/pT2b. T2b/pT2b is used only for grossly or histologically evident continuous invasion beyond the rnyometrium.

'Frozen pelvis' is a clinical term, which means that the tumour extends to the pelvic wall(s), i.e. T3b/pT3b.

Invasion of the rectal wall or bladder wall (not mucosa) is classified as T3a/pT3a. Mucosal involvement is T4/pT4.

Tumour positive peritoneal fluid, e.g. in the pouch of Douglas, is not considered in the TNM or FIGO classification, but should be separately documented.

### *N Classification*
### Regional Lymph Nodes

In the UICC classification the regional lymph nodes are the paracervical, parametrial, hypogastric (internal iliac, obturator), common and external iliac, pre-sacral and lateral sacral nodes. Para-aortic nodes are not regional, but FIGO has decided to include para-aortic nodes as regional. Therefore the UICC has issued an errata so that the regional nodes are the paracervical, parametrial, hypogastric (internal iliac, obturator), common and external iliac, pre-sacral, lateral sacral nodes and para-aortic nodes.

When nodal metastases are identified it is important to indicate the extent of nodal involvement (pelvic lymph nodes and/or para-aortic lymph nodes) and the methodology by which diagnosis was established (pathologic or radiologic).

### Note.

In the 7th edition the para-aortic nodes were considered to be metastatic but to be consistent with advice from FIGO the para-aortic nodes are now classified as regional.

### *M Classification*

Distant metastasis (M1) including peritoneal spread, involvement of supraclavicular or mediastinal lymph nodes, lung, liver or bone but excluding metastasis to vagina, pelvic serosa and adnexa.

## Uterus – Endometrium

The definitions of TNM and the Stage Grouping for these tumours reflect new staging proposals adopted by the International Federation of Gynaecology and Obstetrics and others [89–91].

A separate staging schema has been adopted by FIGO for uterine sarcomas.

## Summary – *Uterus Endometrium*

| TNM | Endometrium | | FIGO |
|-----|-------------|--|------|
| T1 | Confined to uterus (includes cervical glands) | | I |
| | T1a | Tumour limited to the endometrium or less than half of myometrium | IA |
| | T1b | One-half or more of myometrium | IB |
| T2 | Invades cervix | | II |
| T3 | Local or regional as specified below or N1/N2 | | III |
| | T3a | Serosa/adnexa | IIIA |
| | T3b | Vaginal/parametrial | IIIB |
| N1 | Regional lymph node metastasis to pelvic lymph nodes | | IIIC1 |
| N2 | Regional lymph node metastasis to para-aortic lymph nodes with or without positive pelvic lymph nodes | | IIIC2 |
| T4 | Mucosa of bladder/bowel | | IVA |
| M1 | Distant metastasis (excluding metastasis to vagina, pelvic serosa or adnexae, including metastasis to inguinal lymph nodes, intra-abdominal lymph nodes other than para-aortic or pelvic nodes) | | IVB |

### *T Classification*

There may be a small number of patients with T1 corpus carcinoma who will be treated primarily with radiation therapy. For these cases FIGO recommends clinical classification according to the former FIGO schedule (IA, uterine cavity 8 cm or less in length; 1B, uterine cavity more than 8 cm in length); the use of this staging system must be stated.

Foci of carcinoma in the myometrium, which are surrounded by non-neoplastic endometrial stroma, should not be considered invasion of the myometrium. Mostly, these tumours are classified as T1a [92, 93].

Extension of endometrial carcinoma along tongue-like extension into the myometrium should not be considered as 'true' invasion of the myometrium and should not be considered in the classification [93, 94].

T3a or FIGO IIIA includes discontinuous involvement of adnexae or serosa within the pelvis. Invasion of parametria is classified as T3a (FIGO IIIA).

Invasion of the rectal wall or bladder wall (not mucosa) is classified as T3b. Mucosal involvement is T4.

'Frozen pelvis' is a clinical term, which means that the tumour extends to the pelvic wall(s), i.e. T3b.

### Stage – Endometrium

| | | | |
|---|---|---|---|
| Stage I | T1 | N0 | M0 |
| Stage IA | T1a | N0 | M0 |
| Stage IB | T1b | N0 | M0 |
| Stage II | T2 | N0 | M0 |
| Stage IIIA | T3a | N0 | M0 |
| Stage IIIB | T3b | N0 | M0 |
| Stage IIIC | T1, T2, T3 | N1, N2 | M0 |
| Stage IIIC1 | T1, T2, T3 | N1 | M0 |
| Stage IIIC2 | T1, T2, T3 | N2 | M0 |
| Stage IVA | T4 | Any N | M0 |
| Stage IVB | Any T | Any N | M1 |

### G – Histopathological Grading

For histopathological grading use G1, G2 or G3 as outlined in the FIGO Annual Report No. 26 [91]. Cases of carcinoma of the corpus should be grouped with regard to the degree of differentiation of the adenocarcinoma as follows:

G1   <5% of a non-squamous or non-morular solid growth pattern
G2   6–50% of a non-squamous or non-morular solid growth pattern
G3   >50% of a non-squamous or non-morular solid growth pattern

### Notes.

- Nuclear atypia, inappropriate for the architectural grade, raises the grade of a Grade 1 or Grade 2 by 1.
- In serous and clear cell adenocarcinomas, nuclear grading takes precedent.
- Adenocarcinomas with squamous differentiation are graded according to the nuclear grade of the glandular component.

## Uterine Sarcomas

This classification applies to leiomyosarcoma, endometrial stromasarcoma and adenosarcoma [95, 96]. Presently, there are recommendations on how to classify undifferentiated stromal sarcomas.

The anatomical subsites are ICD-O-3 53, 54, 54.1, 54.2.

### Summary – *Uterine Sarcomas*

| | |
|---|---|
| T1 | Confined to uterus |
| T2 | Within pelvis |
| T3 | Abdominal tissues |
| T4 | Bladder/rectum mucosa |

| | | | |
|---|---|---|---|
| Leiomyosarcoma, | T1a | IA | ≤5 cm |
| endometrial stromal sarcoma | T1b | IB | >5 cm |
| Adenosarcoma | T1a | IA | Endometrium/endocervix |
| | T1b | IB | <half of the myometrium |
| | T1c | IC | ≥half of the myometrium |

Stage IC does not apply for leiomyosarcoma and endometrial stromal sarcoma.

**Note.**
Simultaneous tumours of the uterine corpus and ovary/pelvis in association with ovarian/pelvic endometriosis should be classified as independent primary tumours.

## Ovarian, Fallopian Tube and Primary Peritoneal Carcinoma

The classification applies to malignant ovarian neoplasms (ICD-O-3 C56) of both epithelial and stromal origin, including those of borderline malignancy or of low malignant potential corresponding to 'common epithelial tumours' of the earlier terminology [94].

The classification also applies to carcinoma of the fallopian tubes (ICD-O-3 C57) and to the carcinomas of the peritoneum (ICD-O-3 C48.1, 2, 8) (Müllerian origin) [97].

Cases should be separated by histologic type and borderline or invasive nature.

The FIGO stages are based on surgical staging (TNM stages are based on clinical and/or pathological classification).

### Regional Lymph Nodes

The regional lymph nodes are the hypogastric (obturator), common iliac, external iliac, lateral sacral, para-aortic and retroperitoneal nodes.

**Note.**
Including intra-abdominal nodes such as greater omental nodes.

**Summary – *Ovary, Fallopian Tube and Primary Peritoneal Carcinoma***

| TNM | Ovary | | FIGO |
|---|---|---|---|
| T1 | Limited to the ovaries (one/both) or fallopian tubes | | I |
| | T1a | One ovary or fallopian tube, capsule intact, no tumour on surface *or* fallopian tube surface, no malignant cells ascites or peritoneal washings | IA |
| | T1b | Both ovaries or fallopian tubes, capsule intact, no tumour on surface ovarian or fallopian tube surface, no malignant cells in ascites or peritoneal washings | IB |

| | | | |
|---|---|---|---|
| | T1c | One or both ovaries or fallopian tubes | IC |
| | T1c1 | Surgical spill | IC1 |
| | T1c2 | Capsule ruptures before surgery, tumour on ovarian IC2 or fallopian surface | |
| | T1c3 | Malignant cells in ascites or peritoneal washings | IC3 |
| T2 | | One or both ovaries or fallopian tubes with pelvic extension *or* primary peritoneal carcinoma | II |
| | T2a | Extension and/or implants uterus, fallopian tube(s), ovaries | IIA |
| | T2b | Other pelvic tissues including bowel within the pelvis | IIB |
| T3 and/ or N1 | | One or both ovaries or fallopian tubes *or* primary peritoneal carcinoma (with cytologically/histologically confirmed spread to the peritoneum outside the pelvis) and/or metastasis to the retroperitoneal (intraabdominal) lymph nodes | III |
| N1 | | Retroperitoneal lymph node metastasis only | |
| | N1a | Lymph node metastasis $\leq$ 10 mm | IIIA1i |
| | N1b | Lymph node metastasis > 10 mm | IIIA1ii |
| | T3a | Microscopic extrapelvic peritoneal involvement with or without retroperitoneal lymph node involvement, including bowel involvement | IIIA2 |
| | T3b | Macroscopic peritoneal metastasis beyond pelvic brim 2 cm or less including bowel involvement outside the pelvis, with or without retroperitoneal lymph node metastasis | IIIB |
| | T3c | Macroscopic peritoneal metastasis beyond pelvic brim *and/or* retroperitoneal lymph node metastasis | IIIC |
| M1 | | Distant metastasis (excludes peritoneal metastasis) | IV |
| | M1a | Pleural effusion with positive cytology | IVA |
| | M1b | Parenchymal metastasis and metastasis to extra-abdominal organs (including inguinal lymph nodes and lymph nodes outside the abdominal cavity) | IVB |

## Note.
T3c ncludes extension of the tumour to a capsule of the liver and spleen without parenchymal involvement of either organ.

### *T Classification*

T3/pT3 Peritoneal metastasis outside the pelvis includes involvement of the omentum.

T3/pT3 Includes multifocal involvement of the peritoneum in borderline tumours.

Neither in the FIGO nor in the UICC/AJCC TNM classification is there a separation between invasive or non-invasive implants in the omentum.

In the case of peritoneal metastasis the greatest horizontal diameter is considered in the classification, not the thickness of the metastasis.

Microscopic confirmation of a single peritoneal metastasis beyond the pelvic brim, irrespective of the size of the metastasis, is required for T3/pT3. For the subdivision, size alone is relevant. Therefore, T3c is appropriately based on the macroscopic assessment by the surgeon even if microscopic confirmation was of a smaller metastasis only.

In the ovary, peritoneal metastasis is not considered as distant metastasis; it is classified as T3.

**Stage – Ovary, Fallopian Tube and Primary Peritoneal Carcinoma**

| Stage I | T1 | N0 | M0 |
|---|---|---|---|
| Stage IA | T1a | N0 | M0 |
| Stage IB | T1b | N0 | M0 |
| Stage IC | T1c | N0 | M0 |
| Stage II | T2 | N0 | M0 |
| Stage IIA | T2a | N0 | M0 |
| Stage IIB | T2b | N0 | M0 |
| Stage IIIA1 | T1, T2 | N1 | M0 |
| Stage IIIA2 | T3a | N0, N1 | M0 |
| Stage IIIB | T3b | N0, N1 | M0 |
| Stage IIIC | T3c | N0, N1 | M0 |
| Stage IV | Any T | Any N | M1 |
| Stage IVA | Any T | Any N | M1a |
| Stage IVB | Any T | Any N | M1b |

## Gestational Trophoblastic Tumours

The classification for gestational trophoblastic tumours is based on that of the FIGO adopted in 1992 and updated in 2002 [98]. The definitions of the T and M categories correspond to the FIGO stages.

The following histopathologic types are included:

- Choriocarcinoma (9100/3)
- Invasive hydatiforme mole (9100/1)
- Hydatiforme mole (complete, partial) (9100/0)
- Placental site trophoblastic tumour (9104/1)

Histopathological grading is not applicable.

The German TNM Committee [99] recommended the use of the TNM classification of gestational trophoblastic tumours for epithelioid trophoblastic tumours (ICD-O M9105/3).

## Summary – *Gestational Trophoblastic Tumours*

| TM and risk | gestational trophoblastic tumours | Stage |
|---|---|---|
| T1 | Confined to uterus | I |
| T2 | Other genital structures | II |
| M1a | Metastasis to lung(s) | III |
| M1b | Other distant metastasis | IV |

**Risk Categories**

| | |
|---|---|
| Total prognostic score 6 or less = low risk | IA–IVA |
| Total prognostic score 7 or more = high risk | IB–IVB |

**Prognostic Score**

| Prognostic factor | 0 | 1 | 2 | 4 |
|---|---|---|---|---|
| Age | $<40$ | $\geq 40$ | | |
| Antecedent pregnancy | H. mole | Abortion | Term pregnancy | |
| Months from index pregnancy | $<4$ | 4–6 | 7–12 | $>12$ |
| Pre-treatment serum ßhCG (IU/ml) | $<10^3$ | $10^3 - <10^4$ | $10^4 - <10^5$ | $\geq 10^5$ |
| Largest tumour size including uterus | $<3$ cm | 3–5 cm | $>5$ cm | |
| Sites of metastasis | Lung | Spleen, kidney | Gastrointestinal tract | Liver, brain |
| Number of metastasis | | 1–4 | 5–8 | $>8$ |
| Previous failed chemotherapy | | | Single drug | Two or more drugs |

**Note.**
Serum beta HCG could be used as well as urinary beta HCG.

# Urological Tumours

## Penis
Minor changes have been introduced since the 7th edition [17, 24].

## Summary – *Penis*

| | |
|---|---|
| Tis | Penile intraepithelial neoplasia |
| Ta | Non-invasive localized squamous cell carcinoma |

T1 Glans: lamina propria
Foreskin: dermis, lamina propria, Dartos fascia
Shaft: connective tissue between epidermis and corpora regardless of location
  T1a  Without lymphovascular or perineural invasion, not G3–G4
  T1b  With lymphovascular and/or perineural invasion, or G3–G4
T2 Corpus spongiosum (glans or ventral shaft) +/- urethral invasion
T3 Corpora cavernosa (including tunica albuginea) +/- urethral invasion
T4 Other adjacent structures (i.e. scrotum, prostate, pubic bone)

| N1 | Palpable mobile unilateral inguinal | pN1 | 1 or 2 inguinal |
|---|---|---|---|
| N2 | Palpable mobile ≥ 2 unilateral inguinal | pN2 | ≧ 2 inguinal or bilateral inguinal |
| N3 | Fixed inguinal nodal mass or pelvic lymphadenopathy | pN3 | Pelvic lymph node(s), unilateral or bilateral, extranodal extension |

### *T Classification*
Erythroplasia of Queyrat is classified as carcinoma in situ (Tis).

## Prostate
There have been minor changes in this tumour from the 7th edition [17, 24].

## Summary – *Prostate*

T1 Clinically inapparent, not palpable
  T1a  ≤5%
  T1b  >5%
  T1c  Needle biopsy
T2 Confined within prostate
  T2a  ≤ one half of one side
  T2b  More than one half of one lobe
  T2c  Both lobes
T3 Extends through the prostatic capsule
  T3a  Extraprostatic extension (unilateral or bilateral), microscopic bladder involvement
  T3b  Seminal vesicle(s)

T4     Fixed or invades adjacent structure: external sphincter, rectum, levator muscles, pelvic wall

N1     Regional lymph nodes

M1     Distant metastasis
     M1a     Non-regional lymph node(s)
     M1b     Bone(s)
     M1c     Other site(s)

**Note.**
For M1a, when more than one site of metastasis is present, the most advanced category is used. pM1c is the most advanced category.
For M1c, other site(s) are with or without bone metastasis.

### T Classification

The pT classification requires a radical prostatectomy. A transurethral resection is considered to be part of the clinical assessment. There is no pT1 category because there is insufficient tissue to assess the highest pT category.

Similarly, there are no subcategories of pT2.

The prostate capsule is a network of smooth muscle and collagen-rich soft tissue around the prostate. There is no clear fascia.

The prostate includes a right lobe, a left lobe and a middle lobe according to the anatomic literature. Involvement of the right lobe and the middle lobe can be considered as T2 (according to the TNM rule number 4).

Extraprostatic extension with microscopic bladder neck invasion is included in T3a.

The presence of fatty or muscle tissue in a needle biopsy is not in itself evidence of invasion through the capsule into adjacent fatty tissue and thus may not be classified as T3/pT3.

Prostate carcinoma with invasion of M. sphincter internus is classified as T4/pT4.

According to newer anatomical results there are two sphincters:

M. sphincter urethrae externus = M. sphincter urethrae (diaphragmaticae)
M. sphincter urethrae internus = M. sphincter vesicae

The invasion of the M. sphincter urethrae as well as the invasion of the M. sphincter vesicae would be equivalent to an invasion of the bladder neck and should be classified as T4.

When a tumour is an incidental finding in a TUR specimen and after the first TUR a repeated TUR (re-TUR) is performed within 2 months as part of the definitive primary treatment (without a radical prostatectomy), the subdivision into T1a and T1b should be based on the findings of both TURs.

### Examples

1. First TUR: < 5% of tissue resected involved by carcinoma. re-TUR with the same amount of tissue: 10% of tissue involved. Classify as cT1b.
2. First TUR: 10% of tissue resected involved by carcinoma. re-TUR including a threefold amount of tissue: no further tumour found. Classify cT1a.

Transitional cell carcinoma of the prostate (prostatic urethra) is classified under urethra; see page 208 of the TNM 8th edition [14].

If a prostate resection specimen is limited to the prostate and does not include the capsule or parts of the capsule (in the apex region), the pT classification cannot be used unless the tumour is clearly surrounded by non-tumorous prostate tissue.

Involvement of the prostatic urethra is not considered in the T classification.

'Frozen pelvis' is a clinical term, which means that the tumour extends to the pelvic wall(s) and is fixed. It is classified as T4.

### *M Classification*

If a patient has been diagnosed with non-regional lymph node metastasis and bone metastasis then the most advanced category should be used, e.g. M1c/pM1. When more than one site of metastasis is present, the category M1c/pM1c should be used. The impact of the site of metastases on survival in patients with metastatic prostate cancer has been shown [100].

### G Histopathological Grade Group

The Gleason score (2014 criteria) [101, 102] and the WHO Grade Group should both be reported [102].

| Grade group | Gleason score | Gleason pattern |
| --- | --- | --- |
| 1 | ≤6 | ≤3+3 |
| 2 | 7 | 3+4 |
| 3 | 7 | 4+3 |
| 4 | 8 | 4+4 |
| 5 | 9–10 | 4+5, 5+4, 5+5 |

## Clinical Stage – Prostate

| Stage I | T1, T2a | N0 | M0 |
|---|---|---|---|
| Stage II | T2b, T2c | N0 | M0 |
| Stage III | T3 | N0 | M0 |
| Stage IV | T4 | N0 | M0 |
| | Any T | N1 | M0 |
| | Any T | Any N | M1 |

## Proposal for a Pathological Stage – Prostate

| Stage II | pT2 | N0 | M0 |
|---|---|---|---|
| Stage III | pT3 | N0 | M0 |
| Stage IVA | pT4 | N0 | M0 |
| Stage IVB | Any pT | N1 | M0 |
| Stage IVC | Any pT | Any N | M1 |

The AJCC also publishes Prognostic Stage Groups [10].

## Testis

The definitions of TNM and Stage Grouping for this tumour have not changed from the 7th edition [17, 24].

## Summary – *Testis*

| | |
|---|---|
| pTis | Germ cell neoplasia in situ (GCNIS) (intratubular germ cell neoplasia) |
| pT1 | Testis and epididymis, tunica albuginea but not tunica vaginalis, no vascular/lymphatic invasion |
| pT2 | Testis and epididymis with vascular or lymphatic invasion or extension through tunica albuginea with involvement of tunica vaginalis |
| pT3 | Spermatic cord, +/- vascular/lymphatic invasion |
| pT4 | Scrotum, +/- vascular/lymphatic invasion |

| N1 | $\leq 2$ cm or multiple $\leq 2$ cm | pN1 | $\leq 2$ cm or $\leq 5$ nodes $\leq 2$ cm |
|---|---|---|---|
| N2 | $> 2$–5 cm or multiple $\geq 2$–5 cm | pN2 | $> 2$–5 cm or $> 5$ nodes $< 5$ cm or extranodal extension |
| N3 | Lymph node mass $> 5$ cm | pN3 | $> 5$ cm |
| M1 | Distant metastasis | | |
| M1a | Non regional lymph nodes or lung | | |
| M1b | Other sites | | |

### T Classification

In the case of mixed germ cell tumours, the pT classification is determined by the total tumour. The different components should not be classified separately for pT categorization.

Synchronous bilateral tumours should be staged separately as independent primary tumours.

The AJCC [10] proposes a subdivision for pT1 into pT1a (< 3 cm size) and pT1b (≥ 3 cm in size) only for pure seminomas.

Epididymal invasion is considered as pT2 rather than pT1.

Hilar soft tissue invasion is considered as pT2.

pT2:    Invasion beyond the tunica albuginea includes invasion of any of the following: cremaster muscle, cremaster fascia, testicular portion of the internal or external spermatic fascia, i.e. invasion of the scrotum without the skin. Invasion beyond these structures into the subcutis or cutis of the scrotum is classified as pT4.

pT3:    Invasion of the spermatic cord refers to direct extension. Invasion of lymph vessels or blood vessels means unequivocal vessels lined by an endothelium.

The plexus pampiniformis belongs to the spermatic cord, so invasion should be classified as pT3.

Discontinuous involvement of the spermatic cord by vascular/lymphatic invasion represents M1 disease.

### Prognostic Group – Testis

| Stage 0 | pTis | N0 | M0 | S0 |
|---|---|---|---|---|
| Stage I | pT1–4 | N0 | M0 | SX |
| Stage IA | pT1 | N0 | M0 | S0 |
| Stage IB | pT2–4 | N0 | M0 | S0 |
| Stage IS | Any pT/TX | N0 | M0 | S1–S3 |
| Stage II | Any pT/TX | N1–N3 | M0 | SX |
| Stage IIA | Any pT/TX | N1 | M0 | S0 |
| | Any pT/TX | N1 | M0 | S1 |
| Stage IIB | Any pT/TX | N2 | M0 | S0 |
| | Any pT/TX | N2 | M0 | S1 |
| Stage IIC | Any pT/TX | N3 | M0 | S0 |
| | Any pT/TX | N3 | M0 | S1 |
| Stage III | Any pT/TX | Any N | M1a | SX |
| Stage IIIA | Any pT/TX | Any N | M1a | S0 |
| | Any pT/TX | Any N | M1a | S1 |

| | | | | |
|---|---|---|---|---|
| Stage IIIB | Any pT/TX | Any N | M0 | S2 |
| | Any pT/TX | Any N | M1a | S2 |
| Stage IIIC | Any pT/TX | N1–N3 | M0 | S3 |
| | Any pT/TX | Any N | M1a | S3 |
| | Any pT/TX | Any N | M1b | Any S |

## Kidney

Some minor changes have been introduced in this tumour since the 7th edition [17, 24].

### Summary – *Kidney*

T1   ≤7 cm; limited to the kidney
   T1a   ≤4 cm
   T1b   >4–7 cm
T2   >7 cm; limited to the kidney
   T2a   >7–10 cm
   T2b   >10 cm
T3   Into major veins or perinephric tissues but not into the ipsilateral adrenal gland and not beyond Gerota fascia
   T3a   Tumour extends into the renal vein or its segmental branches *or* tumour invades the pelvicalyceal system *or* tumour invades perirenal and/or renal sinus fat (peripelvic) but not beyond Gerota fascia
   T3b   Tumour extends into the vena cava below the diaphragm
   T3c   Tumour extends into the vena cava above the diaphragm or invades the wall of the vena cava
T4   Beyond Gerota fascia including contiguous extension into the ipsilateral adrenal gland
N1   Regional lymph node metastasis

### T/pT Classification

The reason for subdivision of T1 is the selection of patients for partial nephrectomy.

T2 tumours have been divided into T2a (greater than 7 cm but less than or equal to 10 cm) and T2b (> 10 cm).

Invasion of the pelvicalyceal system has been additionally introduced and is classified as T3a/pT3a.

Bulging of a tumour in the sense of changing the contour of the kidney is not sufficient to be classified as T3 or pT3. Penetration of the kidney capsule is needed to classify as T3 or pT3, which should be particularly searched for in the peripelvic fatty tissue.

Invasion of the wall of the vena cava above the diaphragm is T3c.

Ipsilateral involvement of the adrenal gland is classified as T4/pT4 if contiguous invasion and M1 if not contiguous.

Gerota fascia (renal fascia) includes the pre- and retrorenal fascia. Invasion of the peritoneum is invasion beyond the Gerota fascia (prerenal fascia) and is classified as T4.

**Stage – Kidney**

| Stage I | T1 | N0 | M0 |
|---|---|---|---|
| Stage II | T2 | N0 | M0 |
| Stage III | T1, T2 | N1 | M0 |
| | T3 | N0, N1 | M0 |
| Stage IV | T4 | Any N | M0 |
| | Any T | Any N | M1 |

# Renal Pelvis and Ureter

The definitions of TNM and the stages for these tumours have only slightly changed from the 7th edition in the definition of the N/pN categories [17, 24].

**Summary – *Renal Pelvis and Ureter***

| Ta | Non-invasive papillary |
|---|---|
| Tis | In situ |
| T1 | Subepithelial connective tissue |
| T2 | Muscularis |
| T3 | *Renal pelvis:* Beyond muscularis into peripelvic fat or renal parenchyma |
| | *Ureter:* Beyond muscularis into periureteric fat |
| T4 | Adjacent organs, through the kidney into perinephric fat |
| N1 | Single regional, ≤ 2 cm |
| N2 | Single regional, > 2 cm, or multiple |

## *T Classification*

Direct extension into the urinary bladder in the region of the ostium is classified by the depth of greatest invasion in any of the involved organs.

In tumours of the ureter, adjacent organs include the parietal peritoneurn.

The prognosis of T3 in the ureter is worse than in the renal pelvis and corresponds approximately to T4 renal pelvis tumours. Therefore, separate analysis of the ureter and renal pelvis carcinoma is recommended [103].

For classification of multiple synchronous primary tumours the renal pelvis and ureter are considered as a single organ. Therefore, in cases of synchronous tumours in the renal pelvis and the ureter, the tumour with the highest T category should be classified and the multiplicity or the number of tumours should be indicated in parentheses, e.g. T2(m) or T3(2).

In contrast, in the case of synchronous tumours in the renal pelvis and the urinary bladder, both tumours should be classified independently.

In the case of multifocal tumours of the renal pelvis and ureter with Ta and Tis tumours, Tis should be classified.

### Grading

In the urothelial tumours a low- and high-grade designation is used to match the current WHO/ISUP recommended grading system [104].

## Urinary Bladder

The classification applies not only to carcinomas (non-invasive or invasive) but also to 'Papillary urothelial (transitional cell) neoplasm of low malignant potential' (PUNLMP) [105].

AJCC excludes papilloma and PUNLMP from the Ta category [10].

### Summary – *Urinary Bladder*

| | | |
|---|---|---|
| Ta | Non-invasive papillary | |
| Tis | In situ 'flat' tumour | |
| T1 | Subepithelial connective tissue | |
| T2 | Tumour invades muscularis propria | |
| | T2a | Superficial muscle (inner half) |
| | T2b | Deep muscle (outer half) |
| T3 | Tumour invades perivesical tissue | |
| | T3a | Microscopically |
| | T3b | Macroscopically |
| T4 | Prostate stroma, seminal vesicles, uterus, vagina, pelvic wall, abdominal wall | |
| | T4a | Prostate stroma, seminal vesicles, uterus, vagina |
| | T4b | Pelvic wall, abdominal wall |
| N1 | Single regional | |
| N2 | Multiple regional | |
| N3 | Common iliac | |
| M1 | Distant | |
| | M1a | Non-regional lymph nodes |
| | M1b | Other distant |

## T Classification

In the case of multifocal tumours of the urinary bladder with Ta and Tis tumours, Tis should be classified.

In some cases (up to 50%) a lamina muscularis mucosae has been described. Invasion of 'muscularis' means lamina muscularis propria.

If the pathology specimen does not contain muscle, the category T1 is applicable (see General Rule No. 4). However, the pathology report should state the absence of muscle to allow the clinician to consider repeating the biopsy.

In the case of transurethral resection, differentiation between T2a and T2b is possible only if the surgeon submits the material as superficial (inner) and deep (outer) portions and histological examination is performed separately. Otherwise, the case is classified as T2.

Direct invasion of the distal ureter is classified by the depth of greatest invasion in any of the involved organs.

Uncommonly, carcinomas of the bladder show an associated in situ component extending into the prostatic ducts and sometimes into the prostatic glands (or ureter) without any invasion in the prostate. Such cases are classified according to the depth of bladder wall invasion. The extension of the associated in situ component into the prostate does not qualify for classification as T4. It may be indicated by the suffix '(is)', e.g. T2(is). It may be further indicated by the suffix '(is pu)' (extension into the prostatic urethra) or '(is pd)' (extension into the prostatic ducts), e.g. T2(is pu) or T2 (is pd).

Invasion of the prostatic urethra (extension of invasive urinary bladder carcinoma into the prostatic urethra with invasion of the latter) is included in prostatic invasion and is therefore classified as T4a.

Direct invasion of the large or small intestine should be classified as T4a. The same applies to invasion through the peritoneum covering the bladder.

Invasion of seminal vesicles by bladder tumours should be classified as T4a.

## Recurrent Carcinoma after Cystectomy and Ureterosigmoidostomy

A recurrent transitional carcinoma in the region of an ureterosigmoidostomy may invade only the subepithelial connective tissue of the ureter and the adjacent mucosa and submucosa of the sigmoid colon. In this case the invasion of the colon should not be considered as invasion of an adjacent organ. For the T classification the rules for ureter and colon should be applied, i.e. rT1 is the correct classification.

## N Classification

Paravesical lymph nodes should be considered as lymph nodes of the true pelvis and metastasis and therefore should be classified as pN1.

## Grading

In the urothelial tumours a low- and high-grade designation is used to match the current WHO/ISUP recommended grading system [101].

### Stage – Urinary Bladder

| | | | |
|---|---|---|---|
| Stage 0a | Ta | N0 | M0 |
| Stage 0is | Tis | N0 | M0 |
| Stage I | T1 | N0 | M0 |
| Stage II | T2a, T2b | N0 | M0 |
| Stage IIIA | T3a, T3b, T4a | N0 | M0 |
| | T1, T2, T3, T4a | N1 | M0 |
| Stage IIIB | T1, T2, T3, T4a | N2, N3 | M0 |
| Stage IVA | T4b | Any N | M0 |
| | Any T | Any N | M1a |
| Stage IVB | Any T | Any N | M1b |

# Urethra

**Summary – *Urethra***

### Urethra – Male and Female

| | |
|---|---|
| Ta | Non-invasive papillary, polypoid or verrucous |
| Tis | In situ |
| T1 | Subepithelial connective tissue |
| T2 | Corpus spongiosum, prostate, periurethral muscle |
| T3 | Corpus cavernosum, beyond prostatic capsule, anterior vagina, bladder neck (extraprostatic extension) |
| T4 | Other adjacent organs |

### Urothelial (transitional cell) carcinoma of the prostate

| | |
|---|---|
| Tis | In situ, involvement or prostatic urethra, periuretheral or prostatic ducts without stromal invasion |
| T1 | Subepithelial connective tissue (tumours of prostatic urethrae only) |
| T2 | Any of the following: prostatic stroma, corpus spongiosum, periurethral muscle |
| T3 | Any of the following: corpus cavernosum, beyond prostatic capsule, anterior vagina, bladder neck (extraprostatic extension) |
| T4 | Other adjacent organs (i.e. bladder, rectum |
| N1 | Single lymph node |
| N2 | Multiple lymph nodes |

### T Classification
In urethral diverticular carcinoma, a differentiation between T2 and T3 is not possible [106]. In this case T2 is used (according to TNM rule number 4).

### N Classification
The N3 category from the 7th edition [17, 24] has been collapsed into N2.

### Grading
In the urothelial tumours a low- and high-grade designation is used to match the current WHO/ISUP recommended grading system [104].

## Adrenal Cortex Tumours
### Summary – *Adrenal Cortical Carcinoma*

| | |
|---|---|
| T1 | ≤5 cm, no extra-adrenal invasion |
| T2 | >5 cm, no extra-adrenal invasion |
| T3 | Local invasion |
| T4 | Adjacent organs |
| N1 | Regional |

### T Classification
Adjacent organs include kidney, diaphragm, great vessels, pancreas, and liver.

### Stage – Adrenal Cortex Carcinoma

| Stage I | T1 | N0 | M0 |
|---|---|---|---|
| Stage II | T2 | N0 | M0 |
| Stage III | T1, T2 | N1 | M0 |
| | T3, T4 | N0, N1 | M0 |
| Stage IV | Any T | Any N | M1 |

## Ophthalmic Tumours

There have been changes in the classification of several ophthalmic tumour sites from the 7th edition [17, 24].

### Carcinoma of the Conjunctiva
This classification applies to carcinoma of the palpebral and bulbar conjunctiva and the conjunctival fornix.

T1 and T2 definitions have been revised from the 7th to the 8th edition to include invasion of the conjunctival basement membrane.

## Summary – *Conjunctiva Carcinoma*

| | |
|---|---|
| T1 | ≤5 mm, through basement membrane |
| T2 | >5 mm, through basement membrane without invasion of adjacent structures |
| T3 | Adjacent structures |
| T4 | Orbit and beyond |
| | T4a Orbital soft tissues without bone invasion |
| | T4b Bone |
| | T4c Adjacent paranasal sinuses |
| | T4d Brain |
| N1 | Regional |

### Note.

Adjacent structures include the cornea (3, 6, 9 or 12 clock hours), intraocular compartments, forniceal conjunctiva (lower and/or upper), palpebral conjunctiva (lower and/or upper), tarsal conjunctiva (lower and/or upper), lacrimal punctum and canaliculi (lower and/or upper), plica, caruncle, posterior eyelid lamella, anterior eyelid lamella, and/or eyelid margin (lower and/or upper).

### *T Classification*

Carcinomas of the posterior surface of the eyelid are considered under tumours of the conjunctiva.

## Malignant Melanoma of Conjunctiva

There have been some changes from the 7th edition [17, 24].

T categories have been changed to describe circumferential extent.

### Summary – *Malignant Melanoma of Conjunctiva*

| | | | | |
|---|---|---|---|---|
| T1 | Bulbar conjunctiva | pT1 | Bulbar conjunctiva | |
| T1a | ≤1 quadrant | pT1a | ≤2.0 mm, substantia propria | |
| T1b | >1–2 quadrants | pT1b | >2.0 mm, substantia propria | |
| T1c | >2–3 quadrants | | | |
| T1d | >3 quadrants | | | |
| T2 | Non-bulbar conjunctiva, palpebral, forniceal and/or caruncular | pT2 | Palpebral, forniceal, caruncular conjunctiva forniceal and/or caruncular | |
| T2a | Non-caruncular ≤1 quadrant | pT2a | ≤2.0 mm, substantia propria | |
| T2b | Non-caruncular >1 quadrant | pT2b | >2.0 mm, substantia propria | |
| T2c | Caruncular ≤1 quadrant | | | |
| T2d | Caruncular >1 quadrant | | | |
| T3 | Local invasion into | pT3 | Eye, eyelid, nasolacrimal system, orbit | |

| | | | | |
|---|---|---|---|---|
| T3a | Globe | pT3a | Globe |
| T3b | Eyelid | pT3b | Eyelid |
| T3c | Orbit | pT3c | Orbit |
| T3d | Paranasal sinuses, nasolacrimal duct, and/or lacrimal gland | pT3d | Paranasal sinuses, nasolacrimal duct and/or lacrimal sac |
| T4 | CNS | pT4 | CNS |
| N1 | Regional | pN1 | Regional |

**Note.**

1. Melanoma in situ (includes the term primary acquired melanosis) with atypia replacing greater than 75% of the normal epithelial thickness with cytologic features of epithelial cells, including abundant cytoplasm, vesicular nuclei or prominent nucleoli, and/or the presence of an intraepithelial nest of atypical cells.
2. Quadrants are defined by clock hour, starting at the limbus (e.g. 6, 9, 12, 3), extending from the central cornea to and beyond the eyelid margins. This will bisect the caruncle.

### T Classification

This classification applies to malignant melanoma of the bulbar conjunctiva as well as non-bulbar conjunctiva (palpebral, forniceal and/or caruncular).

Involvement of the eyelid is defined as invasion beyond the tarsal plate into the anterior part of the eyelid (T3b/pT3b).

## Malignant Melanoma of Uvea
### Summary – *Uvea Malignant Melanoma*

### Iris Malignant Melanoma

- T1   Limited to iris
  - T1a   ≤3 clock hours
  - T1b   >3 clock hours
  - T1c   With secondary glaucoma
- T2  Tumour confluent with or extending into the ciliary body/choroid, or both
  - T2a   Confluent with or extending into the ciliary body without glaucoma
  - T2b   Confluent with or extending into the choroid without glaucoma
  - T2c   Confluent with or extending into the ciliary body/choroid/both with glaucoma
- T3   Confluent with or extending into the ciliary body, choroid, or both, with scleral extension
- T4   Extrasceral extension
  - T4a   ≤5 mm in diameter
  - T4b   >5 mm in diameter

**Note.**

Iris melanoma originate from, and are predominantly located in, this region of the uvea. If less than half of the tumour volume is located within the iris, the tumour may have originated in the ciliary body and consideration should be given to classify accordingly.

### Ciliary Body and Choroid Malignant Melanoma

A primary ciliary body and choroidal melanomas are classified according to the four tumour size categories (Figure 1 in the TNM 8th edition).

| | | |
|---|---|---|
| T1 | Category 1 | |
| | T1a | Without ciliary body involvement and extraocular extension |
| | T1b | With ciliary body involvement |
| | T1c | Without ciliary body involvement but with extraocular extension $\leq 5$ mm |
| | T1d | With ciliary body involvement and with extraocular extension $\leq 5$ mm |
| T2 | Category 2 | |
| | T2a | Without ciliary body involvement and extraocular extension |
| | T2b | With ciliary body involvement |
| | T2c | Without ciliary body involvement but with extraocular extension $\leq 5$ mm |
| | 2d | With ciliary body involvement and with extraocular extension $\leq 5$ mm |
| T3 | Category 3 | |
| | T3a | Without ciliary body involvement and extraocular extension |
| | T3b | With ciliary body involvement |
| | T3c | Without ciliary body involvement but with extraocular extension $\leq 5$ |
| | T3d | With ciliary body involvement and with extraocular extension $\leq 5$ mm |
| T4 | Category 4 | |
| | T4a | Without ciliary body involvement and extraocular extension |
| | T4b | With ciliary body involvement |
| | T4c | Without ciliary body involvement but with extraocular extension $\leq 5$ mm |
| | T4d | With ciliary body involvement and extraocular extension $\leq 5$ mm |
| | T4e | Any tumour size category with extraocular extension $> 5$ mm in diameter |

### All sites

| | | |
|---|---|---|
| N1 | Regional | |
| M1 | Distant | |
| | M1a | Large metastasis $\leq 3$ cm |
| | M1b | Large metastasis $> 3 - 8$ cm |
| | M1c | Large metastasis $> 8$ cm |

**Notes.**
In clinical practice, the largest tumour basal diameter may be estimated in optic disc diameters (dd, average: 1 dd = 1.5 mm). Tumour thickness may be estimated in diopters (average: 2.5 diopters = 1 mm). However, techniques such as ultrasonography and fundus photography are used to provide more accurate measurements. Ciliary body involvement can be evaluated by the slit-lamp, ophthalmoscopy, gonioscopy and transillumination. However, high-frequency ultrasonography (ultrasound biomicroscopy) is used for a more accurate assessment. Extension through the sclera is evaluated visually before and during surgery, and with ultrasonography, computed tomography or magnetic resonance imaging.

When histopathologic measurements are recorded after fixation, tumour diameter and thickness may be underestimated because of tissue shrinkage.

## T Classification

Extraocular extension is diagnosed if the tumour grows outside the bulb with invasion of the orbit, the optic nerve, the outer eye muscles, the lacrimal apparatus or conjunctiva. The most frequent finding is invasion of the orbit.

In the case of discrepancies between the greatest diameter and the maximum height the most advanced category should be used.

**Example**
12 mm in greatest diameter, 3 mm maximum height: T2.

Thickness (mm)

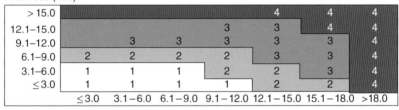

| Thickness (mm) | ≤3.0 | 3.1–6.0 | 6.1–9.0 | 9.1–12.0 | 12.1–15.0 | 15.1–18.0 | >18.0 |
|---|---|---|---|---|---|---|---|
| > 15.0 | | | | | 4 | 4 | 4 |
| 12.1–15.0 | | | | 3 | 3 | 4 | 4 |
| 9.1–12.0 | | 3 | 3 | 3 | 3 | 3 | 4 |
| 6.1–9.0 | 2 | 2 | 2 | 2 | 3 | 3 | 4 |
| 3.1–6.0 | 1 | 1 | 1 | 2 | 2 | 3 | 4 |
| ≤3.0 | 1 | 1 | 1 | 1 | 2 | 2 | 4 |

Largest basal diameter (mm)

(Source: Figure 1, page 222, TNM 8th edition [12])

**Stage**
The stages are for malignant melanoma of the choroid and ciliary body but not of the iris.

# Retinoblastoma
## Summary – Retinoblastoma

| T1 | Confined to the retina with subretinal < 5 mm, without retinal detachment | pT1 | Confined to the eye, no optic nerve/choroidal invasion |
|---|---|---|---|
| | T1a   ≤3 mm or closer than 1.5 mm to the optic nerve or fovea | | |
| | T1b   One tumour > 3 mm or closer than 1.5 mm to the optic nerve/fovea | | |

| | | | | | |
|---|---|---|---|---|---|
| T2 | Vitreous/subretinal seeding or retinal detachment | | pT2 | Tumour with intraocular invasion | |
| | T2a | Subretinal fluid > 5 mm from tumour base | | pT2a | Focal choroidal invasion and pre-/intralaminar invasion of the optic nerve head |
| | T2b | Vitreous/subretinal seeding | | pT2b | Invasion of stroma of iris and/or trabecular meshwork and/or Schlemm's canal |
| T3 | Severe intraocular disease | | pT3 | Significant local invasion | |
| | T3a | Phthisis or prephthisis bulbi | | pT3a | Choroid invasion > 3 mm or multiple foci of invasion > 3mm, any full thickness involvement |
| | T3b | Choroid, pars plana, ciliary body, lens, zonules, iris, anterior chamber | | pT3b | Retrolaminar: optic nerve without invasion transsected end |
| | T3c | Raised intraocular pressure with neovascularization and/or buphthalmos | | pT3c | Partial-thickness involvement sclera (inner 2/3) |
| | T3d | Hyphema and/or vitreous haemorrhage | | pT3d | Full thickness invasion outer 1/3 and/or invasion emissary channels |
| | T3e | Aseptic orbital cellulitis | | | |
| T4 | Extraocular tumour | | pT4 | Extraocular extension | |
| | T4a | Invasion of optic nerve or orbital tissues | | | Tumour involves optic nerve or transsected end, in meningeal space around the optic nerve, full-thickness invasion of the sclera with invasion of the episclera, adipose tissues, extraocular muscle, bone, conjunctiva or eyelid |
| | T4b | Extraocular invasion with proptosis and/or orbital mass | | | |
| N1 | Regional lymph node metastasis | | pN1 | Regional lymph node involvement | |
| M1 | Distant metastasis | | pM1 | Distant metastasis | |
| | M1a | Single/multiple other than CNS/brain | | pM1a | Single/multiple other than CNS |
| | M1b | CNS including brain | | pM1b | CNS parenchyma or CSF fluid |

## Sarcoma of Orbit

There have been minor changes from the 7th edition [17, 24].

### Summary – *Sarcoma or Orbit*

| | |
|---|---|
| T1 | ≤20 mm |
| T2 | >20 mm without invasion of the globe or bony wall |
| T3 | Orbital tissues/bony walls |
| T4 | Globe or periorbital structures: eyelids, temporal fossa, nasal cavity/paranasal sinus(es) and/or central nervous system |
| N1 | Regional |

### Stage

No stages are at present recommended.

## Carcinoma of the Lacrimal Gland

There have been major changes from the 7th edition [24].

### Summary – *Lacrimal Gland Carcinoma*

| | | |
|---|---|---|
| T1 | ≤2 cm, with/without extraglandular extension into orbital soft tissues | |
| | T1a | No periosteal or bone involvement |
| | T1b | Periosteal involvement without bone involvement |
| | T1c | Bone involvement |
| T2 | >2–4 cm | |
| | T2a | No periosteal or bone involvement |
| | T2b | Periosteal involvement without bone involvement |
| | T2c | Bone involvement |
| T3 | >4 cm, extraglandular extension into orbital soft tissue: optic nerve or globe | |
| | T3a | No periosteal or bone involvement |
| | T3b | Periosteal involvement without bone involvement |
| | T3c | Bone involvement |
| T4 | Adjacent structures: sinus(es), temporal fossa, pterygoid fossa, superior orbital fissure, cavernous sinus and/or brain | |
| | T4a | <2 cm |
| | T4b | >2–4 cm |
| | T4c | >4 cm |
| N1 | Regional | |

### Stage

No stages are at present recommended.

# Hodgkin and Non-Hodgkin Lymphomas

A recent consensus conference took place in 2012 in Lugano and suggested an even more simplified system putting together Stages I and II as Limited Stage and Stages III and IV as Advanced Stage lymphoma. The Lugano classification [107], a modification of the Ann Arbor classification, has been published and adopted by the UICC.

### Summary – *Hodgkin and Non-Hodgkin Lymphoma*

| Stage | Hodgkin and Non-Hodgkin Lymphoma |
|---|---|

**Limited Stage**

| | |
|---|---|
| I | Single node region (I) |
| | Localized single extralymphatic organ/site (IE) |
| II | Two or more node regions, same side of diaphragm (II) |
| | Localized single extralymphatic organ/site with its regional lymph nodes, with/without involvement of other contiguous lymph node regions on same side of the diaphragm (IIE) |

**Bulky Stage II**

Stage II disease with a single nodal mass > 10 cm or > 1/3 of the thoracic diameter (CT)

| | |
|---|---|
| III | Lymph node regions both sides of diaphragm (III), +/- spleen involvement (IIIS) |
| IV | Disseminated (multifocal) one or more extralymphatic organs, with/without associated lymph node involvement or non-contiguous extralymphatic organ involvement of lymph node regions on the same or both sides of diaphragm |

**All stages divided into A and B,** absence or presence of defined general symptoms:

1. Unexpected weight loss of more than 10% of the usual body weight in the 6 months prior to the attendance
2. Unexplained fever with temperature above 38°
3. Night sweats

**Note.**
Pruritus alone does not qualify for B classification and nor does a short, febrile illness associated with a known infection.

## Non-Hodgkin Lymphomas

The Lugano classification, a modification of the Ann Arbor classification, is recommended as for Hodgkin lymphoma with the exception of the elimination of the A and B classifications of symptoms.

In Stage II disease, bulk is defined as larger than 6 cm in the greatest dimension in follicular lymphoma and 10 cm in the largest dimension has been recommended for diffuse large cell lymphoma.

## References

[1] O'Sullivan B, Yu E. Staging of nasopharyngeal carcinoma. In *Medical Radiology – Radiation Oncology*, Brady LW, Heilmann HP, Molls M, Nieder C (eds). Volume: Nasopharyngeal Cancer. Multidisciplinary Management, Ju JJ, Cooper JS, Lee AWM (eds). Berlin, Heidelberg: Springer; 2010, pp. 309–322.

[2] Som PM, Dillon WP, Sze G, et al. Benign and malignant sinonasal lesions with intracranial extension: differentiation with MRI imaging. *Radiology* 1989; 172:763–766.

[3] International Anatomical Nomenclature Committee (IANC) (ed.) *Nomina Anatomica*, 5th edn. Baltimore: Williams & Wilkins; 1983, pp. A38–A39.

[4] International Anatomical Nomenclature Committee (IANC) (ed.) *Nomina Anatomica*, 6th edn. Baltimore: Williams & Wilkins; 1989, pp. A43–A44.

[5] Tucker GF, Smith HR. A histological demonstration of the development of laryngeal connective compartments. *Trans Am Acad Ophthalmol Otolaryngol* 1962; 66:308–318.

[6] Tucker GF. Some clinical interferences from the study serial laryngeal sections. *Laryngoscope* 1963; 73:728–748.

[7] Reidenbach MM. The paraglottic space and transglottic cancer. Anatomical considerations. *Clin Anatomy* 1996; 9:244–251.

[8] Maroldi R, Ravanelli M, Farina D. Magnetic resonance for laryngeal cancer. *Curr Opin Otolaryngol Head Neck Surg* 2014; 22:131–139.

[9] Gregoire V, Ang K, Buchach W, et al. Delineation of the neck node levels for head and neck tumors: a 2013 update. DAHANCA, EORTC, HKNPCSG, NCIC CTG, NCRI, RTOG, TROG consensus guidelines. *Radiother Oncol* 2014; 110:172–181.

[10] American Joint Committee on Cancer (AJCC) *Cancer Staging Manual*, 8th edn, Amin MB, Edge SB, Greene FL, et al. (eds). New York: Springer; 2017.

[11] Dralle H, Damm I, Scheumann GFW, et al. Compartment-oriented microdissection of regional lymph nodes in medullary thyroid carcinoma. *Surgery Today* 1994; 24:112–121.

[12] UICC (Union for International Cancer Control) *TNM Classification of Malignant Tumours*, 8th edn, Brierley JD, Gospodarowicz MK, Wittekind C (eds). Oxford: Wiley Blackwell; 2017.

[13] Wreesmann VB, Katabi N, Palmer FL, et al. Influence of extracapsular nodal spread extent on prognosis of oral squamous cell carcinoma. *Head Neck* 2016; 38 Suppl 1:E1192–1199.

[14] UICC (Union for International Cancer Control) *TNM Classification of Malignant Tumours*, 4th edn, 2nd revision, Hermanek P, Sobin LH (eds). Berlin, Heidelberg, New York: Springer; 1992.

[15] UICC (Union for International Cancer Control) *TNM Classification of Malignant Tumours*, 5th edn, Sobin LH, Wittekind C (eds). New York: Wiley; 1997.

[16] UICC (Union for International Cancer Control) *TNM Classification of Malignant Tumours*, 6th edn, Sobin LH, Gospodarowicz MK, Wittekind C (eds). Oxford: Wiley-Blackwell; 2002.

[17] UICC (Union for International Cancer Control) *TNM Classification of Malignant Tumours*, 7th edn, Sobin LH, Gospodarowicz MK, Wittekind C (eds). Oxford: Wiley-Blackwell; 2009.

[18] UICC (Union for International Cancer Control) TNM Supplement. A Commentary on Uniform Use, Wittekind C, Henson DE, Hutter RVP, Sobin LH (eds). Berlin, Heidelberg, New York: Wiley; 2001.

[19] UICC (Union for International Cancer Control) *TNM Supplement 2001. A Commentary on Uniform Use*, 2nd edn, Wittekind C, Henson DE, Hutter RVP, Sobin LH (eds). New York: Wiley; 2001.

[20] UICC (Union for International Cancer Control) *TNM Supplement. A Commentary on Uniform Use*, 3rd edn, Wittekind C, Henson DE, Hutter RVP, Sobin LH (eds). New York; Wiley; 2003.

[21] UICC (Union for International Cancer Control) *TNM Supplement. A Commentary on Uniform Use*, 4th edn, Wittekind Ch, Compton CC, Brierley JD, Sobin LH (eds). Oxford: Wiley-Blackwell; 2012.

[22] Ebrahimi A, Gil Z, Amit M, et al. Primary tumor staging for oral cancer and a proposed modification incorporating depth of invasion: an international multicenter retrospective study. *JAMA Otolaryngol Head Neck Surg* 2014; 14:1138–1148.

[23] *AJCC Cancer Staging Manual*, 6th edn, Greene FL, Page D, Morrow M, et al. (eds). New York: Springer; 2002.

[24] *AJCC Cancer Staging Manual*, 7th edn, Edge SB, Byrd DR, Compton CC, et al. (eds). New York: Springer; 2009.

[25] Kleinsasser O. Revision of classification of laryngeal cancer, is it long overdue? (Proposals for an improved TN-classification) *J Laryngol Otol* 1992; 106:197–204.

[26] Perrier ND, Brierley JD, Tuttle RM. Differentiated and anaplastic thyroid carcinoma: major changes in the American Joint Committee on Cancer eighth edition cancer staging manual. *CA Cancer J Clin* 2018; 68:55–63.

[27] Hamilton SR, Aaltonen LA (eds). Pathology and Genetics of Tumours of the Digestive System. WHO Classification of Tumours. Lyon: IARC Press; 2000.

[28] Siewert JR Stein HJ. Classification of adenocarcinoma of the oesophagogastric junction. *Br J Surg* 1998; 85:1457–1459.

[29] Siewert JR. Adenocarcinoma of the esophagogastric junction. *Gastric Cancer* 1999; 2:87–88.

[30] Sano T, Coit D, Kim HH, for the IGCA Staging Project. Proposal of a new stage grouping of gastric cancer: International Gastric Cancer Association Staging Project. *Gastric Cancer* 2017; 20:217–225.

[31] Barbour AP, Jones M, Gonen M, et al. Refining esophageal cancer staging after neoadjuvant therapy: importance of treatment response. *Ann Surg Oncol* 2008; 15:2894–2902.

[32] Rice TW, Chen L-Q, Hofstetter WL, et al. Worldwide esophageal Cancer Collaboration: pathologic stage data. *Dis Esophagus* 2016; 29:724–733.

[33] Rice TW, Ishwaran H, Blackstone EH, et al. Recommendations for clinical staging (cTNM) of cancer of the esophagus and esophagogastric junction for the 8th edition AJCC/UICC staging manuals. *Dis Esophagus* 2016; 29:913–919.

[34] Rice TW, Ishwaran H, Hofstetter WL, et al. Recommendations for pathologic staging (pTNM) of cancer of the esophagus and esophagogastric junction for the 8th edition AJCC/UICC staging manuals. *Dis Esophagus* 2016; 29:897–905.

[35] Rice TW, Ishwaran H, Kelsen DP, et al. Recommendations for neoadjuvant stage grouping (pTNM) of cancer of the esophagus and esophagogastric junction for the 8th edition AJCC/UICC staging manuals. *Dis Esophagus* 2016; 29:906–912.

[36] Rice TW, Lerut TEMR, Orringer MB, et al. Worldwide esophageal Cancer Collaboration: neoadjuvant staging data. *Dis Esophagus* 2016; 29:715–723.

[37] Japanese Gastric Cancer Association (JGCA) Japanese Classification of gastric carcinoma: 3rd English Edition. *Gastric Cancer* 2011; 14:101–112.

[38] Sano T, Aiko T. New Japanese classification and treatment guidelines for gastric cancer: revision concepts and major revised points. *Gastric Cancer* 2011; 14:97–100.

[39] Japanese Research Society for Gastric Cancer. *Japanese Classification of Gastric Carcinoma*, 1st English edition, Nishi M, Omori Y, Miwa K (eds). Kanehara: Tokyo; 1995.

[40] Japanese Gastric Cancer Association (JGCA). *Japanese Classification of Gastric Carcinoma*, 2nd English edition. *Gastric Cancer* 1998; 1:10–24.

[41] Alakus H, Hölscher AH, Grass G, et al. Extracapsular lymph node spread: a new prognostic factor in gastric cancer. *Cancer* 2010; 116:309–315.

[42] Fukagawa T, Sasako M, Ito S, et al. The prognostic significance of isolated tumor cells in the lymph nodes of gastric cancer patients. *Gastric Cancer* 2010; 13:191–196.

[43] Jeuck TLA, Wittekind C. Gastric carcinoma: stage migration by immuno-histochemically detected lymph node micrometastases. *Gastric Cancer* 2015; 18:100–108.

[44] Ikoma N, Blum M, Estrella JS, et al. Evaluation of the American Joint Committee on Cancer 8th edition staging system for gastric cancer patients after preoperative therapy. *Gastric Cancer* 2018; 21:74–83.

[45] In H, Ravetch E, Langdon-Embry M, et al. The newly proposed clinical and post-neoadjuvant treatment staging classifications for gastric adeno-carcinoma for the American Joint Committee on Cancer (AJCC) staging. *Gastric Cancer* 2018; 21:1–9.

[46] Fielding LP, Arsenault PA, Chappuis PH, et al. Clinicopathological staging for colorectal cancer: An International Documentation System (IDS) and an International Comprehensive Anatomical Terminology (ICAT). *J Gastroenenterol Hepatol* 1991; 6:325–344.

[47] Soreide O, Norstein J, Fielding LP, et al. International standardization and documentation of the treatment of rectal cancer. In *Rectal Cancer Surgery*, Soreide O, Norstein J (eds). Berlin, Heidelberg, New York: Springer; 1997, pp. 405–455.

[48] *SEER Program: Code Manual*, Cunningham I, Ries L, Hankey B, et al. (eds), NIH Publication No. 92 – 1999. Bethesda: National Cancer Institute; 1992.

[49] Zeng Z, Cohen AM, Hajdu S, et al. Serosal cytology study to determine free mesothelial penetration by intraperitoneal colon cancer. *Cancer* 1992; 70:737–740.

[50] Vauthey JN, Lauwers GY, Esnaola NF, et al. Simplified staging of hepatocellular carcinoma. *J Clin Oncol* 2002; 20:1527–1536.

[51] Sindoh J, Aretxabala X, Aloia TA, et al. Tumor location is a strong predictor of tumor progression and survival in T2 gallbladder cancer: an international multicenter study. *Ann Surg* 2015; 261: 733–739.

[52] Hong SM, Pawlik TM, Cho H, et al. Depth of tumour invasion better predicts prognosis than the current American Joint Committee on Cancer T classification for distal bile duct carcinoma. *Surgery* 2009; 146:250–257.

[53] Saka B, Balci S, Basturk O, et al. Pancreatic ductal adenocarcinoma is spread to the peripancreatic soft tissue in the majority of resected cases, rendering the AJCC T-Stage Protocol (7th edition) inapplicable and insignificant: a size-based staging system (pT1: ≤2, pT2: >2–≤4, pT3: >4 cm) is more valid and clinically relevant. *Ann Surg Oncol* 2016; 23:2010–2018.

[54] Lloyd RV, Osamura RY, Klöppel G, Rosai J. *WHO Classification of Tumours of Endocrine Organs*. Lyon: IARC Press; 2017.

[55] Bosman FT, Carneiro F, Hruban RH, Theise ND (eds) *WHO Classification of Tumours of the Digestive System*, 4 edn, Lyon: IARC Press; 2010.

[56] Travis WD, Brambilla E, Burke AP, et al. *WHO Classification of Tumours of the Lung, Pleura, Thymus and Heart*. Lyon: IARC Press; 2015.

[57] Rami-Porta R, Bolejack V, Giroux DJ, et al. The IASLC Lung Cancer Staging Project: the new database to inform the 8th edition of the TNM classification of lung cancer. *J Thorac Oncol* 2014; 9:1618–1624.

[58] Rami-Porta R, Bolejack V, Crowley, J, et al. The IASLC Lung Cancer Staging Project: proposals for the revisions of the T descriptors in the forthcoming 8th edition of the TNM classification for lung cancer. *J Thorac Oncol* 2015; 10:990–1003.

[59] Asamura H, Chansky K, Crowley J, et al. The IASLC Lung Cancer Staging Project: proposals for the revisions of the N descriptors in the forthcoming 8th edition of the TNM classification for lung cancer. *J Thorac Oncol* 2015; 10:1675–1684.

[60] Eberhardt WEE, Mitchell A, Crowley, J, et al. The IASLC Lung Cancer Staging Project: proposals for the revisions of the M descriptors in the forthcoming 8th edition of the TNM classification for lung cancer. *J Thorac Oncol* 2015; 10:1515–1522.

[61] Goldstraw P, et al. The IASLC Lung Cancer Staging Project: proposals for the revision of the stage grouping in the forthcoming 8th edition of the TNM classification of lung cancer. *J Thorac Oncol* 2016; 11:39–51.

[62] Nicholson AG, Chansky K, Crowley J, et al. The IASLC Lung Cancer Staging Project: proposals for the revision of the clinical and pathologic staging of small cell lung cancer in the forthcoming 8th edition of the TNM classification for lung cancer. *J Thorac Oncol* 2016; 11:300–311.

[63] Travis WD, Asamura H, Bankier H, et al. The IASLC Lung Cancer Staging Project: proposals for coding T categories for subsolid nodules and assessment of tumour size in part-solid tumours in the forthcoming 8th edition of the TNM classification of lung cancer. *J Thorac Oncol* 2016; 11:1204–1223.

[64] Detterbeck FC, Franklin WA, Nicholson AG, et al. The IASLC Lung Cancer Staging Project: proposed criteria to distinguish separate primary lung cancers from metastatic foci in patients with two lung tumours in the forthcoming 8th edition of the TNM classification of lung cancer. *J Thorac Oncol* 2016; 11:651–665.

[65] Detterbeck FC, Bolejak V, Arenberg DA, et al. The IASLC Lung Cancer Staging Project: proposals for the classification of lung cancer with separate tumour nodules in the forthcoming 8th edition of the TNM classification of lung cancer. *J Thorac Oncol* 2016; 11:681–692.

[66] Detterbeck FC, Marom EM, Arenberrg DA, et al. The IASLC Lung Cancer Staging Project: proposals for the application of TNM staging rules to lung cancer presenting as multiple nodules with ground glass or lepidic features or a pneumonic-type of involvement in the forthcoming 8th edition of the TNM classification of lung cancer. *J Thorac Oncol* 2016; 11:666–680.

[67] Detterbeck FC, Nicholson AG, Franklin WA, et al. The IASLC Lung Cancer Staging Project: proposals for the revisions of the classifications of lung cancers with

multiple pulmonary sites of involvement in the forthcoming 8th edition of the TNM classification of lung cancer. *J Thorac Oncol* 2016; 11:651–666.

[68] Detterbeck FC, Franklin WA, Nicholson AG, et al. The IASLC Lung Cancer Staging Project: proposed criteria to distinguish separate primary lung cancers from metastatic foci in patients with two lung tumours in the forthcoming 8th edition of the TNM classification of lung cancer. *J Thorac Oncol* 2016; 11:639–650.

[69] Detterbeck FC, Groome P, Bolejack V, et al. The IASLC Lung Cancer Staging Project: methodology and validation used in the development of proposals for revision in the stage classification of non-small cell lung cancer in the forthcoming 8th edition of the TNM classification of lung cancer. *J Thorac Oncol* 2016; 11:1433–1466.

[70] Travis WD, Brambilla E, Rami-Porta R, et al. Visceral pleural invasion: pathologic criteria and use of elastic stains: proposals for the 7th edition of the TNM classification for lung cancer. *J Thorac Oncol* 2008; 3:1384–1390.

[71] Rami-Porta R (Executive ed.) *Staging Manual in Thoracic Oncology*, 2nd edn. Fort Myers: IASLC Publication; 2016.

[72] Travis WD, Brambilla E, Nicholson AG, et al. The 2015 World Health Organization Classification of Lung Tumours: Impact of genetic, clinical and radiological advances since the 2004 classification. *J Thorac Oncol* 2015; 10:1243–1260.

[73] Travis WD, Giroux DJ, Chansky K, et al. The IASLC Lung Cancer Staging Project: bronchopulmonary carcinoid tumours in the forthcoming (seventh) edition of the TNM Classification of Lung Cancer. *J Thorac Oncol* 2008; 3:1213–1223.

[74] The Japan Lung Cancer Society *Classification of Lung Cancer: First English Edition*, 1st edn. Chiba: Kanehara and Co; 2000.

[75] Hammar SP. Common tumours. In *Pulmonary Pathology*, 2nd edn, Dail DH, Hammar SP (eds). New York: Springer; 1994, pp. 11–38.

[76] Lim E, Clough R, Goldstraw P, et al. Impact of positive pleural lavage cytology on survival of patients having lung resection for non-small cell lung cancer: an international individual patient data metaanalysis. *J Thorac Cardiovac Surg* 2010; 139:1441–1446.

[77] Gagliasso M, Migliaretti G, Ardissone F. Assessing the prognostic impact of the International Association for the Study of Lung Cancer proposed definitions of complete, uncertain, and incomplete resection in non-small cell lung cancer surgery. *Lung Cancer* 2017; 111:124–130.

[78] Rusch VW, Venkatraman E. The importance of surgical staging in the treatment of malignant pleural mesothelioma. *J Thorac Surg* 1996; 111: 815–825.

[79] Rusch VW. A proposed new international TNM staging system for malignant pleural mesothelioma from the International Mesothelioma Interest Group. *Lung Cancer* 1996; 14:1–12.

[80] Nicholson AG, Detterbeck FC, Marino M, et al. The IASLC/ITMIG Thymic Epithelial Tumors Staging Project: proposals for the T component for the forthcoming (8th) edition of the TNM classification of malignant tumors. *J Thorac Oncol* 2014; 9:73–80.

[81] Kondo K, Van Schil P, Detterbeck FC, et al. The IASLC/ITMIG Thymic Epithelial Tumors Staging Project: proposals for the N and M components for the forthcoming (8th) edition of the TNM classification of malignant tumors. *J Thorac Oncol* 2014; 9:81–87.

[82] Detterbeck FC, Stratton K, Giroux D, et al. The IASLC/ITMIG Thymic Epithelial Tumors Staging Project: proposal for an evidence-based stage classification system for the forthcoming (8th) edition of the TNM classification of malignant tumors. *J Thorac Oncol* 2014; 9:65–72.

[83] Marchevsky AM, McKenna Jr RJ, Gupta R. Thymic epithelial neoplasms: a review of current concepts using an evidence-based pathology approach. *Oncol Clin North Am* 2008; 22:543–562.

[84] *WHO Classification of Tumours of Bone and of Tissues*, Fletcher CDM, Bridge J, Hogendoorn PCW, Mertens F (eds). Lyon: IARC Press; 2013.

[85] LeBoit PE, Burg G, Weedon D, Sarasin A. *The World Health Organization Classification of Tumours. Pathology and Genetics. Skin Tumours.* Lyon: IARC Press; 2006.

[86] Weiss A, Chavez-MacGregor M, Lichtensztajn DY, et al. Validation Study of the American Joint Committee on Cancer Eighth Edition Prognostic Stage Compared with the Anatomic Stage in Breast Cancer. *JAMA Oncol* 2018; 4:203–209.

[87] FIGO Annual Report on the Results of Treatment in Gynecological Cancer. 24th vol. Pecorelli S, Beller U, Heintz APM, Benedet JL, Creasman WT, Pettersson F, eds. *J Epidemiol Biostatist* 2001; 6:1–184.

[88] FIGO Committee on Gynecologic Cancer. Revised FIGO staging for carcinoma of the vulva, cervix, and endometrium. *Int J Gynecol Obstet* 2009; 105:103–106.

[89] Zaino RJ. Glandular lesions of the uterine cervix. *Mod Pathol* 2000; 13:261–274.

[90] Boronow RC, Morrow CP, Creasman WT, et al. Surgical staging in endometrial cancer: clinical pathological findings of a prospective study. *Obstet Gynecol* 1984; 63:825–832.

[91] Creasman WT, Odicino F, Maisonneuve P, et al. Carcinoma of the corpus uteri. FIGO 26th Annual Report on the results of treatment in gynecologic cancer. *Int J Gynecol Obstet* 2006; 95; Suppl 1:105–143.

[92] Hall JB, Young RH, Nelson Jh. The prognostic significance of adenomyosis in endometrial carcinoma. *Gynecol Oncol* 1984; 17:32–40.

[93] Maassen V, Kindermann G, Lampe B. Zur kontinuierlichen und diskontinuierlichen Ausbreitung des Endometriumkarzinoms. *Verh Dt Gesell Pathol* 1991; 75:383.

[94] Tavassoli FA, Devilee P (eds) *WHO Classification of Tumours. Pathology and Genetics. Tumours of the Breast and Female Genital Organs.* Lyon: IARC Press; 2003.

[95] Prat J. FIGO staging for uterine sarcomas. *Int J Gynaecol Obstet* 2009; 104:177–178.

[96] FIGO Committee on Gyn Onc Report. FIGO staging for uterine sarcoma. *Int J Gynaecol Obstet* 2009; 104:179.

[97] Prat J. FIGO Committee on Gynecologic Oncology. Staging classification for cancer of the ovary, fallopian tube, and peritoneum. *Int J Gynaecol Obstet* 2014; 124:1–5.

[98] Ngan HYS, Bender H, Benedet JL, et al. Committee on Gynecologic Oncology Gestational trophoblastic neoplasia. *Int J Gynecol Obstet* 2002; 77:285–287.

[99] Wittekind Ch, Bootz F, Meyer HJ. *UICC TNM-Klassifikation maligner Tumoren*, 6 Auflage. Berlin, Heidelberg: Springer; 2002.

[100] Gandaglia G, Karakiewicz PI, Briganti A, et al. Impact of the site of metastases on survival in patients with metastatic prostate cancer. *Eur Urol* 2015; 68:325–334.

[101] Epstein JL, Egevad L, Amin MB, et al. The 2014 International Society of Urological Pathology (ISUP) Consensus Conference on Gleason Grading of Prostatic Carcinoma: definition of grading patterns and proposal for new grading system. *Am J Surg Pathol* 2016; 40:244–252.

[102] Humphrey PA, Egevad L, Netto GJ, et al. Tumours of the prostate. In *WHO Classification of Tumours of the Urinary System and Male Genital Organs*, Moch

H, Humphrey PA, Ulbright TM, Reuter VE (eds). Lyon: IARC Press; 2015, pp. 135–183.

[103] Guinan P, Sobin LH, Algaba F, et al. TNM Staging of Renal Cell Carcinoma. Report of Workgroup 3. *Cancer* 1997; 80:992–993.

[104] Grignon DJ, Lloreta J, Al-Ahmadie H, et al. Urothelial tumours. Infiltration urothelial carcinoma. In *WHO Classification of Tumours of the Urinary System and Male Genital Organs*, Moch H, Humphrey PA, Ulbright TM, Reuter VE (eds). Lyon: IARC Press; 2015, pp. 81–98.

[105] UICC (International Union for Cancer Control) *TNM Supplement. A Commentary on Uniform Use*, 3rd edn. Wittekind Ch, Henson DE, Hutter RVP, Sobin LH, eds. New York: Wiley; 2003.

[106] Clayton M, Siami F, Guinan P. Urethral diverticular carcinoma. *Cancer* 1992; 70:665–670.

[107] Cheson BD, Fisher BJ, Barrington SF, et al. Recommendations for initial evaluation, staging and response assessment of Hodgkin and non-Hodgkin lymphoma: the Lugano classification. *J Clin Oncol* 2014;32:3059–3068.

CHAPTER 3

# SITE-SPECIFIC REQUIREMENTS FOR pT AND pN

## Introduction

This chapter is an expansion to the following general rules of the TNM system (*TNM Classification*, 8th edition [1, 2], pp. 3–5):

---

2b) Pathological assessment of the primary tumour (pT) entails a resection of the primary tumour or biopsy adequate to evaluate the highest pT category.

   The pathological assessment of the regional lymph nodes (pN) entails removal of nodes adequate to validate the absence of regional lymph node metastasis (pN0).

   An excisional biopsy of a lymph node without pathological assessment of the primary tumour is insufficient to evaluate the pN category and is a clinical classification.

   If fine needle aspiration (FNA) or core biopsy is performed in the absence of complete dissection of the nodal basin the N category should have the f suffix, e.g. pN0(f).

   The pathological assessment of distant metastasis (pM1) entails microscopic examination.

3) After assigning T, N and M and/or pT, pN and pM categories, these may be grouped into stages. The TNM classification and stages, once established, must remain unchanged in the medical records.

   Clinical and pathological data may be combined when only partial information is available either in the pathological classification or the clinical classification.

4) If there is doubt concerning the correct T, N or M category to which a particular case should be allotted, then the lower (i.e. less advanced) category should be chosen.

---

*TNM Supplement: A Commentary on Uniform Use*, Fifth Edition.

Edited by Christian Wittekind, James D. Brierley, Anne Lee and Elisabeth van Eycken.

© 2019 UICC. Published 2019 by John Wiley & Sons Ltd.

**Table 3.1** Minimal number of lymph nodes usually examined in lymph node dissection specimens to classify pN0 [1]

| Site | Number | |
|---|---|---|
| Oral cavity | | |
| Pharynx | | |
| Larynx | 10 | Selective neck dissection |
| Nasal cavity/paranasal sinuses | 15 | Radical or modified radical neck dissection |
| Major salivary glands | | |
| Unknown primary – cervical nodes | 10 | Selective neck dissection |
| | 15 | Radical or modified radical neck dissection |
| Melanoma – upper aerodigestive tract | 10 | Selective neck dissection |
| Thyroid gland | 6 | |
| Oesophagus including oesophagogastric junction | 7 | |
| Stomach | 16 | |
| Small intestine | 6 | |
| Appendix carcinoma | 12 | |
| Colon and rectum | 12 | |
| Anal canal | 12 | Perirectal–pelvic lymphadenectomy |
| | 6 | Inguinal lymphadenectomy |
| Liver – HCC | 3 | |
| Liver – ICC | 6 | |
| Gallbladder | 6 | |
| Extrahepatic bile ducts, perihilar | 15 | |
| Extrahepatic bile ducts, distal | 12 | |
| Ampulla of Vater | 12 | |
| Pancreas | 12 | |
| Neuroendocrine tumours of the GI tract | No recommendation | |
| Lung | 6 | |
| Pleural mesothelioma | No recommendation | |
| Thymic tumours | No recommendation | |
| Carcinoma of skin | 6 | |
| Malignant melanoma of skin | 6 | |

| | | |
|---|---|---|
| Merkel cell carcinoma of skin | 6 | |
| Breast | 6 | |
| Vulva | 6 | |
| Vagina | 6 | Pelvic lymphadenectomy |
| | 6 | Inguinal lymphadenectomy |
| Cervix uteri | 6 | |
| Corpus uteri – endometrium | 6 | |
| Ovary | 6 | |
| Fallopian tube | 6 | |
| Ophthalmic tumours | 6 | |

**Note.**
With regards to the lung, histopathological examination of hilar and mediastinal lymphadenectomy specimen(s) will ordinarily include 6 or more lymph nodes/stations. Three of these lymph nodes/stations should be mediastinal, including the subcarinal lymph node (No. 7) and three from N1 lymph nodes/stations.

Adequate N staging is generally considered to include sampling or dissection of lymph nodes from stations 2R, 4R, 7, 10R and 11R for right-sided tumours and stations 5, 6, 7, 10L and 11L for left-sided tumours. Station 9 lymph nodes should also be evaluated for lower lobe tumours. The more peripheral stations 12–14 are usually evaluated by the pathologist in lobectomy or pneumonectomy specimen but may be separately removed when sublobar resections (e.g. segmentectomy) are performed.

The numbers of lymph nodes given in the different tumour sites are considered adequate for staging.

If the examined lymph nodes are negative, and the number ordinarily resected is not met, classify as pN0.

The number of lymph nodes examined and the number involved by tumour should be recorded in the pathology report [3–10].

This information may also be added in parentheses, e.g. for colorectal carcinoma pN0(0/11) or pN1b(3/16).

In many tumour sites, the number of involved regional lymph nodes indicates differences in prognosis. For details see TNM Supplement, 1st edition [11].

A correlation exists between the number of examined lymph nodes and the pN classification. With an increasing number of examined lymph nodes a higher frequency of lymph node-positive cases is found and – in tumour sites where more than one positive pN category is provided – a greater proportion of higher pN categories can be observed [12–16]. Therefore, the number of examined lymph nodes reflects the reliability of the pN classification.

### Importance of removed and examined lymph nodes

The importance of the number of nodes resected and examined has been described in many malignancies including cancers of the head and neck, thyroid, oesophagus, colon and rectum, pancreas, lung, breast and bladder. Given that the number of nodes examined is dependent on both the extent of surgery and the extent of the pathological examination to overcome any confounding effect, many researchers have investigated the prognostic significance of the lymph node ratio – the number of nodes involved/number of lymph nodes resected (LNR). In a review of the literature performed by the UICC TNM Literature Watch (unpublished data) in numerous tumour sites, the LNR was been found to be a significant prognostic factor. However, even among the same tumour sites different authors reported different LNR at which the prognosis changes. At the present time the UICC TNM Prognostic Factors Committee does not endorse the use of LNR in determining stage but recommends reporting both the number of nodes involved and the number resected independently.

## Head and Neck Tumours

## pT – Primary Tumour

| Site | Requirements |
|---|---|
| All sites (except anaplastic thyroid carcinoma) | pT3 or less<br>Pathological examination of the primary carcinoma with no gross tumour at the margins of resection (with or without microscopic involvement) |
| Oral cavity | pT4a<br>Microscopic confirmation of invasion through cortical bone into maxilla or mandible, maxillary sinus or skin of face |
| Oral cavity | pT4b<br>Microscopic confirmation of invasion of the masticator space, pterygoid plates, or skull base or encases the internal carotid artery |
| Oropharynx (p16-negative or without p16-immunohisto-chemistry) | pT4a<br>Microscopic confirmation of invasion of any of the following: larynx (see note below), deep/extrinsic muscle of the tongue (M. genioglossus, M. hyoglossus, M. palatoglossus, M. styloglossus), medial pterygoid, hard palate, mandible |

**Note.**
Mucosal extension to the lingual surface of the epiglottis from primary tumours of the base of the tongue and vallecula does not constitute invasion of the larynx.

pT4b
Microscopic confirmation of invasion of any of the following: lateral pterygoid muscle, pterygoid plates, lateral nasopharynx, skull base or encases the carotid artery

Oropharynx
(p16-positive)

pT4
Microscopic confirmation of invasion of any of the following: larynx (see note below), deep/extrinsic muscle of the tongue (M. genioglossus, M. hyoglossus, M. palatoglossus, M. styloglossus), medial pterygoid, hard palate, mandible, lateral pterygoid muscle, pterygoid plate, lateral nasopharynx skull base or encases the carotid artery

**Note.**
Mucosal extension to the lingual surface of epiglottis from primary tumours of the base of the tongue and vallecula does not constitute invasion of the larynx.

Hypopharynx

pT4a
Microscopic confirmation of invasion of any of the following: thyroid/ cricoid cartilage, hyoid bone, thyroid gland, oesophagus, central compartment of soft tissue

pT4b
Microscopic confirmation of invasion of prevertebral fascia, invasion of mediastinal structures or encasement of carotid artery

Nasopharynx

pT4
Microscopic confirmation of intracranial extension and/or involvement of cranial nerves, hypopharynx, orbit, parotid gland and/or infiltration beyond the lateral surface of the lateral pterygoid muscle

**Larynx**
Supraglottis

pT4a
Microscopic confirmation of invasion through the thyroid cartilage and/or invasion of tissues beyond the larynx, e.g. trachea, soft tissues of the neck including deep/extrinsic muscle of the tongue (M. genioglossus, M. hyoglossus, M. palatoglossus, M. styloglossus), strap muscles, thyroid, oesophagus

|  | pT4b<br>Microscopic confirmation of invasion of prevertebral space or encases carotid artery, mediastinal structures |
|---|---|
| Glottis | pT4a<br>Microscopic confirmation of invasion through the outer cortex of the thyroid cartilage and/or invasion of tissues beyond the larynx, e.g. trachea, soft tissues of the neck including deep/extrinsic muscle of the tongue (M. genioglossus, M. hyoglossus, M. palatoglossus, M. styloglossus), strap muscles, thyroid, oesophagus |
|  | pT4b<br>Microscopic confirmation of invasion of pre-vertebral space or encases the carotid artery, mediastinal structures |
| Subglottis | pT4a<br>Microscopic confirmation of invasion of cricoid or thyroid cartilage and/or invasion of tissues beyond the larynx, e.g. trachea, soft tissues of neck including deep/extrinsic muscle of tongue (M. genioglossus, M. hyoglossus, M. palato-glossus, M. styloglossus) strap muscles, thyroid, oesophagus |
|  | pT4b<br>Microscopic confirmation of invasion of prevertebral space or encases the carotid artery, mediastinal structures |
| Maxillary sinus | pT4a<br>Microscopic confirmation of invasion of any of the following: anterior orbital contents, skin of cheek, pterygoid plates, infratemporal fossa, cribriform plate, sphenoid or frontal sinuses |
|  | pT4b<br>Microscopic confirmation of invasion of any of the following: orbital apex, dura, brain, middle cranial fossa, cranial nerves other than V2, nasopharynx, clivus |
| Nasal cavity and ethmoid sinus | pT4a<br>Microscopic confirmation of invasion of any of the following: anterior orbital contents, skin of nose or |

|                                      | cheek, minimal extension to anterior cranial fossa, pterygoid plates, sphenoid or frontal sinuses |
|--------------------------------------|---|
|                                      | pT4b<br>Microscopic confirmation of invasion of any of the following: orbital apex, dura, brain, middle cranial fossa, cranial nerves other than V2, nasopharynx or clivus |
| Malignant melanoma of upper aerodigestive tract | pT4a<br>Microscopic confirmation of invasion of deep soft tissue, cartilage, bone, overlying skin |
|                                      | pT4b<br>Microscopic confirmation of invasion of any of the following: brain, dura, skull base, lower cranial nerves (IX, X, XI, XII), masticator space, carotid artery, prevertebral space, mediastinal structures |
| Major salivary glands                | pT4a<br>Microscopic confirmation of invasion of skin, mandible, ear canal and/or facial nerve |
|                                      | pT4b<br>Microscopic confirmation of invasion of the base of the skull, and/or pterygoid plates, and/or encases the carotid artery |
| Thyroid gland (except anaplastic carcinoma) | pT4a<br>Microscopic confirmation of invasion beyond thyroid capsule and invasion of any of the following: subcutaneous soft tissues, larynx, trachea, oesophagus, recurrent laryngeal nerve |
|                                      | pT4b<br>Microscopic confirmation of invasion of prevertebral fascia, mediastinal vessels, encases carotid artery |

## pN – Regional Lymph Nodes

The pathological assessment of the regional lymph nodes (pN) entails removal of the lymph nodes adequate to validate the absence of regional lymph node metastasis (pN0) or sufficient to evaluate the highest pN category.

An excisional biopsy of a lymph node without pathological assessment of the primary is insufficient to fully evaluate the pN category and is a clinical classification.

The site-specific recommendations regarding the number of lymph nodes for diagnosis of pN0 for all sites of head and neck tumours have been incorporated in the 5th to 7th editions [17–20] and have been modified in the 8th edition [1].

When size is a criterion for pN classification, measurement is made of the metastasis, not of the entire lymph node.

| Site | Requirements |
|---|---|
| All sites except thyroid gland, nasopharynx, and upper aerodigestive tract malignant melanoma | pN1<br>Microscopic confirmation of a metastasis in a single ipsilateral lymph node, 3 cm or less in greatest dimension without extranodal extension<br><br>pN2a<br>Microscopic confirmation of metastasis in a single ipsilateral lymph node 3 cm or less with extranodal extension or more than 3 cm but not more than 6 cm in greatest dimension without extranodal extension<br><br>pN2b<br>Microscopic confirmation of a metastasis in multiple ipsilateral lymph nodes, none more than 6 cm in the greatest dimension without extranodal extension<br><br>pN2c<br>Microscopic confirmation of metastasis in bilateral or contralateral lymph nodes, none more than 6 cm in the greatest dimension without extranodal extension<br><br>pN3a<br>Microscopic confirmation of a lymph node metastasis more than 6 cm in the greatest dimension without extranodal extension |

pN3b
Microscopic confirmation of a regional lymph node metastasis more than 3 cm in the greatest dimension with extranodal extension or multiple ipsilateral, or any contralateral or bilateral lymph node(s) with extranodal extension

| | |
|---|---|
| Nasopharynx | pN1<br>Microscopic confirmation of metastasis in unilateral cervical lymph node(s) and/or metastasis in unilateral or bilateral retropharyngeal lymph nodes, 6 cm or less in the greatest dimension, above the caudal border of cricoid cartilage |
| | pN2<br>Microscopic confirmation of metastasis in bilateral cervical lymph nodes, 6 cm or less in the greatest dimension, above the caudal border of cricoid cartilage |
| | pN3<br>Microscopic confirmation of metastasis in lymph node(s) greater than 6 cm in dimension and/or extension below the caudal border of the cricoid cartilage |
| Melanoma upper aerodigestive tract | pN1<br>Microscopic confirmation of regional lymph node metastasis |
| Thyroid gland | pN1a<br>Microscopic confirmation of lymph node metastasis in pretracheal, paratracheal, prelaryngeal/Delphian lymph nodes or upper/superior mediastinal lymph nodes |
| | pN1b<br>Microscopic confirmation of lymph node metastasis in other unilateral, bilateral or contralateral cervical or retropharyngeal |

## Digestive System Tumours

## pT – Primary Tumour

| Site | Requirements |
| --- | --- |

### pT – Primary Tumour

Oesophagus, oesophagogastric junction, stomach, small intestine, appendix carcinoma, colon and rectum, anal canal

|  | pT3 or less<br>Pathological examination of the surgically removed primary tumour with no gross tumour at the circumferential (deep, radial, lateral), proximal and distal margins of resection (with or without microscopic involvement) or pathologically examination of endoscopically removed primary tumours with histologically tumour-free resection margins |
| --- | --- |
| Oesophagus and oesophagogastric junction | pT4a<br>Microscopic confirmation of invasion of pleura, pericardium, azygos vein, diaphragm, peritoneum |
|  | pT4b<br>Microscopic confirmation of invasion of other adjacent structures such as: aorta, vertebral body, trachea |
| Stomach | pT4a<br>Pathological confirmation of perforation of the serosa |
|  | pT4b<br>Microscopic confirmation or invasion of adjacent structures: spleen, transverse colon, liver, diaphragm, pancreas, abdominal wall, adrenal gland, kidney, small intestine, retroperitoneum |
| Small intestine | pT4<br>Microscopic confirmation of perforation of the visceral peritoneum or microscopic confirmation of invasion of other organs or structures (including other loops of small intestine, mesentery or retroperitoneum and abdominal wall by way of serosa)<br>(For duodenum only: invasion of pancreas) |

| Appendix carcinoma | pT4a<br>Microscopic confirmation of perforation of the visceral peritoneum, including mucinous peritoneal tumour or acellular mucin on the serosa of the appendix or mesoappendix |
|---|---|
| | pT4b<br>Microscopic confirmation of direct invasion of other organs/structures |
| Colon and rectum | pT4a<br>Microscopic confirmation of perforation of the visceral peritoneum |

**Note.**

This may be achieved from biopsies or resection specimens or by cytology of specimens obtained from the serosa overlying the primary tumour [21].

pT4b
Microscopic confirmation of direct invasion of other organs/structures including microscopic confirmation of invasion of other segments of the colorectum by way of the serosa or for tumours in a retroperitoneal or subperitoneal location, microscopic confirmation of direct invasion of other organs and structures by virtue of extension beyond the muscularis propria

| Anal canal and anal skin | pT4<br>Microscopic confirmation of invasion of adjacent organs, e.g. vagina, urethra, bladder |
|---|---|

Liver – HCC, liver – ICC, gallbladder, extrahepatic bile ducts (perihilar, distal), ampulla of Vater, pancreas

pT2 or less
Pathological examination of the surgically removed primary tumour with no gross tumour at the margins of resection (with or without microscopic involvement)
or for the ampulla of Vater
Pathological examination of the endoscopically removed primary tumour with histologically tumour-free margins of resection

| | |
|---|---|
| Liver<br>HCC | pT3<br>Microscopic confirmation of multiple tumours (any macroscopically > 5 cm)<br><br>pT4<br>Microscopic confirmation of invasion of a major branch of the portal or hepatic vein or microscopic invasion of direct invasion of adjacent organ(s) (including the diaphragm) other than the gallbladder or microscopic confirmation of tumour(s) with perforation of the visceral peritoneum |
| Liver<br>ICC | pT3<br>Microscopic confirmation of tumour(s) with perforation of the visceral peritoneum<br><br>pT4<br>Microscopic confirmation of invasion of local extrahepatic structures |
| Gallbladder | pT3<br>Microscopic confirmation of perforation of the serosa (visceral peritoneum) and/or direct invasion of the liver and/ or invasion of at least one adjacent organ or structure (stomach, duodenum, colon, pancreas, omentum, extrahepatic bile ducts)<br><br>pT4<br>Microscopic confirmation of invasion of main portal vein or hepatic artery, or invasion of two or more extrahepatic organs or structures |
| Extrahepatic bile ducts, perihilar | pT3<br>Microscopic confirmation of invasion of unilateral branches of the portal vein or proper hepatic artery<br><br>pT4<br>Microscopic confirmation of invasion of the main portal vein or its branches bilaterally or the common hepatic artery or the second-order biliary radicals bilaterally or unilateral second-order biliary radicals with contralateral portal vein or hepatic artery involvement |
| Extrahepatic bile ducts, distal | pT3<br>Microscopic confirmation of invasion of bile duct wall >12 mm |

|  | pT4<br>Microscopic confirmation of invasion of the coeliac axis, the superior mesenteric artery or the common hepatic artery |
|---|---|
| Ampulla of Vater | pT3<br>Microscopic confirmation of invasion into the pancreas or peripancreatic tissue |
|  | pT3a<br>Microscopic confirmation of invasion into the pancreas ≤0.5 cm |
|  | pT3b<br>Microscopic confirmation of invasion into the pancreas >0.5 cm or microscopic confirmation of invasion into peripancreatic tissue or duodenal serosa (without involvement of coeliac axis/mesenteric artery/common hepatic artery) |
|  | pT4<br>Microscopic confirmation of involvement of coeliac axis/ mesenteric artery/common hepatic artery |
| Pancreas | pT3<br>Microscopic confirmation of tumour >4 cm in greatest dimension |
|  | pT4<br>Microscopic confirmation of invasion of coeliac axis or superior mesenteric artery/common hepatic artery |

## Well-Differentiated Neuroendocrine Tumours of the Gastrointestinal Tract

| Site | Requirements |
|---|---|

**pT – Primary Tumour**

Gastric, duodenum/ampullary, jejunum/[leum, appendix, colon/rectum, pancreas

|  | pT3 or less<br>Pathological examination of the surgically removed primary tumour with no gross tumour at the circumferential (deep, radial, lateral), proximal and distal margins of resection (with or without microscopic involvement) or pathologically examination of endoscopically removed primary tumours with histologically tumour-free resection margins |
|---|---|

| Stomach | pT4<br>Microscopic confirmation of perforation of the visceral peritoneum (serosa) or invasion of other organs/adjacent structures |
|---|---|
| Duodenal/<br>ampullary<br>tumours | pT4<br>Microscopic confirmation of perforation of the visceral peritoneum (serosa) or microscopic confirmation of invasion of other organs |
| Jejunum/ileum | pT4<br>Microscopic confirmation of perforation of the visceral peritoneum (serosa) or microscopic confirmation invasion of other organs/adjacent structures |
| Appendix | pT4<br>Microscopic confirmation of perforation of the peritoneum or microscopic confirmation invasion of other organs/adjacent structures (other than direct mural extension to adjacent subserosa, e.g. abdominal wall and skeletal muscle) |
| Colon and rectum | pT4<br>Microscopic confirmation of perforation of the visceral peritoneum or microscopic confirmation invasion of other organs |
| Pancreas | pT4<br>Microscopic confirmation of invasion of other organs (stomach, spleen, colon, adrenal gland) or microscopic confirmation of invasion of the wall of large vessels (coeliac axis or the superior mesenteric artery) |

## pN – Regional Lymph Nodes

| Site | Requirements |
|---|---|
| Oesophagus including oesophago-gastric junction | pN1<br>Microscopic confirmation of metastasis in 1 or 2 regional lymph node(s)<br><br>pN2<br>Microscopic confirmation of metastasis in 3 to 6 regional lymph nodes |

pN3
Microscopic confirmation of metastasis in 7 or more regional lymph nodes

Stomach

pN1
Microscopic confirmation of metastasis in 1 or 2 regional lymph node(s)

pN2
Microscopic confirmation of metastasis in 3 to 6 regional lymph nodes

pN3a
Microscopic confirmation of metastasis in 7 to 15 regional lymph nodes

pN3b
Microscopic confirmation of metastasis in 16 or more regional lymph nodes

Small intestine

pN1
Microscopic confirmation of metastasis in 1 to 2 regional lymph node(s)

pN2
Microscopic confirmation of metastasis in 3 or more regional lymph nodes

Appendix carcinoma

pN1
Microscopic confirmation of metastasis in 1 to 3 regional lymph node(s)

pN1a
Microscopic confirmation of metastasis in 1 regional lymph node

pN1b
Microscopic confirmation of metastasis in 2–3 regional lymph nodes

pN1c
Microscopic confirmation of tumour deposit(s) in subserosa or in non-peritonealized pericolic tissue without regional lymph node metastasis

pN2
Microscopic confirmation of metastasis in 4 or more regional lymph nodes

| | |
|---|---|
| Colon and rectum | **pN1a**<br>Microscopic confirmation of metastasis in 1 regional lymph node |
| | **pN1b**<br>Microscopic confirmation of metastasis in 2–3 regional lymph nodes |
| | **pN1c**<br>Microscopic confirmation of tumour deposit(s) in subserosa or non-peritonealized pericolic or perirectal tissue without regional lymph node metastasis |
| | **pN2a**<br>Microscopic confirmation of metastasis in 4–6 regional lymph nodes |
| | **pN2b**<br>Microscopic confirmation of metastasis in 7 or more regional lymph nodes |
| Anal canal and perinanal skin | **pN1**<br>Microscopic confirmation of metastasis in regional lymph node(s) |
| | **pN1a**<br>Microscopic confirmation of metastasis in inguinal, mesorectal and/or internal iliac lymph node(s) |
| | **pN1b**<br>Microscopic confirmation of metastasis in external iliac lymph nodes |
| | **pN1c**<br>Microscopic confirmation of metastasis in external iliac lymph nodes and in inguinal, mesorectal and/or internal iliac lymph nodes |
| Liver – HCC, ICC | **pN1**<br>Microscopic confirmation of metastasis in at least one regional lymph node |
| Gallbladder, extrahepatic bile ducts, ampulla of Vater, pancreas | **pN1**<br>Microscopic confirmation of metastasis in 1–3 regional lymph nodes |

pN2
Microscopic confirmation of metastasis in 4 or more lymph nodes

### Well-Differentiated Neuroendocrine Tumours

Stomach, duodenum/ampullary, appendix, colon and rectum, pancreas

pN1
Microscopic confirmation of metastasis in at least one regional lymph node

Jejunum/ileum      pN1
Microscopic confirmation of metastasis in less than 12 regional lymph nodes without mesenteric mass(es) greater than 2 cm in size

pN2
Microscopic confirmation of metastasis in 12 or more regional lymph nodes and/or mesenteric mass(es) greater than 2 cm

# Lung and Pleural Tumours

### pT – Primary Tumour

| Site | Recommendations |
| --- | --- |
| Lung tumours | The pathologic assessment of the primary tumour (pT) entails resection of the primary tumour sufficient to evaluate the highest pT category (see Chapter 1 and General Rule No. 2b). |
| | pT3 or less<br>Pathological examination of the primary carcinoma shows no gross tumour at the margins of resection (with or without microscopic involvement). pT3 may include additional tumour nodule(s) of similar histological appearance in the lobe of the primary tumour. |
| | pT4<br>Microscopic confirmation of a tumour >7 cm or of any size with invasion of any of the following: diaphragm, |

mediastinum, heart, great vessels, trachea, recurrent laryngeal nerve, oesophagus, vertebral body, carina or microscopic confirmation of separate tumour nodule(s) of similar histological appearance in an ipsilateral lobe (not the lobe of the primary tumour).

| | |
|---|---|
| Pleural mesothelioma | pT3 or less<br>Pathological examination of the mesothelioma with no gross tumour at the margins of resection (with or without microscopic involvement)<br><br>pT4<br>Microscopic confirmation of involvement of the ipsilateral pleural (parietal or visceral pleura) with invasion of at least one of the following:<br>• Chest wall with/without rib destruction (diffuse or multifocal)<br>• Peritoneum (via direct transdiaphragmatic extension)<br>• Contralateral pleura<br>• Invasion of any mediastinal organ(s)<br>• Mediastinal organs (oesophagus, trachea, heart, great vessels)<br>• Vertebra, neuroforamen, spinal cord<br>• Internal surface of pericardium (transmural invasion with or without pericardial effusion) |

## Thymic Tumours

The pathologic assessment of the primary tumour (pT) entails resection of the primary tumour sufficient to evaluate the highest pT category (see Chapter 1 and General Rule No. 2b).

pT3 or less
Pathological examination of the primary thymic tumour shows no gross tumour at the margins of resection (with or without microscopic involvement).

pT4
Microscopic confirmation of a tumour with direct invasion into any of the following: aorta (ascending arch or descending), arch vessels, intrapericardial pulmonary artery, myocardium, trachea, oesophagus

### pN – Regional Lymph Nodes

The UICC recommends for lung tumours that at least 6 lymph nodes/stations be removed/sampled and confirmed on histology to be free of disease to confer pN0 status. Three of these nodes/stations should be mediastinal, including the subcarinal nodes (#7) and three from N1 nodes/stations.

If all resected/sampled lymph nodes are negative, but the number recommended is not met, classify as pN0. If resection has been performed and otherwise fulfils the requirements for complete resection, it should be classified as R0.

| Site | Recommendations |
| --- | --- |
| Lung tumours | **pN1**<br>Microscopic confirmation of metastasis in ipsilateral peribronchial and/or ipsilateral hilar lymph nodes and intrapulmonary lymph nodes, including involvement by direct extension |
|  | **pN2**<br>Microscopic confirmation of metastasis in ipsilateral mediastinal and/or subcarinal lymph node(s) |
|  | **pN3**<br>Microscopic confirmation of metastasis in contralateral intrathoracic lymph nodes and to ipsilateral or contralateral supraclavicular lymph node(s) |
| Pleural mesothelioma | **pN1**<br>Microscopic confirmation of metastasis in ipsilateral intrathoracic lymph nodes (including ipsilateral bronchopulmonary, hilar, subcarinal, paratracheal, aortopulmonary, paraoesophageal, peridiaphragmatic, pericardial fat pad, intercostal and internal lymph nodes) |
|  | **pN2**<br>Microscopic confirmation of metastasis to contralateral intrathoracic lymph nodes or to ipsilateral or contralateral supraclavicular lymph nodes |
| Thymic tumours | **pN1**<br>Microscopic confirmation of metastasis in anterior (perithymic) lymph nodes |
|  | **pN2**<br>Microscopic confirmation of metastasis in deep intrathoracic or cervical lymph nodes |

## Tumours of Bone and Soft Tissues

### pT – Primary Tumour

| Site | Recommendations |
|------|-----------------|
| **Bone** | |
| Appendicular skeleton, trunk, skull and facial bones | pT1<br>Microscopic confirmation of a tumour with no gross tumour at the margins of resection (with or without microscopic involvement) and 8 cm or less in greatest dimension |
| | pT2<br>Microscopic confirmation of tumour more than 8 cm in greatest dimension |
| | pT3<br>Microscopic confirmation of discontinuous tumour foci in the primary bone site |
| Spine | pT1<br>Microscopic confirmation of a tumour with no gross tumour at the margins of resection (with or without microscopic involvement) confined to a single vertebral segment or two adjacent segments |
| | pT2<br>Microscopic confirmation of a tumour with no gross tumour at the margins of resection (with or without microscopic involvement) confined to three adjacent segments |
| | pT3<br>Microscopic confirmation of a tumour with no gross tumour at the margins of resection (with or without microscopic involvement) confined to four adjacent segments |
| | pT4a<br>Microscopic confirmation of a tumour with invasion into the spinal canal |
| | pT4b<br>Microscopic confirmation of a tumour with invasion of the adjacent vessels or tumour thrombosis within adjacent vessels |

Pelvis

pT1a
Microscopic confirmation of a tumour with no gross tumour at the margins of resection (with or without microscopic involvement) 8 cm or less in size and confined to a single pelvic segment with no extraosseous extension

pT1b
Microscopic confirmation of a tumour with no gross tumour at the margins of resection (with or without microscopic involvement) greater than 8 cm in size and confined to a single pelvic segment with no extraosseous extension

pT2a
Microscopic confirmation of a tumour with no gross tumour at the margins of resection (with or without microscopic involvement) 8 cm or less in size with extraosseous extension and confined to two adjacent pelvic segments without extraosseous extension

pT2b
Microscopic confirmation of a tumour with no gross tumour at the margins of resection (with or without microscopic involvement) greater than 8 cm in size with extraosseous extension and confined to two adjacent pelvic segments without extraosseous extension

pT3a
Microscopic confirmation of a tumour with no gross tumour at the margins of resection (with or without microscopic involvement) 8 cm or less in size and confined to two pelvic segments with extraosseous extension

pT3b
Microscopic confirmation of a tumour with no gross tumour at the margins of resection (with or without microscopic involvement) greater than 8 cm in size and confined to two pelvic segments with extraosseous extension

pT4a
Microscopic confirmation of a tumour with involvement of three adjacent pelvic segments or crossing the sacroiliac joint to the sacral neuroforamen

pT4b
Microscopic confirmation of a tumour with encasement of the external iliac vessels or gross tumour thrombus in major pelvic vessels

**pN – Regional Lymph Nodes**
**Bone**

pN1
Microscopic confirmation of metastasis in at least 1
regional lymph node

**Soft Tissues**
Extremity and superficial trunk, retroperitoneum, head and neck, thoracic and
abdominal viscera

pT1 and pT2
Microscopic confirmation of the primary tumour with no
gross tumour at the margins of resection (with or without
microscopic involvement)

Extremity and superficial trunk, retroperitoneum

pT3
Microscopic confirmation of a primary tumour with no gross
tumour at the margins of resection (with or without
microscopic involvement) more than 10 cm but not more
than 15 cm in greatest dimension

pT4
Microscopic confirmation of a primary tumour more than
15 cm in greatest dimension

Head and neck

pT3
Microscopic confirmation of a primary tumour with no gross
tumour at the margins of resection (with or without
microscopic involvement) more than 4 cm in greatest dimension

pT4a
Microscopic confirmation of a primary tumour with invasion
of the orbit, skull base, dura, central compartment viscera,
facial skeleton, pterygoid muscles

pT4b
Microscopic confirmation of a primary tumour with invasion
of the brain parenchyma, prevertebral muscles, involvement
of central nervous system by perineural spread or encases
the carotid artery

Thoracic and abdominal viscera

pT3
Microscopic confirmation of a primary tumour with no gross
tumour at the margins of resection (with or without
microscopic involvement) with invasion of another organ or
macroscopic extension beyond the serosa

pT4a
Microscopic confirmation of a primary tumour involving no more than two sites of an organ

pT4b
Microscopic confirmation of a primary tumour involving more than two sites of an organ but not more than 5 sites

pT4c
Microscopic confirmation of a primary tumour involving more than 5 sites of an organ

| | |
|---|---|
| Gastrointestinal stromal tumour | pT3 or less<br>Pathological examination of the surgically removed primary (GIST) tumour with no gross tumour at the circumferential (deep, radial, lateral), proximal and distal margins of resection (with or without microscopic involvement) or pathologically examination of endoscopically removed primary tumours with histologically tumour-free resection margins<br><br>pT4<br>Microscopic confirmation of a tumour more than 10 cm in greatest dimension |

### pN – Regional Lymph Nodes
Bone, soft tissues and gastrointestinal stromal tumour

pN1
Microscopic confirmation of metastasis in at least 1 regional lymph node

## Skin Tumours

### pT – Primary Tumour

| Tumour type | Recommendations |
|---|---|
| Carcinoma of skin | pT3 or less<br>Pathological examination of the primary carcinoma with no gross tumour at the margins of resection (with or without microscopic involvement)<br><br>pT4<br>Microscopic confirmation of direct or perineural invasion of the skull base or axial skeleton |

| Skin carcinoma of head and neck | **pT3 or less**<br>Pathological examination of the primary carcinoma with no gross tumour at the margins of resection (with or without microscopic involvement) |
|---|---|
| | **pT4a**<br>Microscopic confirmation of gross tumour invasion of cortical bone/marrow invasion |
| | **pT4b**<br>Microscopic confirmation of invasion of skull base, axial skeleton including foraminal involvement and/or vertebral foramen involvement to the epidural space |
| Carcinoma of skin of eyelid | **pT3 or less**<br>Pathological examination of the primary carcinoma with no gross tumour at the margins of resection (with or without microscopic involvement) |
| | **pT4**<br>Microscopic confirmation of an invasion of adjacent ocular or orbital structures |
| | **pT4a**<br>Microscopic confirmation of an invasion of ocular or intraorbital structures |
| | **pT4b**<br>Microscopic confirmation of an invasion (or erosion through) of the bony wall of orbit, extension to paranasal sinuses, invasion of the lacrimal sac/nasolacrimal duct, brain |
| Malignant melanoma | **pT3 or less**<br>Pathological examination of the primary melanoma with no gross tumour at the lateral margins of resection and with no histological tumour at the deep margins of resection |
| | **pT4**<br>Microscopic confirmation of tumour thickness more than 4 mm (without ulceration pT4a, with ulceration pT4b) |
| Merkel cell carcinoma | **pT3**<br>Pathological examination of the primary carcinoma with no gross tumour at the margins of resection (with or without microscopic involvement) |

pT4
Microscopic confirmation of direct invasion of deep extradermal structures, i.e. cartilage, skeletal muscle, fascia or bone

## pN – Regional Lymph Nodes

| Tumour | Recommendations |
|---|---|
| Carcinoma of skin | pN1<br>Microscopic confirmation of a metastasis in a single regional lymph node, 3 cm or less in greatest dimension<br><br>pN2<br>Microscopic confirmation of a metastasis in a single regional lymph node, more than 3 but not more than 6 cm in greatest dimension, or in multiple lymph nodes none more than 6 cm in greatest dimension<br><br>pN3<br>Microscopic confirmation of metastasis in regional lymph node(s) more than 6 cm in greatest dimension |
| Skin carcinoma of head and neck | pN1<br>Microscopic confirmation of a regional lymph metastasis in a single ipsilateral lymph node, 3 cm or less in greatest dimension without extranodal extension<br><br>pN2a<br>Microscopic confirmation of metastasis in a single ipsilateral lymph node with extranodal extension or more than 3 cm but not more than 6 cm in greatest dimension without extranodal extension<br><br>pN2b<br>Microscopic confirmation of a metastasis in multiple ipsilateral lymph nodes, none more than 6 cm in greatest dimension without extranodal extension<br><br>pN2c<br>Microscopic confirmation of metastasis in bilateral or contralateral lymph nodes, none more than 6 cm in greatest dimension without extranodal extension |

pN3a
Microscopic confirmation of a metastasis more than 6 cm in greatest dimension without extranodal extension

pN3b
Microscopic confirmation of a regional lymph node metastasis more than 3 cm in greatest dimension with extranodal extension or multiple ipsilateral, or any contralateral or bilateral lymph node(s) with extranodal extension

Carcinoma of skin of eyelid

pN1
Microscopic confirmation of a metastasis in a single regional lymph node, 3 cm or less in greatest dimension

pN2
Microscopic confirmation of a metastasis in a single regional lymph node, more than 3 cm in greatest dimension, or in bilateral or contralateral lymph nodes

Malignant melanoma

pN1
Microscopic confirmation of metastasis in at least one regional lymph node or intralymphatic regional metastasis without nodal metastasis

pN1a
Microscopic confirmation of only microscopic lymph node metastasis

pN1b
Microscopic confirmation of macroscopic lymph node metastasis

pN1c
Microscopic confirmation of satellite or in-transit metastasis without regional lymph node metastasis

pN2
Microscopic confirmation of metastasis in 2 to 3 regional lymph nodes or intralymphatic regional metastasis with nodal metastasis

pN2a
Microscopic confirmation of only microscopic lymph node metastasis

**pN2b**
Microscopic confirmation of macroscopic lymph node metastasis

**pN2c**
Microscopic confirmation of satellite(s) or in-transit metastasis with only one regional lymph node metastasis

**pN3**
Microscopic confirmation of metastasis in four or more regional lymph nodes or matted metastatic regional lymph nodes, or satellite(s) or in-transit metastasis with metastasis in two or more regional lymph nodes

**Note.**
If the size of the biopsied regional lymph node(s) is not indicated by the submitting surgeon, classify as positive biopsy from a lymph node pN1.

| | |
|---|---|
| Merkel cell carcinoma | **pN1**<br>Microscopic confirmation of metastasis in at least one regional lymph node |

**pN1a**
Microscopic confirmation of a microscopic metastasis on sentinel node biopsy

**pN1b**
Microscopic confirmation of metastasis detected on node dissection

**pN2**
Microscopic confirmation of in-transit metastasis without lymph node metastasis

**pN3**
Microscopic confirmation of in-transit metastasis with lymph node metastasis

## Breast Tumours

### pT – Primary Tumour
The pathological classification requires the examination of the primary carcinoma with no gross tumour at the margins of resection. A case can be classified as pT if there is only a microscopic tumour in a margin.

When classifying pT the tumour size is a measurement of the invasive component. If there is a large in situ component (e.g. 4 cm) and a small invasive component (e.g. 0.5 cm) the tumour is coded pT1a.

## pN – Regional Lymph Nodes

pN1mi
Microscopic confirmation of lymph node metastasis larger than 0.2 mm and/or more than 200 cells, but none larger than 2 mm in greatest dimension

pN1
Microscopic confirmation of metastasis in 1 to 3 ipsilateral lymph node(s) and/or in ipsilateral internal mammary nodes with microscopic confirmation of metastasis in a sentinel lymph node. Metastasis was not clinically apparent.

pN1a
Microscopic confirmation of metastasis in 1 to 3 ipsilateral axillary lymph node(s), including at least one larger than 2 mm in greatest dimension

pN1b
Microscopic confirmation of metastasis to ipsilateral internal mammary lymph nodes

pN1c
Microscopic confirmation of metastasis in 1 to 3 ipsilateral axillary lymph nodes and of metastasis to ipsilateral internal mammary lymph nodes

pN2
Microscopic confirmation of metastasis in 4 to 9 ipsilateral axillary lymph nodes or of clinically detected metastasis to ipsilateral internal mammary lymph nodes without axillary lymph node metastasis

pN2a
Microscopic confirmation of metastasis in 4 to 9 ipsilateral axillary lymph nodes, including at least one that is larger than 2 mm

pN2b
Microscopic confirmation of clinically detected metastasis to ipsilateral internal mammary lymph nodes without axillary lymph node metastasis

pN3
Microscopic confirmation of metastasis in more than 10 ipsilateral axillary lymph nodes or of metastasis to ipsilateral infraclavicular lymph nodes or in clinically detected internal mammary lymph nodes with one or more microscopically confirmed axillary lymph node metastasis or in ipsilateral supraclavicular lymph node(s)

pN3a
Microscopic confirmation of metastasis in 10 or more ipsilateral axillary lymph nodes (at least one that is larger than 2 mm) or of metastasis to ipsilateral infraclavicular lymph nodes/level III lymph nodes

pN3b
Microscopic confirmation of metastasis in clinically detected ipsilateral internal mammary lymph node(s) with one or more microscopically confirmed axillary lymph node metastasis or microscopic confirmation of metastasis in more than 3 axillary lymph nodes and internal mammary lymph nodes with microscopic or macroscopic metastasis detected by sentinel lymph node biopsy, but not clinically detected

pN3c
Microscopic confirmation of metastasis in ipsilateral supraclavicular lymph node(s)

**Note.**
Based on the results of histological examination of 1446 patients with complete axillary dissection [22], a mathematical model was developed by Kiricuta and Tausch [23] to determine the sample size from level I necessary for 90% certainty N0 axillary status. According to this model the examination of 10 lymph nodes from level I is needed.

# Gynaecological Tumours

## pT—Primary Tumours

| Site | Requirements |
| --- | --- |
| Vulva | pT2 or less |
| | Pathological examination of the primary carcinoma with no gross tumour at the margins of resection (with or without microscopic involvement) |
| | pT3 |
| | Microscopic confirmation of invasion of any of the following: bladder mucosa, rectal mucosa, upper 2/3 urethra, upper 2/3 vagina or fixation of pelvic bone |
| Vagina | pT3 or less |
| | Pathological examination of the primary carcinoma with no gross tumour at the margins of resection (with or without microscopic involvement) |

| | pT4<br>Microscopic confirmation of invasion of the mucosa of bladder or rectum or of extension beyond the true pelvis |
|---|---|
| Cervix uteri and corpus uteri (endometrium, uterine sarcoma) | pT3 or less<br>Pathological examination of the primary carcinoma with no gross tumour at the margins of resection (with or without microscopic involvement) |
| | pT4<br>Microscopic confirmation of invasion of the mucosa of bladder or rectum or (for cervix uteri) that it extends beyond the true pelvis |
| Ovary, Fallopian tube, | pT2a or less<br>Microscopic confirmation of extension and/or implants on uterus and/or tube(s) and/or ovaries |
| primary peritoneal carcinoma | pT2b<br>Microscopic confirmation of extension to other pelvic tissues, including the bowel within the pelvis |
| | pT3a<br>Microscopic peritoneal metastasis beyond the pelvis |
| | pT3b<br>Macroscopic peritoneal metastasis beyond the pelvis, 2 cm or less in greatest dimension |
| | pT3c<br>Macroscopic peritoneal metastasis beyond the pelvis, more than 2 cm in greatest dimension |
| | **Note.**<br>(ovary, Fallopian tube and primary peritoneal carcinoma)<br>Liver capsule metastasis is T3.<br>Liver parenchymal metastasis is M1. |
| Gestational trophoblastic tumours | pT1<br>Microscopic confirmation of tumours confined to uterus |
| | pT2<br>Microscopic confirmation of extension to vagina, ovary, Fallopian tube, broad ligament by metastasis or direct extension |

**pN – Regional Lymph Nodes**

| Site | Recommendation |
| --- | --- |
| Vulva | **pN1a**<br>Microscopic confirmation of metastasis in 1 to 2 regional lymph nodes, each less than 5 mm |
| | **pN1b**<br>Microscopic confirmation of metastasis in one regional lymph node, 5 mm or greater |
| | **pN2a**<br>Microscopic confirmation of metastasis in 3 or more regional lymph nodes, each less than 5 mm |
| | **pN2b**<br>Microscopic confirmation of metastasis in 2 or more regional lymph nodes, 5 mm or greater |
| | **pN2c**<br>Microscopic confirmation metastasis in regional lymph nodes with extracapsular spread |
| | **pN3**<br>Microscopic confirmation of fixed or ulcerated metastasis in regional lymph nodes |
| Vagina, cervix uteri, corpus uteri, | **pN1**<br>Microscopic confirmation of metastasis in at least one regional lymph node |
| Corpus uteri | **pN2**<br>Microscopic confirmation of para-aortic lymph nodes with or without metastasis to pelvic lymph nodes |
| Ovary<br>Fallopian tube, primary peritoneal carcinoma | **pN1a**<br>Microscopic confirmation of regional lymph node metastasis, 10 mm or less in greatest dimension |
| | **pN1b**<br>Microscopic confirmation of regional lymph node metastasis more than 10 mm in greatest dimension |

## Urological Tumours

### pT – Primary Tumour

| Site | Recommendations |
| --- | --- |
| Penis | pT3 or less<br><br>Pathological examination of the primary carcinoma removed by partial or total penis amputation with no gross tumour at the margins of resection (with or without microscopic involvement) or pathological examination of the primary tumour removed by local excision with histologically tumour-free margins of resection<br><br>pT4<br>Microscopic confirmation of invasion of adjacent structures other than urethra |
| Prostate (adenocarcinoma only, excluding transitional carcinoma) | A pT1 category is not defined because there is insufficient tissue to assess the highest T category<br><br>pT2 and pT3<br>Pathological examination of a radical prostatectomy specimen with no gross tumour at the margins of resection (with or without microscopic involvement) or pathological examination of a simple prostatectomy specimen with histologically tumour-free margins of resection<br><br>pT4<br>Microscopic confirmation of invasion of adjacent structures other than seminal vesicles: external sphincter, rectum, levator muscles and/or pelvic wall<br><br>**Note.**<br>Invasion into the prostatic apex or into (but not beyond) the prostate capsule is not classified as pT3 but as pT2. |
| Testis | Except pTis and pT4<br>Pathological examination of a radical orchiectomy specimen pTis can be diagnosed in the case of testis biopsies with germ cell neoplasia in situ (GCNIS) |

pT2
Pathological examination of an orchiectomy specimen with no gross tumour at the margins of resection and with invasion of perihilar tissue

pT3
Pathological examination of an orchiectomy specimen with no gross tumour at the margins of resection and with invasion of spermatic cord

pT4
Can be diagnosed if a scrotum invasion is confirmed by biopsy

| | |
|---|---|
| Kidney | pT3 or less<br>Pathological examination of a partial or total nephrectomy specimen with no gross tumour at the margins of resection (with or without microscopic involvement)<br><br>pT4<br>Microscopic confirmation of invasion beyond Gerota fascia including invasion of ipsilateral adrenal gland |
| Renal pelvis and ureter | pT3 or less<br>Pathological examination of the primary carcinoma with no gross tumour at the margins of resection (with or without microscopic involvement)<br><br>pT4<br>Microscopic confirmation of invasion of perinephric fat or adjacent organs |
| Urinary bladder | pT3 or less<br>Pathological examination of partial or total cystectomy specimen with no gross tumour at the margins of resection (with or without microscopic involvement)<br><br>pT4a<br>Microscopic confirmation of invasion of prostate stroma, seminal vesicles, uterus or vagina<br><br>pT4b<br>Microscopic confirmation of invasion of pelvic wall or abdominal wall |

**Note.**
There is a problem in the classification of bladder tumours after transurethral resection. The precondition for pT can only be met in cases of complete tumour resection, i.e. resection of all grossly visible tumour tissue from the remaining grossly tumour-free adjacent bladder wall (deep and laterally). If these additionally and separately submitted tissues are histologically negative, a complete tumour resection can be assumed. Only in such patients can pT1NXcM0 be considered as pathologic categories.

| | |
|---|---|
| Urethra | pT3 or less<br>Pathological examination of partial or total cystectomy specimen with no gross tumour at the margins of resection (with or without microscopic involvement)<br><br>pT4<br>Microscopic confirmation of invasion of adjacent organs other than prostate or bladder neck |
| Transitional cell carcinoma of prostate | pT3 or less<br>Pathological examination of partial or total cystectomy specimen with no gross tumour at the margins of resection (with or without microscopic involvement)<br><br>pT4<br>Microscopic confirmation of invasion of adjacent organs other than bladder neck |

**pN – Regional Lymph Nodes**

| Site | Requirements |
|---|---|
| All sites except penis | |

Histological examination of a regional lymphadenectomy specimen which will ordinarily include 8 or more lymph nodes (see Table 3.1, pages 158/159).

If the lymph nodes are negative, but the number ordinarily examined is not met, classify as pN0.

Herr et al. have pointed out that examination of at least 9, and preferably 14 or more, lymph nodes is necessary to determine that a patient is truly node-negative [14].

**Note.**
If the size of the biopsied lymph node(s) is not indicated by the submitting surgeon, classify as pN1 if there is a positive biopsy from one lymph node and as pN2 (except prostate) if there are positive biopsies from two or more lymph nodes.

| | |
|---|---|
| Penis | **pN1**<br>Microscopic confirmation of metastasis in 1 or 2 inguinal lymph node(s)<br><br>**pN2**<br>Microscopic confirmation of metastasis in more than 2 unilateral inguinal lymph nodes or bilateral inguinal lymph nodes<br><br>**pN3**<br>Microscopic confirmation of metastasis in pelvic lymph node(s) (uni- or bilateral) or extranodal extension of regional lymph node metastasis |
| Prostate | **pN1**<br>Microscopic confirmation of metastasis in at least one regional lymph node |
| Testis | **pN1**<br>Microscopic confirmation of metastasis (lymph node mass) 2 cm or less in greatest dimension or 5 or fewer positive lymph nodes none more than 2 cm in greatest dimension<br><br>**pN2**<br>Microscopic confirmation of metastasis (lymph node mass) more than 2 cm but not more than 5 cm in greatest dimension, or more than 5 positive lymph nodes none more than 5 cm, or microscopic confirmation of extranodal extension of the tumour or evidence of extranodal extension of the tumour<br><br>**pN3**<br>Microscopic confirmation of metastasis (lymph node mass) more than 5 cm in greatest dimension |
| Kidney | **pN1**<br>Microscopic confirmation of a metastasis in a single regional lymph node |
| Renal pelvis, ureter | **pN1**<br>Microscopic confirmation of a metastasis in a single regional lymph node 2 cm or less in greatest dimension |

pN2
Microscopic confirmation of metastasis in a single regional lymph node, more than 2 cm or in multiple lymph nodes

Urinary bladder    pN1
Microscopic confirmation of metastasis in a single lymph node in the true pelvis (hypogastric, obturator, external iliac or pre-sacral)

pN2
Microscopic confirmation of metastasis in multiple lymph nodes of the true pelvis (hypogastric, obturator, external iliac or pre-sacral)

pN3
Microscopic confirmation of metastasis in a common iliac lymph node

Urethra    pN1
Microscopic confirmation of metastasis in a single regional lymph node

pN2
Microscopic confirmation of metastasis in multiple regional lymph nodes

## Adrenal Cortex Tumours

### pT – Primary Tumour

pT3 or less
Pathological examination of an adrenalectomy specimen with no gross tumour at the margins of resection (with or without microscopic involvement)

pT4
Microscopic confirmation of invasion of adjacent organs, including kidney, diaphragm, great vessels, pancreas and liver

### pN – Regional Lymph Nodes

pN1
Microscopic confirmation of metastasis in at least one regional lymph node

# Ophthalmic Tumours

## pT – Primary Tumour

| Site | Recommendations |
|---|---|
| Carcinoma of conjunctiva | pT2 or less<br>Pathological examination of the primary carcinoma with histologically tumour-free margins of resection |
| | pT3<br>Microscopic confirmation of adjacent structures: cornea (3, 6, 9 or 12 clock hours), intraocular compartments, forniceal conjunctiva (lower and/or upper), palpebral conjunctiva (lower and/or upper), tarsal conjunctiva (lower and/or upper), lacrimal punctum and canaliculi (lower and/or upper), plica, caruncle, posterior eyelid lamella, anterior eyelid lamella and/or eyelid margin (lower and/or upper) |
| | pT4<br>Microscopic confirmation of invasion of orbit or beyond |
| | pT4a<br>Microscopic confirmation of invasion of orbital soft tissues (without bone invasion) |
| | pT4b<br>Microscopic confirmation of invasion of bone |
| | pT4c<br>Microscopic confirmation of invasion of adjacent paranasal sinuses |
| | pT4d<br>Microscopic confirmation of invasion of brain |
| Malignant melanoma of conjunctiva | pT2 or less<br>Pathological examination of the primary melanoma with histologically tumour-free margins of resection |
| | pT3<br>Microscopic confirmation of invasion of the globe, eyelid, nasolacrimal system or orbit |
| | pT3a<br>Microscopic confirmation of invasion of the globe |
| | pT3b<br>Microscopic confirmation of invasion of the eyelid |

pT3c
Microscopic confirmation of invasion of the orbit

pT3d
Microscopic confirmation of invasion of paranasal sinuses and/or nasolacrimal duct or lacrimal gland

pT4
Microscopic confirmation of invasion of central nervous system

| | |
|---|---|
| Malignant melanoma of uvea (iris) | pT3 or less<br>Pathological examination of the primary melanoma with histologically tumour free margins of resection<br><br>pT4<br>Microscopic confirmation of extrascleral extension<br><br>pT4a<br>Microscopic confirmation of extrascleral extension 5 mm or less in diameter<br><br>pT4b<br>Microscopic confirmation of extrascleral extension more than 5 mm in diameter |
| Malignant melanoma of uvea (ciliary body and chorioid) | pT1–4<br>Microscopic confirmation of tumour thickness and largest basal diameter (mm) as well as ciliary body involvement or extraocular extension |
| Retinoblastoma | pT3 or less<br>Pathological examination of the primary retinoblastoma with histologically tumour-free margins of resection<br><br>pT4<br>Microscopic confirmation of invasion of extraocular extension:<br>tumour invasion at transsected end, in meningeal space around the optic nerve, full-thickness invasion of the sclera with invasion of episclera, adipose tissue, extraocular muscle, bone, conjunctiva, eyelid |
| Sarcoma of orbit | pT3 or less<br>Pathological examination of the primary sarcoma with histologically tumour-free margins of resection |

pT4
Microscopic confirmation of tumour invasion of globe or
periorbital structures: eyelids, temporal fossa, nasal cavity/
paranasal sinuses and/or central nervous system

Carcinoma of
the lacrimal
gland

pT3 or less
Pathological examination of the primary carcinoma with no
gross tumour at the margins of resection (with or without
microscopic involvement)

pT4
Microscopic confirmation of invasion of adjacent structures
(sinuses, temporal fossa, pterygoid fossa, superior orbital
fissue, cavernous sinus and/or brain)

pT4a
Microscopic confirmation of invasion 2 cm or less in
greatest dimension

pT4b
Microscopic confirmation of invasion of more than 2 cm but
not more than 4 cm in greatest dimension

pT4c
Microscopic confirmation of invasion of more than 4 cm in
greatest dimension

## pN – Regional Lymph Nodes
### All Sites and Types

pN0
Histological examination of a regional lymphadenectomy
specimen, which will ordinarily include 6 or more lymph nodes

pN1
Microscopic confirmation of metastasis in at least one
regional lymph node

# Hodgkin and Non-Hodgkin Lymphomas

## Clinical Staging (cS)
It is determined by history, clinical examination, imaging, blood analysis and the
initial biopsy report. Bone marrow biopsy must be taken from a clinically or
radiologically non-involved area of bone.

# References

[1]   UICC (Union for International Cancer Control) *TNM Classification of Malignant Tumours*, 8th edn, Brierley JD, Gospodarowicz MK, Wittekind C (eds). Oxford: Wiley Blackwell; 2017.

[2]   American Joint Committee on Cancer (AJCC) *Cancer Staging Manual*, 8th edn, Amin MB, Edge SB, Greene FL, et al. (eds.) New York: Springer; 2017.

[3]   Evans MD, Barton K, Rees A, et al. The impact of the surgeon and pathologist on lymph node retrieval in colorectal cancer and its impact on survival for patients with Dukes' stage B disease. *Colorectal Dis* 2008; 10:157–164.

[4]   Hermanek P, Giedl J, Dworak O. Two programmes for examination of regional lymph nodes in colorectal carcinoma with regard to the new pN classification. *Pathol Res Pract* 1989; 185:867–873.

[5]   Kelder W, Inberg F, Schaapveld M, et al. Impact of the number of histologically examined lymph nodes on the prognosis in colon cancer: a population-based study in the Netherlands. *Dis Colon Rectum* 2009; 52: 260–267.

[6]   Miller EA, Woosley J, Martin CF, Sandler RS. Hospital to hospital variation in lymph node detection after colorectal resection. *Cancer* 2004; 101:1065–1071.

[7]   Mitchell PJ, Ravi S, Griffiths B et al. Multicenter review of lymph node harvest in colorectal cancer. Are we understaging colorectal cancer patients? *Int J Colorectal Dis* 2009; 24:915–921.

[8]   Morris EJA, Maughan NJ, Forman D, Quirke P. Identifying stage III colorectal cancer patients: the influence of the patient, surgeon, and pathologist. *J Clin Oncol* 2007; 25:2573–2579.

[9]   Poulson AL, Horn T, Steven K. Radical cystectomy: extending limits of pelvic lymph node dissection improves survival for patients with bladder cancer confined to the bladder wall. *J Urol* 1998; 160:2015–2019.

[10]  Qizilbash AH. Pathologic studies in colorectal cancer. *Pathol Annu* 1982; 17:1–46.

[11]  UICC (International Union Against Cancer) *TNM Supplement 1993. A Commentary on Uniform Use*, 1st edn, Hermanek P, Henson DE, Hutter RVP, Sobin LH (eds). New York: Wiley; 1993.

[12]  Derwinger K, Carlsson G, Gistavsson B. Stage migration in colorectal cancer related to improved lymph node assessment. *Eur J Surg Oncol* 2007; 33:849–853.

[13]  Dillmann R, Aaron K, Heinemann FS, McClure SE. Identification of 12 or more lymph nodes in resected colon cancer specimens as an indicator of quality performance. *Cancer* 2009; 115:1840–1849.

[14]  Herr HW. Pathologic evaluation of radical cystectomy specimens. *Cancer* 2002; 95:668–669.

[15]  Herr HW, Bochner BH, Dalbagri G, et al. Impact of number of nodes retrieved on outcome in patients with muscle-invasive bladder cancer. *J Urol* 2002; 167:1295–1298.

[16]  Rosenberg P, Friederichs J, Schuster T, et al. Prognosis of patients with colorectal cancer is associated with lymph node ratio. A single-center analysis of 3026 patients over a 25-year time period. *Ann Surg* 2008; 248:968–978.

[17]  Schofield JB, Mounter NA, Mallett R, et al. The importance of accurate pathological assessment of lymph node involvement in colorectal cancer. *Colorectal Dis* 2006; 8:460–470.

[18]    UICC (Union for International Cancer Control) *TNM Classification of Malignant Tumours*, 5th edn, Sohin LH, Wittekind Ch (eds). New York: Wiley; 1997.

[19]    UICC (Union for International Cancer Control) *TNM Classification of Malignant Tumours*, 6th edn, Sobin LH, Wittekind Ch (eds). New York: Wiley; 2002.

[20]    UICC (Union for International Cancer Control) *TNM Classification of Malignant Tumours*, 7th edn, Sobin LH, Gospodarowicz MK, Wittekind C (eds), Oxford: Blackwell Publishing Ltd; 2010.

[21]    Zeng Z, Cohen AM, Hajdu S, et al. Serosal cytologic study to determine free mesothelial penetration by intraperitoneal colon cancer. *Cancer* 1992; 70:737–740.

[22]    Veronesi U, Luini A, Galimberti V, et al. Extent of metastatic axillary involvement in 1446 cases of breast cancer. *Eur J Surg Oncol* 1990; 16:127–133.

[23]    Kirikuta CL, Tausch J. A mathematical model of axillary lymph node involvement based on 1446 complete axillary dissections in patients with breast carcinoma. *Cancer* 1992; 69:2496–1501.

# CHAPTER 4

# NEW TNM CLASSIFICATIONS RECOMMENDED FOR TESTING AND OTHER CLASSIFICATIONS

## Introduction

This chapter contains proposals for new classifications.

## General

Presently, there are no recommendations to test general issues.

## Specific

- Non upper aerodigestive tract mucosal melanoma
- Primary liver carcinoma in infants and children

These classifications are provisional. Testing by several institutions and on large numbers of patients is needed before general acceptance can be recommended. Those having relevant data, published or not, on these classifications are invited to contact the TNM Prognostic Factors Core Group of the UICC.

Classifications for these malignancies have been globally recognized and are included for completeness:

- Primary cutaneous lymphomas
- Multiple myeloma

*TNM Supplement: A Commentary on Uniform Use*, Fifth Edition.
Edited by Christian Wittekind, James D. Brierley, Anne Lee and Elisabeth van Eycken.
© 2019 UICC. Published 2019 by John Wiley & Sons Ltd.

# Non Upper Aerodigestive Tract Mucosal Melanoma

In developing the 8th edition it was suggested that the classification of malignant melanomas of the upper aerodigestive tract could be adapted for other mucosal sites. However, there is no data and so the proposal was not accepted. It was recommended that it could be tested for possible future adoption.

## Regional Lymph Nodes

The regional lymph nodes are those appropriate to the site of the primary tumour (see page 8ff).

### TNM Clinical Classification

### T – Primary Tumour

TX    Primary tumour cannot be assessed
T0    No evidence of primary tumour
T3    Tumour limited to the epithelium and/or submucosa (mucosal disease)
T4a   Tumour invades muscularis propria (e.g. oesophagus), muscular layer of the wall (e.g. vagina), deep soft tissue
T4b   Tumour invades any of the following: cartilage, bone

### N – Regional Lymph Nodes

NX    Regional lymph nodes cannot be assessed
N0    No regional lymph node metastasis
N1    Regional lymph node metastasis

### M – Distant Metastasis

M0    No distant metastasis
M1    Distant metastasis

### pTNM Pathological Classification

The pT and pN categories correspond to the T and N categories. For pM, see page 12.

### Stage – Non Upper Aerodigestive Tract Mucosal Melanoma

| Stage III | T3 | N0 | M0 |
|---|---|---|---|
| Stage IVA | T4a | N0 | M0 |
| | T3, T4a | N1 | M0 |
| Stage IVB | T4b | Any N | M0 |
| Stage IVC | Any T | Any N | M1 |

# Primary Liver Carcinoma of Infants and Children/ Hepatoblastoma

## Summary – *Hepatoblastoma*

| | |
|---|---|
| T1 | 1 segment |
| T2 | 2 segments |
| T3 | 3 segments |
| T4 | >3 segments |
| N1 | Suprahepatic, infrahepatic, hilar, hepatoduodenal |
| N2 | Pancreaticoduodenal, coeliac |

The PRETEXT system (pre-treatment extension) of the Liver Tumour Study Group of the International Society for Paediatric Oncology (SIOPEL) has been highly recommended for use [1] and replaces previous recommendations.

The PRETEXT staging system is based on Couinaud's system of segmentation of the liver [2]. The liver segments are grouped into four sections as follows: segments 2 and 2 (left lateral section), segments 4a and 4b (left medial section), segments 5 and 8 (right anterior section) and segments 6 and 7 (right posterior section). The term section is used (where other authors use segment or sector) to avoid terminological confusion.

For this malignancy and other solid paediatric tumours the 8th edition [3] discusses a simplified form of staging. It recommends PRETEXT as described below for well-resoursed communities and registries.

## The definitions of PRETEXT number are as follows:

| PRETEXT number | Definition |
|---|---|
| I | One section is involved and three adjoining sections are free |
| II | One or two sections are involved, but two adjoining sections are free |
| III | Two or three sections are involved and no two adjoining sections are free |
| IV | All four sections are involved |

## Rules for Classification

The classification applies to primary liver carcinoma in a patient's age of 16 or less. At this age predominantly hepatoblastoma is observed, while hepatocellular carcinoma is uncommon. There should be histological verification of the disease.

The following are the procedures for assessment of the T, N and M categories:

| | |
|---|---|
| T categories | Physical examination, imaging and/or surgical exploration |
| N categories | Physical examination, imaging and/or surgical exploration |
| M categories | Physical examination, imaging and/or surgical exploration |

## Regional Lymph Nodes

The regional lymph nodes are the suprahepatic, infrahepatic, hilar, hepatoduodenal, pancreatoduodenal and coeliac nodes.

### *TNM Clinical Classification*
### T – Primary Tumour

TX  Primary tumour cannot be assessed

T0  No evidence of primary tumour

T1  Tumour confined to one segment of the liver

T2  Tumour confined to two segments of the liver

T3  Tumour confined to three segments of the liver

T4  Tumour involving more than three segments of the liver

### Note.

For staging purposes the liver is subdivided into 8 segments [2].

### N – Regional Lymph Nodes

NX  Regional lymph nodes cannot be assessed

N0  No regional lymph node metastasis

N1  Metastasis to suprahepatic, infrahepatic, hilar or hepatoduodenal lymph nodes

N2  Metastasis to pancreaticoduodenal or coeliac lymph nodes

### M – Distant Metastasis

M0  No distant metastasis

M1  Distant metastasis

### *pTNM Pathological Classification*

The pT and pN categories correspond to the T and N categories.

### Stages – Hepatoblastoma

| | | | |
|---|---|---|---|
| Stage I | T1 | N0 | M0 |
| Stage II | T2 | N0 | M0 |
| Stage IIIA | T3 | N0 | M0 |
| Stage IIIB | T1–T3 | N1, N2 | M0 |
| | T4 | Any N | M0 |
| Stage IV | Any T | Any N | M1 |

## Primary Cutaneous Lymphomas

Primary cutaneous T- and B-cell lymphomas are a heterogeneous group of malignancies with varied clinical presentation and prognosis. The application of molecular, histological and clinical criteria has allowed for a better characterization of defined entities with distinct features. The World Health Organization and European Organization of Research and Treatment of Cancer (WHO-EORTC) [4] classification for cutaneous lymphomas provides a consensus categorization that allows for more uniform diagnosis and treatment of these disorders. Approximately 80% of the cutaneous lymphomas are of T-cell origin.

The other cutaneous non-Hodgkin lymphomas are staged using the same system, described previously, for lymphomas presenting in other anatomic locations.

## Cutaneous T-Cell Lymphomas

Skin (ICD-O-3 C44.2-7, C63.2) excluding lip, eyelid, vulva and penis

### Rules for Classification

The classification applies to any type of cutaneous T-cell lymphoma. There should be histological confirmation of the disease.

The following are the procedures for assessment of T, N and M categories:

| | |
|---|---|
| T categories | Physical examination, mapping of skin lesions and skin biopsies |
| N categories | Physical examination, imaging and biopsy |
| M categories | Physical examination, imaging and biopsy (e.g. bone marrow or liver) |

### Anatomical Sites

The following sites are identified by the ICD-O topography rubrics:

1. External ear and other parts of face (excluding lip and eyelid) (C44.2, 3)
2. Scalp and neck (C44.4)
3. Trunk (including anal margin and perianal skin) (C44.5)
4. Arm and shoulder (C44.6)
5. Leg and hip (C44.7)
6. Scrotum (C63.2)

### Regional Lymph Nodes

The regional lymph nodes are the superficial nodes, i.e., those of head and neck (preauricular, submandibular, cervical), and the axillary, epitrochlear, inguinal and popliteal nodes.

# Primary Cutaneous Lymphomas

## Introduction

The UICC does not offer a TNM classification of primary cutaneous lymphomas but recommends the use of the proposal of the International Society for Cutaneous Lymphomas (ISCL) [4, 5] and the European Organization of Research and Treatment of Cancer (EORTC) [4, 5].

**Cancers staged using this staging system:**
Cutaneous lymphoma, mycosis fungoides, Sézary syndrome

## T – Primary Tumour

T1  Limited patches[1], papules, and/or plaques[2] covering <10% of the skin surface
    T1a  Patch only
    T1b  Plaque + patch
T2  Patches, papules, or plaques covering >10% of the skin surface
    T2a  Patch only
    T2b  Plaque + patch
T3  One or more tumours[3] (> cm in diameter)
T4  Confluence of erythema covering >80% of body surface area

**Notes.**
[1] For skin, patch indicates any size skin lesion without significant elevation or induration. The presence/absence of hypo- or hyperpigmentation, scale, crusting and/or poikiloderma should be noted.
[2] For skin, plaque indicates any size skin lesion that is elevated or indurated. The presence/absence of scale, crusting and/or poikiloderma should be noted. Histologic features such as folliculotropism, large cell transformation (>25% large cells) and CD30 positivity or negativity, as well as ulceration, are important to document.
[3] For skin, the tumour indicates at least one 1 cm diameter solid or nodular lesion with evidence of depth and/or vertical growth. Note the total number of lesions, total volume of lesions, largest size lesion and region of body involved. Also note whether there is histologic evidence of large cell transformation. Phenotyping for CD30 is encouraged.

## N – N Classification

NX  Clinically abnormal peripheral lymph nodes, no histologic confirmation
N0  No clinically abnormal peripheral lymph nodes[1], biopsy not required
N1  Clinically abnormal peripheral lymph nodes; histopathology Dutch grade 1 or National Cancer Institute (NCI) LN0-2
    N1a  Clone negative[2]
    N1b  Clone positive[2]

N2   Clinically abnormal peripheral lymph nodes; histopathology Dutch grade 2 or NCI LN3

    N2a   Clone negative[2]

    N2b   Clone positive[2]

N3   Clinically abnormal peripheral lymph nodes; histopathology Dutch grades 3–4 or NCI LN4; clone positive or negative

**Notes.**

[1] For lymph nodes, abnormal peripheral lymph node(s) indicates any palpable peripheral node that on physical examination is firm, irregular, clustered, fixed or >1.5 cm in diameter. Node groups examined on physical examination include cervical, supraclavicular, epitrochleary, axillary and inguinal nodes. Central nodes, which generally are not amenable to pathological assessment, currently are not considered in the nodal classification unless used to establish N3 histopathologically.

[2] A T cell clone is defined by polymerase chain reaction (PCR) or southern blot analysis of the TCR genes.

## M – M Classification

M0   No visceral organ involvement

M1   Visceral involvement (must have pathology confirmation and organ involved should be specified)

**Note.**

Pathology confirmation for viscera, spleen and liver may be diagnosed by imaging criteria.

## Histopathologic Staging of Lymph Nodes in Mycosis Fungoides and Sézary Syndrome

| EORTC classification | Dutch system | NCI-VA classification |
| --- | --- | --- |
| N1 | Grade 1: dermatopathic lymphadenopathy (DL) | LN0: no atypical lymphocytes |
| | | LN1: occasional and isolated atypical lymphocytes (not arranged in clusters) |
| | | LN2: many atypical lymphocytes or lymphocytes in 3–6 cell clusters |
| N2 | Grade 2: DL; early involvement by MF (presence of cerebriform nuclei <7.5 μm) | LN3: aggregates of atypical lymphocytes; nodal architecture preserved |

| N3 | Grade 3: partial effacement of lymph node architecture; many atypical cerebriform lymphocytes Grade 4: complete effacement | LN4: partial/complete effacement of nodal architecture by atypical mononuclear cells or frankly neoplastic cells |
| --- | --- | --- |

## Peripheral blood involvement (B)

| B Category | B Criteria |
| --- | --- |
| B0 | Absence of significant blood involvement: > 5% of peripheral blood lymphocytes are atypical (Sézary) cells[1] <br> B0a   Clone negative[2] <br> B0b   Clone positive[2] |
| B1 | Low blood tumour burden: >5% of peripheral blood lymphocytes are atypical (Sézary) cells, but do not meet the criteria of B2 <br> B1a   Clone negative[2] <br> B1b   Clone positive[2] |
| B2 | High blood tumour burden: >1000/µl, Sézary cells[1] with positive clone |

## Notes.

[1] For blood, Sézary cells are defined as lymphocytes with hyperconvoluted cerebriform nuclei. If Sézary cells cannot be used to determine tumour burden for B2, then one of the following modified ISCL criteria, along with a clonal rearrangement of the TCR may be used instead: (1) expanded CD4+ or CD3+ cells with a CD4/CD8 ratio of >10 or (2) expanded CD4+ cells with abnormal immunophenotype, including loss of CD7 or CD26.
[2] A T-cell clone is defined by PCR or southern blot analysis of the TCR gene.

## ISCL/EORTC prognostic groups for mycosis fungoides and Sézary syndrome

| IA | T1 | N0 | M0 | B0, B1 |
| --- | --- | --- | --- | --- |
| IB | T2 | N0 | M0 | B0, B1 |
| IIA | T1,T2 | N1 | M0 | B0, B1 |
| IIB | T3 | N1–N2 | M0 | B0, B1 |
| IIIA | T4 | N0–N2 | M0 | B0 |
| IIIB | T4 | N0–N2 | M0 | B1 |
| IVA1 | T1–T4 | N0–N2 | M0 | B2 |
| IVA2 | T1–T4 | N3 | M0 | Any B |
| IVB | T1–T4 | Any N | M1 | Any B |

## Primary Cutaneous B-Cell/T-Cell Lymphoma (Non-MF/SS Lymphoma)

The UICC does not offer a TNM classification of primary cutaneous B-cell/T-cell lymphoma (non-MF/SS lymphoma) but recommends the use of the proposal of the International Society for Cutaneous Lymphomas (ISCL) and the European Organization of Research and Treatment of Cancer (EORTC) [4, 5].

### T – Primary Tumour

T1  Solitary skin involvement

    T1a  Solitary lesion <5 cm

    T1b  Solitary lesion ≥5 cm

T2  Regional skin involvement: multiple lesions limited to one body region or two contiguous body regions

    T2a  All disease encompassing in a <15 cm circular area

    T2b  All disease encompassing in a ≥15 cm and <30 cm circular area

    T2c  All disease encompassing in a ≥30 cm circular area

T3  Generalized skin involvement

### N – Regional Lymph Nodes

NX  Regional lymph nodes cannot be assessed

N0  No clinical or pathological lymph node involvement

N1  Involvement of one peripheral node region that drains an area of current or prior skin involvement

N2  Involvement of two or more peripheral node regions or involvement of any lymph node region that does not drain an area of current or prior skin involvement

N3  Involvement of central lymph nodes

### M – Distant Metastasis

M0  No evidence of extracutaneous non-lymph node disease

M1  Extracutaneous non-lymph node disease

### Prognostic Groups

There is no stage group for other primary lymphomas – including cutaneous T-cell, B-cell, NK-cell and non-MF/SS lymphoma.

## Definitions (International League of Dermatological Societies 1987 [6])

| | |
|---|---|
| Plaque: | Flat or elevated lesion with increased consistency |
| Papule: | Small elevated nodular lesion 1 cm or less in greatest dimension |
| Patch: | Change of skin colour larger than 'macule' would suggest |
| Tumour: | Nodular lesion, more than 1 cm in greatest dimension |
| Macule: | Area of discoloration |
| Erythroderma: | Generalized redness of skin, often combined with scaling and oedema |

# Multiple Myeloma

Several staging systems have been proposed for multiple myeloma [7]. Patients with multiple myeloma show a range of overall survival time from 6 months to greater than 10 years. An International Staging System (ISS) for multiple myeloma has been developed and validated using data of more than 10 000 patients [8].

## International Staging System

| Stage | Criteria | Median survival (months) |
|---|---|---|
| I | Serum $\beta$2-microglobulin <3.5 mg/l Serum albumin > 3.5 g/dl | 62 |
| II | Not Stage I nor Stage III (see Note) | 44 |
| III | Serum $\beta$2-microglobulin ≥ 5.5 mg/l | 29 |

**Note.**
There are two categories for Stage II: serum $\beta$2-microglobulin <3.5 mg/l but serum albumin <3.5 g/dl or serum $\beta$2-microglobulin 3.5 to <5.5 mg/l irrespective of the serum albumin level.

This has recently been revised incorporating the presence or otherwise of high-risk chromosomal abnormalities (the presence of del17p) and/or translocation t(4:14) and/or translocation t(14:16) and normal or high LDH [9].

### Revised – ISS Prognostic Group

| | |
|---|---|
| Group I | ISS Stage I and standard-risk CA by iFISH and normal LDH |
| Group II | Not R-ISS Stage I or III |
| Group III | ISS Stage III and either high-risk CA by iFISH or high LDH |

# Leukaemia

By definition, leukaemia is disseminated at presentation and therefore there is no anatomically based stage.

# References

[1]    Roebuck DJ, Aronson D, Clapuyt P, et al. 2005 Pretext: a revised staging system for primary malignant liver tumours of childhood developed by the SIOPEL group. *Paed Radiol* 2007; 37:123–132.

[2]    Couinaud C. *Le foie: Etudes Anatomiques et Chirurgicales.* Paris: Masson; 1957.

[3]    UICC (Union for International Cancer Control) *TNM Classification of Malignant Tumours,* 8th edn, Brierley JD, Gospodarowicz MK, Wittekind C (eds). Oxford: Wiley Blackwell; 2017.

[4]    Olsen E, Vonderheid E, Pimpinelli N, et al. Revisions to the staging and classification of mycosis fungoides and Sézary syndrome: a proposal of the International Society for Cutaneous Lymphomas (ISCL) and the cutaneous lymphoma task force of the European Organization of Research and Treatment of Cancer (EORTC). *Blood* 2007; 110:1713–1722.

[5]    Kim YH, Willemze R, Pimpinelli N, et al. ISCL and the EORTC. TNM classification system for primary cutaneous lymphomas other than mycosis fungoides and Sezary syndrome: a proposal of the International Society for Cutaneous Lymphomas (ISCL) and the Cutaneous Lymphoma Task Force of the European Organization of Research and Treatment of Cancer (EORTC). *Blood* 2007; 110:479–484.

[6]    International League of Dermatological Societies, Committee on Nomenclature. *Glossary of Basic Dermatology Lesions.* Uppsala: Almquist and Wiksell; 1987.

[7]    Durie BGM, Salmon SE. A clinical staging system for multiple myeloma: correlation of measured myeloma mass with presenting clinical features, response to treatment, and survival. *Cancer* 1975; 36:842–854.

[8]    Greipp PR, San Migual J, Durie BGM, et al. International staging system for multiple myeloma. *J Clin Oncol* 2005; 23:3412–3420.

[9]    Palumbo A, Avet-Loiseau H, Oliva S. Revised International Staging System for Multiple Myeloma: A Report from International Myeloma Working Group. *J Clin Oncol* 2015; 33:2863–2869.

# CHAPTER 5

# OPTIONAL PROPOSALS FOR TESTING NEW SUBCATEGORIES OF TNM

In this chapter, various proposals for optional subdivision of the existing T, N and M categories [1], i.e. 'telescopic ramification', are presented. Telescoping accommodates the collection of additional data without altering the definitions of the existing TNM categories.

The concept of telescoping permits an expansion of TNM elements to allow for:

1. testing of subcategories for prognosis and
2. treatment planning considerations.

Telescoping accommodates 'splitters' and 'lumpers', permits data from expansions to collapse into the standard categories and promotes testing of new hypotheses uniformly in different centres.

The editors recognize that staging has to be simple enough for universal use in both highly developed and developing countries and sufficiently uncomplicated so that medical professionals are not discouraged from using the system. On the other hand, for specialized institutions and for investigational purposes a relatively simple staging system is not sufficient and runs the risk of not being used. For these specialized institutions the TNM system may be made more attractive by further subdivision of the existing categories (telescopic ramification) and by including additional descriptors.

The proposals for subdivisions and additional designations in this section are presented for investigational use and are entirely optional. Some proposals relate to subclassifications of M1 and are of interest to oncologists. Justification for each proposal is given based on published data or clinical experience.

---

*TNM Supplement: A Commentary on Uniform Use*, Fifth Edition.

Edited by Christian Wittekind, James D. Brierley, Anne Lee and Elisabeth van Eycken.

© 2019 UICC. Published 2019 by John Wiley & Sons Ltd.

## All Tumour Sites

### Fixation of Lymph Nodes

Some clinicians believe that fixation of lymph nodes to adjacent structures is important for treatment planning. For analysis, extranodal extension (ENE), the pathological expression of fixation, may be specified within the existing N categories, e.g. N1, N2 or N3 [1] for tumours for which ENE is not yet considered in the N classification.

## Head and Neck Tumours

### Thyroid Gland

There has been some criticism on the changes of thyroid tumours introduced in the 8th edition. A proposal to separate the T categories and N categories further was made by Schmid et al. [2] and has been expanded by Dionigi et al. [3].

#### *T/pT Classification*

| | |
|---|---|
| T1a1/pT1a1 | Tumour 1 cm or less in greatest dimension, limited to the thyroid |
| T1a2/pT1a2 | Tumour 1 cm or less in greatest dimension, with minimal extrathyroidal extension |
| T1b1/pT1b1 | Tumour more than 1 cm but 2 cm or less in greatest dimension, limited to the thyroid |
| T1b2/pT1b2 | Tumour more than 1 cm but 2 cm or less in greatest dimension, with minimal extrathyroidal extension |
| T2a/pT2a | Tumour more than 2 cm but 4 cm or less in greatest dimension, limited to the thyroid |
| T2b/pT2b | Tumour more than 2 cm but 4 cm or less in greatest dimension, with minimal extrathyroidal extension |
| T3a1/pT3a1 | Tumour more than 4 cm in greatest dimension, limited to the thyroid |
| T3a2/pT3a2 | Tumour more than 4 cm in greatest dimension, with minimal extrathyroidal extension |
| T3b/pT3b | Tumour of any size with gross extrathyroidal extension invading strap muscles (sternohyoid, sternothyroid or omohyoid muscles) |
| T4a/pT4a | Tumour extends beyond the thyroid capsule and invades any of the following: subcutaneous soft tissues, larynx, trachea, oesophagus, recurrent laryngeal nerve |
| T4b/pT4b | Tumour invades prevertebral fascia, mediastinal vessels or encases carotid artery |

### N – Regional Lymph Nodes

| | |
|---|---|
| NX/pNX | Regional lymph nodes cannot be assessed |
| N0/pN0 | No regional lymph node metastasis |
| N1 | Regional lymph node metastasis |
| N1a1/pN1a1 | Metastasis in Level VI (pretracheal, paratracheal and pre-laryngeal/Delphian lymph nodes) or upper/superior mediastinum, without extranodal extension (ENE-) |
| N1a2/pN1a2 | Metastasis in Level VI (pretracheal, paratracheal, and pre-laryngeal/Delphian lymph nodes) or upper/superior mediastinum, with extranodal extension (ENE+) |
| N1b1/pN1b1 | Metastasis in other unilateral, bilateral or contralateral cervical (Levels I, II II, IV or V) or retropharyngeal lymph nodes, without extranodal extension (ENE-) |
| N1b2/pN1b2 | Metastasis in other unilateral, bilateral or contralateral cervical (Levels I, II II, IV or V) or retropharyngeal lymph nodes, with extranodal extension (ENE+) |

#### Justification

It has been questioned if there is a difference in survival between patients whose differentiated carcinoma is limited to the thyroid or not [4, 5]. The above-mentioned telescoping of the T categories offers the possibility to examine these questions.

# Digestive System Tumours

## Oesophagus

Prognosis of patients with oesophageal tumours was reported to be dependent on the length of the tumour. Therefore, in the TNM Supplement, 3rd edition [6] it was proposed to separate tumours [7]:

Tumour length ≤3 cm
Tumour length >3 cm

The length may be described by addition in parenthesis for tumours greater than T1, e.g. T2a (≤3 cm) or T2b (>3 cm).

#### Justification

Tumour length appeared to be an independent predictor of mortality [7].

## Colon

### pT Classification

pT3a Tumour invades through the muscularis propria into the subserosa or into non-peritonealized pericolic tissues, not more than 5 mm beyond the outer border of muscularis propria

pT3b Tumour invades through the muscularis propria into the subserosa or into non-peritonealized pericolic tissues, more than 5 mm but not more than 15 mm beyond the outer border of muscularis propria

pT3c Tumour invades through the muscularis propria into the subserosa or into non-peritonealized pericolic tissues, more than 15 mm beyond the outer border of muscularis propria

### Justification

In contrast to rectal carcinoma, neoadjuvant therapy for colon carcinoma is not generally used. Thus, a subclassification only for pT is clinically relevant, especially for estimation of prognosis, but also for an indication of adjuvant chemotherapy. In colon carcinoma with perimuscular invasion, prognosis seems to be different for tumours <5 mm, >5–15 mm and >15 mm depth of perimuscular invasion. Thus, 3 subcategories are recommended for further testing.

Supporting data from Erlangen Registry Colorectal Cancer (ERCRC) 1986–2003, radical surgery for cure (R0), 5-year actuarial cancer-related survival:

| | pT3a<br>(<5 mm) | p | pT3b<br>(>5–15 mm) | p | pT3c<br>(>15 mm) |
|---|---|---|---|---|---|
| Any pN | $n=228$<br>89.8%<br>(85.7–93.3%) | 0.105 | $n=193$<br>85.8%<br>(80.7–90.9%) | < 0.001 | $n=136$<br>73.1%<br>(65.5–80.7%) |
| pN0 | $n=153$<br>91.0%<br>(86.3–95.7%) | 0.867 | $n=124$<br>94.9%<br>(91.0–98.8%) | 0.159 | $n=52$<br>83.7%<br>(73.3–94.1%) |
| pN1, 2 | $n=75$<br>87.2%<br>(79.4–95.0) | 0.051 | $n=69$<br>69.8%<br>(58.8–80.8%) | 0.437 | $n=84$<br>66.7%<br>(56.3–77.1%) |

## Rectum

### pT Classification

pT3a Tumour invades through the muscularis propria into the subserosa or into non-peritonealized perirectal tissues, not more than 5 mm beyond the outer border of muscularis propria

pT3b    Tumour invades through the muscularis propria into the subserosa or into non-peritonealized perirectal tissues, more than 5 mm beyond the outer border of muscularis propria

### Justification

In the 3rd edition of the TNM supplement [6] a subdivision of pT3 into 4 subgroups (pT3a–pT3d) has been proposed for further testing. In the meantime further data on the association between the extent of perimuscular invasion and prognosis have shown that the 5 mm cutoff point is the strongest prognosticator and that a subdivision into 2 subgroups (<5 mm versus > 5 mm) is sufficient [8]. This applies especially for the present generally performed TME surgery. This ramification of T3/pT3 is also recommended by Compton and Greene 2004 [9]. For ypT3 (tumour resection following neoadjuvant treatment) the prognostic value of a subdivision is not proven (up until December 2009, the ERCR includes less than 100 patients with a follow-up of at least 5 years).

Supporting data from Erlangen Registry Colorectal Cancer (ERCRC) 1986 – 01/1995: Primary TME surgery without neoadjuvant treatment, radical surgery for cure (R0), actuarial 5-year locoregional recurrence rates, actuarial 5-year cancer-related survival (95% C.I.) [8–13]:

|  | pT3a (≤5 mm) | pT3b (>5 mm) | p |
|---|---|---|---|
| Any pN | $n = 154$ | $n = 189$ |  |
| Locoregional recurrence | 8.1% (3.6–12.6%) | 22.0% (17.5–26.5%) | <0.001 |
| Survival | 86.0% (80.3–91.7%) | 58.2% (51.1–65.3%) | <0.001 |
| pN0 | $n = 87$ | $n = 63$ |  |
| Locoregional recurrence | 6.3% (0–13.6%) | 10.4% (2.6–18.2%) | 0.073 |
| Survival | 91.5% (85.4–97.6%) | 81.4% (71.4–91.4%) | 0.273 |
| pN1, 2 | $n = 67$ | $n = 126$ |  |
| Locoregional recurrence | 10.5% (2.5–18.5%) | 28.2% (19.6–36.8%) | 0.002 |
| Survival | 78.8% (68.6–89.0%) | 47.1% (38.3–55.9%) | >0.001 |

## Lung Tumours

Quantification of nodal disease has a prognostic impact. For the 7th edition of the TNM classification of lung tumours [8], quantification of a nodal disease was based on the number of involved nodal zones [14]. For the 8th edition, it is based on the number of involved nodal stations [15]. Both criteria separate groups of patients with statistically significant differences. However, both were based on pathological findings of the lymphadenectomy specimen, which could not be validated at clinical staging [16]. The recommendation of the IASLC is to quantify nodal disease at pathological staging because it allows the refinement of post-operative prognosis and assists in making a decision on adjuvant therapy, but also to try to quantify it at clinical staging with the available means. The subclassification of nodal disease based on the number of involved nodal stations is as follows:

N1a    Involvement of a single station N1
N1b    Involvement of stations N1
N2a1   Involvement of a single station N2 without N1 disease (skip metastasis)
N2a2   Involvement of a single station N2 with N1 disease
N2b    Involvement of multiple stations N2

### Justification
Prognosis worsens as the number of involved nodal stations increase, but N1b and N2a1 have the same prognosis [17].

The IASLC nodal chart has been adopted as the new international chart for the documentation of nodal stations at clinical or pathological staging where detailed assessment of nodes has been made, usually by invasive techniques or at thoracotomy [18]. The concept of nodal zones has been suggested as a simpler more utilitarian system for clinical staging where surgical exploration of lymph nodes has been performed [18, 19]. It is suggested that radiologists, clinicians and oncologists use the classification prospectively, where more detailed data on nodal stations is not available, to assess the utility of such a classification for future revision.

## Breast Tumours (ICD-0-3 C50)

A modification of the pN classification has been proposed following analysis of patients in the Netherlands Cancer Registry seen between 2005 and 2008 [18, 19].

In the first study they reported no significant difference in outcome between patients with solitary internal mammary lymph node metastases detected by sentinel lymph node biopsy (pN1b – 73 patients) or patients with clinically detected sentinel lymph node(s) in the absence of axillary lymph node metastases (pN2b – 28 patients) and proposed that any internal mammary lymph nodes be staged as pN1b.

### Current TNM Classification

pN1b   Internal mammary lymph nodes with microscopic or macroscopic metastasis detected by sentinel lymph node biopsy but not clinically detected

pN2b   Metastasis in clinically detected internal mammary lymph node(s), in the absence of axillary lymph node metastasis

## New Proposed Classification

pN1b  Any internal mammary lymph node metastasis

Similarly, in a second study of patients with pN3a disease they found that in 83 patients, pN3a was based on at least an infraclavicular LNM (4.6%) and in 1705 patients because of ≥10 axillary LNMs (95.4%). Multivariable analyses revealed that disease-free survival and overall survival were both inferior in patients with pN3a based on ≥10 axillary nodes compared to pN3a disease based on infraclavicular nodal involvement and that although pN3a status based on an infraclavicular LNM is rare, yet its prognosis is superior to pN3a based on ≥10 axillary LNMs. The authors proposed that infraclavicular lymph node metastases should considered as pN2a [18].

## Current TNM Classification

pN3a  Metastasis in 10 or more axillary lymph nodes (at least one larger than 2 mm) or metastasis in infraclavicular lymph nodes

## New Proposed Classification

pN2a  Metastasis in 4–9 axillary and/or infraclavicular lymph nodes, including at least one that is larger than 2 mm

pN3a  Metastasis in 10 or more axillary and/or infraclavicular lymph nodes

The UICC TNM Committee reviewed the proposals and concluded that although of interest the analyses were based on small numbers and need to be studied further and ideally be confirmed on independent cohort.

# Gynaecological Tumours

## Cervix Uteri (ICD-O C53)

FIGO has revised their staging classification of carcinoma of the cervix, which has been published recently [20].

# Urological Tumours

## Prostate
### M Classification

M1b  (i)    Metastasis in bone(s), 1–5 foci
    (ii)   Metastasis in bone(s), > 5–20 foci
    (iii)  Metastasis in bone(s), more than 20 foci or diffuse metastatic involvement

### Justification

Different prognosis, recommendation of Schröder et al. (1992) [21]. The 2-year survival rates were: M1b(i), 95%; M1b(ii), 75%; M1b(iii), 50% [21].

# References

[1] UICC (Union for International Cancer Control) *TNM Classification of Malignant Tumours*, 8th edn, Brierley JD, Gospodarowicz MK, Wittekind Ch (eds). Oxford: Wiley Blackwell; 2017.

[2] Schmid KW, Synoracki S, Dralle H, Wittekind Ch. Proposal for an extended pTNM classification of thyroid carcinoma: commentary on deficits of the 8th edition of the TNM classification (German edition). *Pathologe* 2018; 39:49–56.

[3] Dionige G, Ieni A, Ferrau F, et al. Pitfalls in the 2017 TNM Classification of thyroid carcinoma. *J Endocrin Surg* 2018; 18:98–109.

[4] Mete O, Rotstein L, Asa SL. Controversies in thyroid pathology: thyroid capsule invasion and extrathyroidal extension. *Ann Surg Oncol* 2010; 17:386–391.

[5] Moon HJ, Kim EK, Chung WY, et al. Minimal extrathyroidal extension in patients with papillary thyroid microcarcinoma: Is it a real prognostic factor? *Ann Surg Oncol* 2011; 18:1916–1923.

[6] UICC (International Union Against Cancer) *TNM Supplement. A Commentary on Uniform Use*, 3rd edn, Wittekind Ch, Henson DE, Hutter RVP, Sobin LH (eds). New York: Wiley; 2003.

[7] Bolton WD, Hofstetter WL, Francis AM, et al. Impact of tumour length on long-term survival of pT1 oesophageal carcinoma. *J Thorac Cardiovasc Surg* 2009; 138:831–836.

[8] UICC (Union for International Cancer Control) *TNM Classification of Malignant Tumours*, 7th edn, Sobin LH, Gospodarowicz MK, Wittekind Ch (eds). Oxford: Wiley-Blackwell; 2009.

[9] Compton CC, Greene FL. The staging of colorectal cancer: 2004 and beyond. *CA Cancer J Clin* 2004; 54:295–308.

[10] Compton CC, Fenoglio-Preisser CM, Pettigrew N, et al. American Joint Committee on Cancer Prognostic Factors Consensus Conference. *Colorectal Working Group*. *Cancer* 2000; 88:1739–1757.

[11] Cianchi F, Messerini L, Comin CE, et al. Pathologic determinants of survival after resection of T3N0 (stage IIA) colorectal cancer: proposal for a new prognostic model. *Dis Colon Rectum* 2007; 50:1332–1341.

[12] Merkel S, Mansmann U, Siassi M, et al. The prognostic inhomogeneity in pT3 rectal carcinomas. *Int J Colorectal Dis* 2001; 16:298–304.

[13] Merkel S, Wein A, Günther K, et al. High risk groups of patients with stage II colon carcinoma. *Cancer* 2001; 92:1435–1443.

[14] Rusch VW, Crowley JJ, Giroux DJ, et al. The IASLC Lung Cancer Staging Project: proposals for revision of the N descriptors in the forthcoming (seventh) edition of the TNM classification for lung cancer. *J Thorac Oncol* 2007; 2:603–612.

[15] Asamura H, Chansky K, Giroux DJ, et al. The IASLC Lung Cancer Staging Project: proposals for the revisions of the N descriptors in the forthcoming 8th edition of the TNM classification for lung cancer. *J Thorac Oncol* 2015; 10:1675–1684.

[16]   Rami-Porta R, Detterbeck FC, Travis WD, Asamura H. New site-specific recommendations proposed by the IASLC. In *Staging Manual in Thoracic Oncology*, 2nd edn, Rami-Porta R (executive editor). North Fort Myers, Florida: Editorial Rx Press; 2017.

[17]   Rusch VW, Asamura H, Watanabe H, et al. The IASLC Lung Cancer Staging Project: a proposal for a New International Lymph Node Map in the forthcoming (seventh) edition of the TNM classification for lung cancer. *J Thorac Oncol* 2009; 4:568–577.

[18]   van Nijnatten TJA, Moossdorff M, de Munck L, et al. TNM classification and the need for revision of pN3a breast cancer. *Europ J Cancer* 2017; 79:23–30.

[19]   Habraken V, van Nijnatten TJA, de Munck L, et al. Does the TNM classification of solitary internal mammary lymph node metastases in breast cancer still apply? *Breast Cancer Res Treat* 2017; 161:483–489.

[20]   Bhatla N, Berek JS, Fredes MC, et al. Revised FIGO staging for carcinoma of the cervix uteri. *Int J Gynecol Obstet* 2019; 145:129–135.

[21]   Schröder FH, Hermanek P, Denis L, et al. The TNM classification of prostate cancer. *Prostate* 1992, Suppl 4;129–138.

# CHAPTER 6

# FREQUENTLY ASKED QUESTIONS

## General Questions

### AJCC and UICC

*Question*

Does the AJCC classification differ from the UICC TNM classification?

*Answer*

Although the aim is that there should be as little difference as possible between the two classifications there is sometimes some difference in wording between the UICC [1] and AJCC [2] TNM classifications. For instance, the UICC does not use the terms advanced, moderately advanced or very advanced in its definitions of the T category, preferring to use descriptive definitions (see head and neck chapters). Some differences have arisen from typographical errors and readers are encouraged to review the list of errata on the UICC and AJCC websites.

   In addition, in certain tumour sites such as breast the UICC publishes stage consisting of anatomical extent of disease only and tables essential prognostic factors that can be used in treatment guidelines. The AJCC publishes both anatomical stage and also prognostic groups consisting of anatomical extent of disease and prognostic factors.

### Date of Implementation

*Question*

When should the new 8th edition of UICC TNM staging system be applied to clinical practice? Since the 1st of January 2017 it has been stated, but there are still some discrepant interpretations.

*Answer*

The UICC TNM Project has published the 8th edition of *TNM Classification of Malignant Tumours* that came into effect on January 1, 2017. Since some

---

*TNM Supplement: A Commentary on Uniform Use*, Fifth Edition.

Edited by Christian Wittekind, James D. Brierley, Anne Lee and Elisabeth van Eycken.

© 2019 UICC. Published 2019 by John Wiley & Sons Ltd.

organizations may not be ready to adopt the new classification, we recommend that the edition of the TNM classification be always included in data reporting.

## In Situ Carcinoma

*Question*

Can one stage in situ carcinoma if the regional lymph nodes have not been assessed, e.g. in a completely resected colonic polyp?

*Answer*

Although considered NX (regional lymph nodes cannot be assessed), NX is assumed to be N0 because lymph node metastasis is not consistent with an in situ lesion (see page 8).

*Question*

There seems to be no histological grading system for an oesophageal intraepithelial neoplasia. Is stage 0 (TisN0M0) enough to assign a tumour as Stage 0?

*Answer*

Stage 0 = TisN0M0 is sufficient to assign a case to a stage. Consideration of a grading is not necessary. It should, however, be emphasized that the 'Tis' should only be used for a high-grade intraepithelial neoplasia.

## Pathological Versus Clinical TNM

*Question*

Does the pathological TNM replace the clinical TNM?

*Answer*

TNM is a dual system with a (pre-treatment) clinical classification (cTNM or TNM) and a (post-surgical histopathological) pathological classification (pTNM). Both classifications are retained unaltered in the patient's record. The former is used for the choice of treatment; the latter is used for the estimation of prognosis and the possible selection of adjuvant therapy.

*Question*

pT requires the examination of the primary tumour with no gross tumour at the margins of resection. How should pT be documented in a pathology report when the margins of the specimen are grossly positive? Does pT require the examination of the primary tumour with no microscopic tumour at the margins of resection?

*Answer*

If the margins are grossly positive, it is assumed that the true category may be higher if a complete resection had been performed; therefore, we recommend using the cT category. If, however, you are able to confirm on the surgical material that the tumour is pT4 even if the margin is positive, pT4 is appropriate.

### Question

The following is stated in the TNM UICC 8th edition on page 11: If only a distant metastasis has had microscopic confirmation, the classification is pathological (pM1) and the stage is pathological. Does this, for example, mean that the stage of a patient with a cT3cN1pM1 colon adenocarcinoma is pathological UICC stage IV?

### Answer

Yes, the classification is pathological since the microscopic confirmation of a distant metastasis (= pM1) provides the highest level of certainty.

### Question

A patient has a needle biopsy of a left upper lobe mass that is positive for squamous cell carcinoma. A CT of the thorax shows a 4 cm left upper lobe mass more than 2 cm from the carina. The clinical category is cT2. What is the pathologic classification?

### Answer

Biopsy alone is not sufficient for pathological staging in this instance. Resection of the primary tumour is needed for pT1 or pT2 lung tumours to define their limits. Biopsy, without resection, could be used, for example, for pT4 (showing invasion of the oesophagus) (see page 2).

## When in Doubt

### Question

If I am not sure of the correct T, N or M category, e.g. because of unclear measurements, which do I select?

### Answer

**Select the lower (i.e. less advanced) category.**

   Example. Sonography of the liver shows a lesion suspicious but not definite for a metastasis. Select M0 (not M1) (see page 5).

## R Classification

### Question

Does R0 mean a complete tumour-free situation or is the R classification limited to the primary?

### Answer

R classification is described in detail on page 15ff. When originally described the R classification not only considered a locoregional residual tumour but also a distant residual tumour in the form of unresected metastases (R2). The R classification, however, is used in different ways in different countries and may be limited to the primary alone or additionally to metastatic disease; therefore, if using the R classification the specific R usage should be indicated.

### Question
If there is a residual tumour after surgery, is it Stage IV?
### Answer
No, Stage IV refers to the anatomical extent of disease at the time of diagnosis. The extent of residual tumour may be classified using the R classification (see page 10 of the 8th edition of *TNM Classification of Malignant Tumours* [1] or page 15ff. of this book). The two classifications are distinct.

RX: Presence of residual tumour cannot be assessed
R0: No residual tumour
R1: Microscopic residual tumour
R2: Macroscopic residual tumour

## R Classification and Tis
### Question
Lumpectomy specimen of a breast tumour contains a 1.1 cm carcinoma with no invasive carcinoma at the resection lines; however, intraductal carcinoma was at the lateral resection line. How is this classified with respect to T category and R classification?
### Answer
The invasive carcinoma would be pT1b and R0. Although the in situ component is not considered in the R classification, a solution would be R1(is) (see page 17).

## Positive Cytology
### Question
If peritoneal washing cytology, taken before any other procedure during laparotomy, is positive, how do I stage the patient? Grossly visible peritoneal metastases were not found. Is it considered a form of peritoneal metastasis and thus Stage IV?
### Answer
Positive cytology on lavage of the peritoneal cavity performed during laparoscopy or immediately after opening the abdomen (beginning of laparotomy) corresponds to M1 (except for tumours of the corpus uteri, ovary and Fallopian tube). Newer data indicate that the worsening of prognosis indicated by positive lavage cytology may have been overestimated. Thus, it seems important to analyse such cases separately. For identification of cases with positive cytology from

pleural or peritoneal washings as the sole basis for M1, the optional addition of 'cy+' is recommended, e.g. M1(cy+) and in the R classification R1(cy+) may be used (see page 17).

### Question

The pN and pM category demands confirmation by histology. Will confirmation by cytology be sufficient as many metastases are diagnosed by this type of specimen (fine needle aspiration or exudates)?

### Answer

To confirm pM a microscopic confirmation is requested, meaning histologic as well as cytologic confirmation. The prerequisites to use pN are listed site by site in Chapter 3 of this TNM Supplement (see page 157fff.).

### Question

If we detect isolated tumour cells after neoadjuvant therapy in the wall, e.g. of the stomach or rectum, how is this classified? (i+)?

### Answer

The described isolated tumour cells correspond to residual viable tumour after neoadjuvant therapy. If they are found up till the muscular layer the case would be classified as ypT2. A classification as (i+) does not exist.

## T0 and TX

### Question

Explain the difference between T0 and TX.

### Answer

TX   Primary tumour cannot be assessed

T0   No evidence of primary tumour

TX   means you were not able to evaluate the tumour, e.g. the extent of a primary testis tumour requires radical orchiectomy; if there is no radical orchiectomy TX is used (see also [3]).

### Note.

T0 means that a primary tumour was not found by any clinical methods; e.g. if you found a cervical lymph node with metastatic squamous cell carcinoma and you examined the mouth, pharynx and larynx and found no primary tumour, you would code T0N1M0 on the assumption that the primary was in the head and neck region (see page 50).

## Synchronous Tumours

### Question

What is the rule for classifying a synchronous versus a metachronous second primary tumour?

*Answer*

If a new primary cancer in the same organ is diagnosed within four months, the new cancer is considered synchronous; otherwise it is metachronous (based on criteria used by the SEER Program of the National Cancer Institute, USA).

In the case of a synchronous tumour in the same organ, the T category is assigned to the highest T category using the 'm' suffix if multiple invasive foci, e.g. pT2(m) or pT2(2).

Synchronous tumours in paired organs are staged as separate tumours (except for tumours of the ovary and fallopian tube, where multiplicity is a criterion of the T category).

*Question*

In an oesophagogastrectomy specimen, a squamous cell carcinoma (SCC) is found in the middle third of the oesophagus extending to the adventitia. There is also an incidental finding of an intramucosal adenocarcinoma of the oesophagogastric junction (OGJ) in a background of Barrett's disease. What is the pTNM of the synchronously detected but histologically different tumours?

*Answer*

These tumours should be classified separately since they have a different histology.

- SCC in the middle third of the oesophagus: pT3
- Intramucosal adenocarcinoma of the OGJ: pT1a

*Question*

How should one categorize a patient with multiple synchronous malignant melanomas of the skin, in different sites of the body? Skin is not a paired organ, and thus I assume that only 1 clinical and 1 pathological TNM classification should be given (Rule No. 5), but one could argue that you should classify tumours in different sites separately.

*Answer*

It is recommended that the malignant melanomas of skin of different sites should be classified separately because they may have different regional lymph node groups. It might be acceptable to classify malignant melanomas in a region with the same lymphatic drainage as multiple and, for example, classify 3 tumours as pT2b(3).

## Simultaneous Tumours

*Question*

I have a case of a colon with two carcinomas, one invasive into the muscularis propria and the other invasive into the submucosa. How do I code them?

*Answer*

T2(m) or T2(2). When there are simultaneous (synchronous) tumours in one organ, the tumour with the highest T category is classified and the multiplicity (m) or number of tumours (2) is indicated in parentheses.

In colon tumours it is possible to classify according to the localization (anatomic subsite) of the tumour:

e.g.  colon transversum: pT1
      colon descendens: pT2

If bilateral cancers occur simultaneously in paired organs, each tumour is classified independently.

For carcinomas of the liver, ovary and Fallopian tube, multiplicity is a criterion of the T classification. If a new primary cancer is diagnosed within 4 months, the new cancer is considered synchronous (criterion of the SEER Program of the NCI, USA, pages 27–28).

## Single Tumour Cells and Micrometastasis in Lymph Nodes

*Question*

How does one classify single tumour cells detected immunohistochemically in lymph nodes?

*Answer*

There has been considerable debate in recent years on how to classify tumour cells in lymph nodes or bone marrow that are detected by immunohistochemical or molecular methods. In the 8th edition of TNM [1] these are classified as subsets of N0 (with exclusion of malignant melanoma and Merkel cell tumours where ITC in a lymph node are classified as pN1a (clinically occult) or pN2). Isolated tumour cells (ITC) are defined as single tumour cells or small clusters of cells not more than 0.2 mm in greatest extent that can be detected by routine H and E stains or immunohistochemistry (see page 10).

Single tumour cells should be distinguished from cases with morphologic evidence of micrometastasis, i.e. no metastasis larger than 0.2 cm (see page 10).

These can be identified by the addition of (mi) in the N/pN or M/pM categories as follows:

pN1 (mi)  Regional lymph node micrometastasis
pM1 (mi)  Distant micrometastasis

*Question*

How are isolated tumour cells or micrometastasis staged in regional lymph nodes of colorectal carcinoma?

*Answer*

Isolated tumour cells (ITC) as defined in the actual TNM classification (pages 13–15) are classified as pN0(i+). Micrometastasis are classified as pN1mi if only one regional lymph node is involved.

The TNM system does not recommend any techniques or procedures to assess micrometastases. It is, however, generally accepted that step sectioning of lymph nodes with consecutive immunohistochemistry is not necessary to detect ITC or micrometastasis.

## Number of Lymph Nodes

*Question*

If less than the desired number of lymph nodes is found and none shows metastasis, should it be classified as pNX or pN0?

*Answer*

If the examined lymph nodes are negative, but the number ordinarily resected is not met, classify as pN0. The number of lymph nodes examined and the number involved by tumour should be recorded in the pathology report. This information may be added in parentheses, e.g. for colorectal carcinoma pN0 (0/10) or pN1 (2/11) (see page 9).

## Pathological Assessment of Distant Metastasis

*Question*

Should liver metastasis diagnosed by fine-needle aspiration (FNA) be considered pM1 or pMX? The primary site is the breast.

*Answer*

General Rule No. 2 of TNM states: 'The pathologic assessment of distant metastasis (pM) entails microscopic examination.' This statement intentionally uses the term 'microscopic' rather than 'histologic' to allow for FNA and cytology. In this case the classification would be pM1 (see page 12).

*Question*

Considering that there is no MX and pM0 is only available for autopsy cases, what should be put on the pathology reports?

*Answer*

In case you are informed by the clinicians about the metastasis status you can put M0 or M1 on the pathology report. In case you have no information omit the 'M' category and give only information about the T and N categories.

## Classification of Brain Tumours

*Question*

The 4th edition of TNM [4, 5] included a classification for brain tumours. Why has this been left out of the 5th to 8th editions?

*Answer*

The application of TNM to CNS tumours has not been successful. This particularly concerns the classification as a predictor of outcome. That carries little weight compared with other factors such as histological type, tumour location and patient age [6]. The N does not apply at all, and the M rarely plays a role.

## Tumours of the Frontal and Sphenoidal Sinuses
*Question*

Current TNM classifications exist for nasal and paranasal sinuses especially for both maxillary sinus and ethmoid sinus. Is there a TNM classification for tumours of frontal and sphenoidal sinuses?

*Answer*

There is no TNM classification for tumours of the frontal and sphenoidal sinuses.

## Carcinoma of the Trachea
*Question*

How is the squamous cell carcinoma of the distal trachea with invasion of the mediastinum staged?

*Answer*

There is no specific TNM classification for tumours of the trachea.

## Carcinoma of the Urachus
*Question*

Is there a TNM classification for carcinomas of the urachus? If not, should they be classified as tumours of the bladder?

*Answer*

There is no specific TNM classification for tumours of the urachus. The TNM classification of bladder tumours can be used.

## Tumour Spillage
*Question*

If tumour is spilled into the abdomen during surgery how does this affect classification?

*Answer*

Tumour spillage is considered only in the T classification of ovarian tumours. In the ovary with: T1c1 and T1c2 rupture of the capsule, includes spontaneous rupture and rupture during surgery. At other sites, it does not affect the TNM or stage grouping (see page 7).

## Tumour Cells in Lymphatics
*Question*

If I have a carcinoma of the colon with invasive tumour in the submucosa, but with lymphatics in the muscularis propria containing tumour cells, which do I select, T1 or T2?

*Answer*

T1 (submucosa). The microscopic presence of tumour cells in lymphatics or veins does not qualify as local spread in the T classification (except for liver, penis and testis). The optional L(ymphatic) and V(enous) classifications can be used to record such involvement (see page 10, TNM 8th edition [1]).

## Direct Spread

*Question*

Is a tumour that has spread directly from a gastric primary into an adjacent regional lymph node coded in the T or N category?

*Answer*

N category. Direct spread into a regional lymph node is classified as lymph node metastasis; direct spread into an adjacent organ, e.g. the liver from a gastric primary, is recorded in the T classification (see page 7, TNM 8th edition [1]).

## N Versus M

*Question*

For gastric carcinoma, when we find tumour nodules in the omentum, should we classify them as lymph node metastasis?

*Answer*

Unless the nodules are in the lymphatic drainage region (regional lymph nodes) they should be considered distant metastasis and classified M1 or pM1 (see page 62ff).

## Recurrent Tumour

*Question*

How can I classify a patient who had an apparently complete local excision of a carcinoma of the rectum, but was found, 2 years later, to have a recurrent tumour at the same site?

*Answer*

Use the recurrent tumour, r symbol. There must be a documented disease-free interval to use this symbol. For example, rT0N0M0 would designate the status during the disease-free interval and rT1N0M0 would indicate a recurrent tumour at the primary site (estimated clinically and confirmed by biopsy to be in the submucosa). After a second resection the result might be expressed as: rpT-2pN0M0, if the resected tumour was found pathologically to be in the muscularis propria.

In other cases, the recurrence in the area of the primary tumour may be indicated by 'rT+'.

**Example**

Local recurrence after simple mastectomy, 2 cm in greatest dimension, with or without invasion of skin or chest wall: rT+.

**Question**

If a patient has a primary resected colorectal carcinoma classified as pT3pN1bM0 and one year later develops metastatic disease, what is the correct TNM classification? T3N1M1?

**Answer**

The correct staging at the time of recurrence would be rT0N0M1 provided no recurrent primary tumour or regional lymph node metastasis is present. The original TNM status is not considered in a recurrent tumour.

**Question**

If the initial tumour was treated with chemotherapy and had a disease-free interval, should the recurrent tumour be classified as rpT or rypT?

**Answer**

The recurrent tumour could be classified as rcT or rpT.

**Question**

If the recurrent tumour was treated with chemotherapy, should yrpT be used or not?

**Answer**

No. For further discussion see TNM Supplement, page 20.

## Unknown Primary

**Question**

Unknown primary in the head and neck region. Cervical nodes are EBV positive. Histological methods should be used to identify EBV. Is immunohistochemistry EBV-LMP good enough? Is in situ hybridization required?

**Answer**

The UICC recommends the use of immunohistochemical methods to decide on HPV and EBV positivity. Molecular methods are not required [1].

**Question**

How do I classify a patient who has metastatic melanoma in a cervical lymph node less than 3 cm in greatest dimension without a primary or other metastasis?

**Answer**

T0pN1M0, stage III. The staging is based on the regional lymph node and/or distant metastasis status. In this case the site of metastasis is assumed to be regional.

## Sentinel Lymph Node

*Question*

How do I classify sentinel lymph node status?

*Answer*

The following is applicable when sentinel lymph node assessment is attempted:

pNX(sn)   Sentinel lymph node could not be assessed
pN0(sn)   No sentinel lymph node metastasis
pN1(sn)   Sentinel lymph node metastasis

*Question*

A patient underwent sentinel node biopsy prior to neoadjuvant treatment followed by surgery. The sentinel node was positive at that time but at resection the nodes were negative (ypN0 – no fibrosis). However, in view of the previous sentinel biopsy, the final TNM was given as pN1(sn) – is that correct? What would be the final TNM in the case where the original sentinel lymph node was core biopsied only?

*Answer*

A sentinel lymph node biopsy without removal of the primary breast carcinoma should be classified in this case as cN1(sn).

After the neo-adjuvant therapy, the examination of the primary tumour and the axillary regional lymph nodes, the lymph node findings should be classified as ypN0 if negative. The previous cN1(sn) findings should of course be taken into account for a treatment decision but there is no recommendation to have an overall summary classification.

*Question*

To classify a case as V1 or V2 do we have to demonstrate tumour cells in the lumen of the vessel or is an invasion sufficient to classify as V1 or V2?

*Answer*

Invasion of the vessel wall is sufficient to classify as V1 or V2.

## Site-Specific Questions

### Oral Cavity

*Question*

What is the rationale for removing invasion of extrinsic lingual muscles as a criterion for a pT4a oral cavity tumour in the TNM 8th edition [1]?

*Answer*

Extrinsic muscle (M. genioglossus, M. hyoglossus, M. palatoglossus and M. styloglossus) infiltration is no longer a criterion for the T4 category because DOI (depth of invasion) has been shown to be prognostically more important and extrinsic muscle invasion is difficult to assess (clinically and pathologically).

### Question

A 70-year-old male, squamous cell carcinoma, well differentiated, keratinizing variety on lateral border of tongue. Macroscopy: there are two lesions (1.7 × 1.0 cm and 0.5 × 0.5 cm), located very close to each other almost touching. Microsocopy: they are located 2–3 mm apart only. How should the tumour size be measured? Should they be combined or considered separately as done in breast malignancies? DOI is 5.8 mm and Worst Pattern of Invasion (WPOI) type 5 is seen because tumour satellites were seen 1.18 mm away from each other. 0 lymph nodes involved out of 55 lymph nodes examined in a neck dissection specimen.

### Answer

If there is an area of non-tumoural tissue between the two tumours, then it is recommended to classify them as two different tumour entities.

It is recommended to classify this case as pT2(2)pN0(0/55)M0.

### Question

What is the definition of the 'masticator space'?

### Answer

The masticator space (MS) is the lateral anatomic region below the middle cranial fossa and is defined by distinct fascial planes. The main fascial boundary is related to the superficial layer of the deep cervical fascia. This is also known as the investing fascia. The investing fascia is formed when the superficial layer of the deep cervical fascia splits at the lower margin of the body of the mandible and rises to enclose the muscles of mastication. Medially the fascia combines with another fascia, the interpterygoid fascia, and then rises up to the skull base. Laterally, the fascia rises up above the level of the zygomatic arch and covers the temporalis muscle. The zygomatic arch is used to subdivide the MS into a supra-zygomatic MS (portion above the zygomatic arch) and the nasopharyngeal MS (portion below the level of the zygomatic arch). The contents of the MS include the mandibular division of the fifth cranial nerve, the muscles of mastication, sections of the internal maxillary artery, the pterygoid plexus and the ramus and coronoid of the mandible. For lesions related to the lower alveolus, these would be related to the most inferior part of the masticator space that is still enclosed by the investing fascia [7] (see pages 35, 42, Plate 2.1).

### Question

How to stage an oral cavity carcinoma that has infiltrated to the subcutaneous layer of skin but with dermis and epidermis free of tumour?

*Answer*
We consider the subcutaneous layer of the skin as part of the skin and thus oral cavity carcinomas with invasion of this layer should be classified as pT4a.

*Question*
How to measure the depth of invasion in lip and oral cavity tumours in the case of exophytic or ulcerated tumours?

*Answer*
The *AJCC Cancer Staging Manual*, 8th edition [2], page 87, addresses this issue in two figures.

*Question*
In a left modified neck dissection, lymphovascular invasion was found with soft tissue extension but without any evidence of lymphoid tissue, along with other positive lymph nodes (5 in number/73 total lymph nodes) all without any ENE. Should this be reported ENE positive or negative? How should I determine its size as no capsule can be seen? This soft tissue deposit was smaller than other positive lymph nodes in size.

*Answer*
The classification of soft tissue deposits is difficult because we do not know the prognostic importance of these lesions. The UICC recommends considering them as lymph node metastasis. The case you describe could be classified as pN3b, considering the soft tissue deposit as an ENE+ lesion.

*Question*
Should a salivary gland tumour of the floor of the mouth be staged as an oral cavity tumour or as a major salivary gland carcinoma?

*Answer*
According to the 8th edition of the *TNM Classification of Malignant Tumours* [1], page 47, tumours arising in minor salivary glands should be classified at their anatomic site of origin (i.e. oral cavity) and are not included in the classification of major salivary glands.

## Oropharynx

*Question*
Regarding the N3b class criteria in p16-negative oropharyngeal carcinoma:

on page 25 of the 8th edition of the UICC TNM classification it states that N3b includes tumours with 'Metastasis in a single or multiple lymph nodes with CLINICAL extranodal extension'. Under the asterisk it says that 'The presence of skin involvement or soft tissue invasion with deep fixation/tethering to underlying muscle or adjacent structures or clinical signs of nerve involvement is classified as clinical extranodal extension'.

The use of the word 'clinical' here is a bit confusing, since it states in the introduction on page 4 that 'Clinical classification is based on evidence acquired before treatment by imaging, endoscopy, biopsy…', etc.

How should we classify a patient with radiological evidence of extranodal extension e.g. with extension to the sternocleidomastoid muscle but with no suspicion of such involvement in physical examination (palpation)? Should the tumours be classified according to the most accurate modality, i.e. in this case the finding on imaging?

**Answer**

Extranodal extension is poorly assessed by imaging and clinical examination is the most accurate modality. Assessment should be by clinical examination, which can be supported by radiological evidence but cannot be determined by radiological evidence alone, Chapter 2, page 40.

## Hypopharynx

**Question**

For hypopharyngeal cancer, invasion of the oesophagus has been added to the T4a category. However, in T3 extension to the oesophagus is still mentioned. How should this be interpreted?

**Answer**

The difference should be made between mucosal extension to the oesophagus (T3) or invasion of the oesophageal wall (T4a).

## Larynx

**Question**

Are there any changes to classify laryngeal squamous cell cancers in the 8th edition of the *TNM Classification of Malignant Tumours*?

**Answer**

Basically, there are no changes in the definition of the T and M categories for laryngeal cancer. There is an introduction of a separate cN and pN classification and extranodal extension is added as a descriptor in the N categories. We refer to the 8th edition of the UICC *TNM Classification of Malignant Tumours*, page 33 [1].

**Question**

Since the T classification of laryngeal tumours involves assessment of vocal cord fixation, does it mean that pT is not possible without such information given by the clinician?

*Answer*

For pathological classification concerning impaired mobility or fixation of vocal cords the information from the clinical T is used for the pathologic T. This is in accordance with TNM rule number 2: pathological classification 'is based on the evidence acquired before treatment, supplemented or modified by the additional evidence acquired from surgery and from pathological examination' (see page 1).

*Question*

In a total laryngectomy specimen including 6 tracheal rings of cartilage, what would a paratracheal lymph node towards the distal end of the trachea (below the thyroid cartilage and the thyroid) be regarded as? Would this still be considered a cervical lymph node and if so at what level?

*Answer*

This is an unusual situation. In the TNM Supplement (see page 36) the regional lymph nodes of head and neck carcinomas are described and listed. The paratracheal lymph nodes are included and should therefore be considered regional and are classified as level VIa (see Chapter 2, page 36).

*Question*

Regarding the definition of extranodal spread in the pN staging of head and neck SCC: in the AJCC TNM 8th edition description, there is a cutoff at 2 mm extension beyond the lymph node capsule to classify the lymph node as ENE positive. This is not stated in the UICC booklet. Should any extracapsular extension at histology be regarded as pENE+ (i.e. pN3b in most cases) or is there a cutoff at 2 mm as in the AJCC guidelines?

*Answer*

The AJCC recommends that pathologically detected ENE (extranodal extension) should be classified as either ENEmi (≤2 mm) or ENEma (>2 mm) for data collection and further testing purposes only, but both are considered ENE(+) for the definition of pN.

## Unknown Primary – Cervical Nodes

*Question*

Is it correct that (T0), which stands for occult primary, has been deleted for all head and neck TNM subsites except for HPV related and EBV positive neck node metastasis, where the primary tumour has not been found despite all diagnostic methods? Does that mean that we can only use TX for HPV and EBV negative neck node metastasis without any signs of primary tumour using all diagnostic methods (based on the assumption that the primary tumour can still be anywhere in the body/head and neck region)?

*Answer*

For unknown primary tumours with cervical lymph node metastasis of a squamous cell carcinoma (without HPV or EBV positivity in the neck nodes), a specific staging system for cN/pN/M has been introduced in the 8th TNM edition (see pages 40–44) and T0 is appropriate for these cases (and not TX).

Patients with HPV or EBV positive cervical nodes are staged according to their oropharyngeal or nasopharyngeal cN/pN/M categories, respectively. Also in these cases, T0 should be used.

## Thyroid Gland

*Question*

How do I stage a papillary carcinoma of the thyroid that has a small lymph node attached to the thyroid and focally involved by the papillary carcinoma?

*Answer*

The problem is addressed in the TNM booklet, 8th edition [1], page 7. Direct extension of the primary tumour into lymph nodes is classified as lymph node metastasis. Thus the case is classified as pN1a. If it is not evident from the resection specimen the surgeon has to mark the removed lymph node(s) to allow the pathologist to distinguish between pN1a and pN1b.

*Question*

Has the minimal extension beyond the thyroid gland disappeared in category T3 for thyroid gland cancer? If a tumour is less than 4 cm but shows minimal extension beyond the thyroid gland, is that a pT2?

*Answer*

Minor extrathyroidal extension was indeed intentionally removed from the definition of T3 disease. As a result, minor extrathyroidal extension does not affect either the T category or stage. The case should indeed be classified as pT2.

*Question*

Should a papillary carcinoma of the thyroid infiltrating anterior soft tissues be classified as pT4a?

*Answer*

According to the 8th edition of the TNM classification, the definition of a T4a/pT4a is that the tumour extends beyond the thyroid capsule and invades any of the following: subcutaneous soft tissues, larynx, trachea, oesophagus, recurrent laryngeal nerve. An invasion of subcutaneous soft tissues indeed justifies a T4a/pT4a classification.

*Question*

How do we classify a thyroid carcinoma with gross extrathyroidal extension into the sternothyroid muscle? Is this a pT4a?

*Answer*

According to the 8th edition of the *TNM Classification of Malignant Tumours* [1], invasion of the sternothyroid muscle is included in the definitions of T3b/pT3b.

*Question*

Is it correct that in the 8th edition the upper mediastinal lymph node metastases were changed from N1b into N1a?

*Answer*

The upper/superior mediastinal lymph nodes are indeed now in the 8th edition classified as N1a/pN1a (and were previously classified as N1b/pN1b).

*Question*

A poorly differentiated thyroid carcinoma in which a vascular invasion in the perithyroid muscle tissue is found. Should we consider this vascular invasion as an invasion of the perithyroid muscle tissue (i.e. T3b) or just a vascular invasion itself?

*Answer*

The findings of vascular invasion (L1 or V1) are not considered in the T or N categories of thyroid cancer. The case should be classified according to the T criteria.

*Question*

Thyroid cancer: there is no statement regarding involvement of parathyroid glands. A current case has a 3.5 cm papillary thyroid carcinoma with gross (can be seen on the slide with the naked eye) involvement of a parathyroid gland that is partly within and partly outside the thyroid gland. What would the staging be under TNM8? Is it pT2 or pT3b?

*Answer*

That is correct. An invasion of the parathyroid glands by a thyroid carcinoma is not explicitly mentioned or defined in the T categories. We would propose to classify this case as T4a.

## Oesophagus

*Question*

Is a tumour of the oesophagus with invasion of perioesophageal fatty tissue without infiltration of adjacent structures classified as pT3 or pT4? Does the perioesophageal fatty tissue belong to the mediastinum and thus to adjacent structures?

*Answer*

The described situation is classified as pT3. The fatty tissue belongs to the adventitia and not to adjacent structures such as bronchus, heart, pericardial sac and aorta.

## Question

The present definition of regional lymph nodes in oesophageal cancer is not very precise. How are the lymph nodes enumerated according to the Japanese nomenclature classified with regard to regional lymph nodes or distant metastasis? Are supraclavicular nodes considered regional lymph nodes or distant metastasis?

## Answer

A list of the lymph nodes with numbers of the Japanese classification and the proposal to classify involved lymph nodes as regional or distant metastasis is shown on page 47 of the Supplement, 4th edition and page 56 of the 5th edition. They are also listed in detail in the *AJCC Cancer Staging Manual*, 8th edition, pages 189–190. In general, the regional lymph nodes of the oesophagus, irrespective of the site of the primary tumour, are those in the oesophagus drainage area, including coeliac axis nodes and paraoesophageal nodes in the neck above the clavicle, but not non-paraoesophageal supraclavicular nodes as they are considered distant metastasis.

The problem was addressed in AJCC 8th edition [2], page 189:

'The nomenclature for cervical regional nodes follows that of head and neck chapters (see Chapter 6) and are located in periesophageal levels VI and VII. Lymph nodes in continuity with the esophagus would be considered regional.'

On page 59 of the 8th edition, Figure 5.1 and Table 5.1 clarify this definition. Supraclavicular lymph nodes are in boundary levels IV and VB. Since they are not in levels VI and VII (which are perioesophageal) they are not regional lymph nodes for the esophagus. They are distant metastasis.

## Question

How do we classify small tumour cell-complexes in regional lymph nodules of an oesophageal carcinoma after neoadjuvant therapy? Some lymph nodes have several small tumour cell complexes (each < 0.1 cm) and some are only identified by immunohistochemistry.

## Answer

According to the description, the tumour cell complexes could be considered as isolated tumour cells (ITCs). We suggest classifying the findings as ypN0(i+) and to document in how many regional lymph nodes these ITC could be detected. Data to understand the prognostic impact of these findings are needed.

## Question

An oesophagogastrectomy specimen (adenocarcinoma of the lower oesophagus, status after neo-adjuvant therapy) with the tumour classified as ypT2N0 are, according to the TNM 8th edition, shows the presence of two malignant glands in the capsule of a bronchial lymph node. The other 20 nodes are negative. There are no regression changes in any of the lymph nodes. Should this be classified as ypN0, ypN1 or ypN1mi?

*Answer*
The case should be classified as ypT2pN1cM0. If the glands measure less than 2 mm you might add a 'mi', ypT2pN1micM0.

*Question*
Should we use the prefix 'y' for tumours in oesophagectomy specimens, which have previously been treated by endomucosal resection (EMR)?

*Answer*
Endomucosal resection does not qualify for using the prefix 'y'.

The 'y' symbol should be used in cases in which classification is performed during or following multimodality therapy. EMR should be considered as a biopsy assuming the margins are positive. If the margins are negative the pathology from the EMR can be used to determine the pT category.

*Question*
Do you classify coeliac axis or left gastric artery nodes as M1 or N for an oesophageal cancer that involves the lower 5 cm of the oesophagus and spreads to the proximal 2 cm of the stomach with no other sites of disease apart from perioesophageal or perigastric nodes?

*Answer*
Direct spread to the stomach by an oesophageal tumour makes the lymph nodes of the stomach regional and therefore they should be classified in the N category (depending on number of involved lymph nodes) and not as M1/pM1.

## Stomach

*Question*
Are tumours of the cardia whose epicentre is within 2 cm of the oesophagogastric junction (OGJ), but in which there is no involvement of the OGJ, staged according to gastric cancer TNM?

*Answer*
According to the 8th edition of the *TNM Classification of Malignant Tumours*, cardia cancers not involving the OGJ are classified as stomach tumours.

*Question*
A post-chemotherapy gastrectomy case with signet ring cell carcinoma shows one clearly positive lymph node. Immunohistochemistry showed one positive cell in 5 other regional lymph nodes?

*Answer*

The one positive regional lymph node is classified as ypN1. It seems difficult to classify the other findings. Strictly, these findings should be classified as isolated tumour cells (ITCs) and should not be considered in the N classification. On the other hand, this might represent regressive changes of lymph node metastasis after chemotherapy and should then be classified as ypN2.

Rule no. 4 should be applied; 'if in doubt use the lower stage', i.e. ypN1.

*Question*

How should I classify the N or M category in the case of supraclavicular lymph node metastasis of a signet-ring cell carcinoma of the stomach?

*Answer*

The supraclavicular lymph node metastasis is classified as pM1 LYM.

*Question*

What will be the stage in stomach cancer with omental deposits?

*Answer*

Omental deposits correspond to peritoneal metastasis and should therefore be classified as M1/pM1 (Stage IV). In rare cases, these deposits are lymph node metastases and might be considered regional lymph node metastases if they are located in lymph nodes number 4a or 4b, according to the Japanese Nomenclature.

*Question*

A gastric cardia carcinoma infiltrates the subserosa of the stomach and extends to the muscularis propria and adventitia of the oesophagus (resection margin). Should this be classified as T4b?

*Answer*

Intramural extension of a gastric tumour into the duodenum or oesophagus is classified by the depth of greatest invasion in any of these sites including the stomach. In this case, the extension of the stomach adenocarcinoma into the oesophagus should be classified as pT3 and not as T4b.

If the carcinoma was demonstrated in the circumferential resection margin, the addition of the R1 classification (oesophagus) would be appropriate.

*Question*

Radical gastrectomy specimen with a part of the left lobe of the liver and the gallbladder, adherent to the posterior surface of the stomach. On microscopy, the serosal layer of the stomach is involved and the liver parenchyma is free. However, the serosal layer of the gallbladder is microscopically involved by the tumour. What should be the pTNM stage – pT4a M1 or pT4b?

*Answer*

We would suggest classifying the stomach tumour as pT4b, provided this is a direct invasion by serosa of the stomach into the serosa of the gallbladder.

## Colon and Rectum

*Question*

In carcinoma of the colon is a tumour that has reached the serosal surface classified as pT3 or pT4? What is the definition of reaching the serosa? In some places it is taken to be a tumour that is within 1 mm of the serosal surface.

*Answer*

T3 covers tumours in the subserosa, i.e. those beneath the serosal surface.

   T4 applies to tumours that 'perforate visceral peritoneum', i.e. the serosal surface (see page 71).

*Question*

I have a carcinoma of the sigmoid colon extending in the submucosa. In a vein in the pericolic fat there is a tumour thrombus. Metastasis is present in 1 of 8 regional lymph nodes. How should this case be staged?

*Answer*

The case is classified as pT1pN1a(1/8)cM0, V1. Venous invasion is neither considered in the T or in the N category (see page 24).

*Question*

If only 4 negative lymph nodes are found in a rectal cancer specimen post-neoadjuvant chemoradiotherapy, will the nodal stage be ypN0 or ypNX?

*Answer*

The case should be classified as ypN0(0/4) and should be separately evaluated.

*Question*

How should we classify the following case: a pT4a colorectal cancer with extensive omental deposits, M1b representing a peritoneal metastasis? Or pT4b if it should be viewed as direct extension into an adjacent structure?

*Answer*

According to the UICC TNM 8th edition [1], the omental deposits should be classified as peritoneal metastasis, pM1.

*Question*

In a patient with adenocarcinoma of colon there was full thickness penetration of the wall, 13 positive nodes and also a 'free-floating' focus of carcinoma in the peritoneal cavity. No other peritoneal tumour was found. Should that be staged as T0, TX or T1?

*Answer*

The case should be considered as pM1, because there was tumour in the peritoneal cavity separate from the primary. The primary tumour would be classified as pT3, or if it penetrated the serosa, pT4a, and pN2b because of the number of nodes involved.

*Question*

How do I classify a carcinoma in a diverticulum of the sigmoid colon with penetration of the muscularis propria and penetration into the pericolic fat? The diverticulum is lined by a thin fibrous membrane. There are 31 regional lymph nodes without metastasis and no distant metastasis.

*Answer*

The case should be classified as pT3pN0(0/31)M0.

*Question*

In the 6th and 7th editions of the TNM classification [8, 9], tumour deposits (TDs) are recorded as a site-specific factor. It appears they do not affect the N classification unless no lymph nodes are involved, in which case it is designated as N1c. How would you classify a tumour that has three involved lymph nodes and four tumour deposits without lymphoid tissue? Would it be N1bTD4?

*Answer*

The case is classified as pN1b. The TDs should be separately counted (see page 72). It may sometimes be difficult to count TDs correctly. For that issue I may refer you to the TNM booklet [9], page 103. In addition, you need to be sure that TDs are not lymph node metastasis.

*Question*

Do pericolic tumour deposits (TDs) correspond to positive regional lymph nodes in colorectal carcinoma or is N1c/pN1c used only in the absence of lymph node metastasis?

*Answer*

N1c/pN1c is used only in the absence of regional lymph node metastasis.

*Question*

I have a case of colon carcinoma with discontinuous extramural extension and with two regional lymph node metastases. How do classify this case? pN1b or pN1c?

*Answer*

The case you describe is classified as pN1b and pT3 because of the discontinuous extension of the primary tumour. pN1c is only applicable if there are no regional lymph node metastases.

## Question

Is a rectal carcinoma that extends into the anus a T3 or a T4?

## Answer

The TNM supplement states that: 'Intramural direct extension from one subsite (segment) of the colon to an adjacent one is not considered in the T classification. The same applies to intramural direct extension from the rectum to the anal canal'. The T category is determined by the depth of penetration (see page 71).

## Question

Is a rectal carcinoma infiltrating the levators to be considered as T3 or a T4?

## Answer

We suggest a rectal carcinoma infiltrating the levators is classified as T4b (invasion of adjacent structures). This is based on:

- The poor prognosis
- Difficulty in achieving an R0 state (no residual tumour)
- Radical surgery required

## Question

I have a rectal carcinoma below the peritoneal reflection that perforates the mesorectal fascia but does not affect peritoneal serosa. Is this a pT3 or pT4 tumour?

## Answer

pT3 seems to be correct.

We have no data to classify the perforation of the mesorectal fascia as T4/pT4.

## Question

A colorectal carcinoma of the coecum presented at surgery with adhesions to segments of the small intestine and the bladder dome. Parts of the bladder wall and the small intestine were resected. However, in the embedded material there is a tumour close to the perivesical fat but not in the perivesical fat or muscular bladder wall; in fact the adhesions showed only extensive acute inflammation and granulation tissue. Should this still be called a tumour, which infiltrates pericolic fat, pT3 or pT4 due to the fact that it is difficult to tell due to the inflamed fibrotic tissue in the adhesions where the pericolic fat ends?

## Answer

Please see page 74 of the UICC TNM book, 8th edition [1]: a tumour that is adherent to other organs or structures, macroscopically, is classified as cT4b. However, if no tumour is present in the adhesion, microscopically, the classification should be pT1–3 (pT3 in your case), depending on the anatomical depth of wall invasion.

## Question

Does a serosal penetration in a colonic adenocarcinoma influence R classification? There are no known clinical metastases and more than 1 mm to mesocolic resection.

## Answer

The perforation of a colorectal carcinoma is not considered in the R classification; e.g. if other tumour margins are without tumour invasion the case can be classified as R0.

## Question

I received a colon tumour that is a moderately differentiated adenocarcinoma and approximately 50% at most mucinous. I was able to find multiple mesenteric lymph nodes that are negative for the tumour. However, three of the lymph nodes had mucinous pools in them. Despite multiple serial sections of at least three levels, I could find no atypical cells. I feel that I cannot call these pools of mucin metastatic tumour even though I believe the mucin is from the lesion. I have made note of the mucin in the report, but I am unsure how to classify these lymph node findings. What is the current consensus concerning this type of lesion under these circumstances?

## Answer

The TNM approach depends on whether there has been neoadjuvant therapy. If the surgery was done after neoadjuvant therapy, mucin pools without tumour cells in the bowel wall or lymph nodes are not considered positive for tumour. If there has been no neoadjuvant therapy, mucin pools are considered positive for tumour.

## Question

What is UICC's position on whether a post-treatment metastatic lymph node containing no viable tumour cells should be regarded as positive? Current guidance from the Royal College of Pathologists is that a lymph node is only regarded as positive if viable malignant cells are present at the time of resection; if not it is designated yN0.

## Answer

Such findings in a regional lymph node in the drainage area of CRC should be classified as ypN0.

The post-neoadjuvant therapy pathological N category (ypN) must be based on the largest continuous focus of residual cancer in the lymph nodes.

## Question

We have a patient who had a mucinous adenocarcinoma of the rectum. After neoadjuvant therapy we only could find mucinous masses in the intestinal wall and in 3 of 19 regional lymph nodes, there was no distant metastasis clinically. How is this case classified according to TNM?

*Answer*

This case (after neoadjuvant therapy) is classified as ypT0pN0(0/19)M0. Mucinous masses without viable tumour cells are not considered in the ypTanypN classification.

*Question*

I have a rectal mucinous adenocarcinoma (pT3) and metastasis to one of 16 regional lymph nodes (pN1a). An additional lymph node with metastasis was received located at the pelvic wall. Should this lymph node metastasis be considered among the regional lymph nodes or is it a distant metastasis?

*Answer*

If the lymph node localization is interpreted as lateral sacral or mesorectal, this lymph node metastasis being regional would change the classification to pT3pN1b(2/17)M0, Stage IIIB. However, if it was an external iliac lymph node it would be considered to be pM1.

*Question*

In a colon carcinoma with invasion of the Gerota fascia but not the kidney, is this T3 or T4?

*Answer*

Gerota's fascia should be considered an adjacent structure and should therefore be classified as T4b/pT4b.

*Question*

For rectal adenocarcinoma that is invading beyond the muscularis propria but not involving lymph nodes, would invasion of the anal skin (undermining the anal squamous epithelium close to the distal excision margin) upstage the tumour from pT3 to pT4?

*Answer*

If no sphincter structures are involved the case should be classified as T3/pT3.

*Question*

Which R classification is appropriate to describe intraoperative tumour perforation in resection of rectal cancer, if macroscopically and microscopically the tumour is completely removed?

*Answer*

It is classified as R0. The T category is not implied by perforation. Perforation should be documented separately because of the poorer prognosis.

## Question

A previous version of the TNM classification stated that if there is colon perforation from a colorectal cancer, it should be classified as T4. Does this still hold true or do you need to see tumour at the serosa regardless of whether there is perforation?

## Answer

The definition of T4a/pT4a in the 8th edition of TNM is:

T4a    Tumour perforates visceral peritoneum.

This means that tumour cells have to be demonstrable at the peritoneal surface of the perforation site. If you have a tumour with invasion of muscularis propria and perforation, then this case should be classified as pT2.

## Question

Which TNM classification should be used for a mixed adenoneuroendocrine carcinoma (MANEC) of the colon – the classification for carcinomas of the colon or the one for gastrointestinal neuroendocrine tumours?

## Answer

The MANECs should be classified according to the TNM classification of colon carcinoma.

## Question

Is there a classification for malignant melanomas of the rectum? Can they be classified according to the TNM of the skin?

## Answer

There has been no specific TNM classification for malignant melanomas of the rectum. There are not enough data to propose a TNM classification. The TNM for skin melanoma cannot be used for this situation.

## Question

In a right hemicolectomy for colonic cancer 15 tumour-free lymph nodes are found and one completely necrotic lymph node metastasis (round focus, very much reminiscent). In the necrosis, some immunohistochemical positivity is found for pancytokeratin but no vital tumour at all. Should I integrate this finding into the TNM classification, and, if yes, how?

## Answer

Provided no neoadjuvant therapy has been administered to this patient, the findings in one out of 16 regional lymph nodes should be classified as pN1a(1/16).

*Question*

How should we classify an adenocarcinoma of the colon ascendens with meso-colonic infiltration, infiltration per continuitatem in mesenterial fat and appendix vermiformis?

*Answer*

The case should be classified as pT4b.

*Question*

We have no consensus in our team about the pT category of an adenocarcinoma of colon descendens with infiltration of the lateral abdominal wall.

*Answer*

This type of invasion is considered 'invasion of an adjacent structure' and should therefore be classified as pT4b. If you have an extension of a carcinoma of the caecum within the bowel wall to the ileum, this should be classified as pT2 if the depth of invasion is limited to muscularis propria. If you have a perforation of the serosa by a caecal carcinoma with invasion of the ileum via serosa this should be classified as pT4b.

*Question*

How to classify the following situation? A right hemicolectomy specimen en block with a Whipple resection. There is a tumour arising in the right colon invading directly into the duodenum and peripancreatic fat. There is metastatic carcinoma in a single lymph node at the head of the pancreas (i.e. classically regarded as a non-regional lymph node for a colorectal tumour) – for staging purposes is this still counted as non-regional lymph node involvement (M1a)? Or since the tumour has directly invaded this region are the peripancreatic lymph nodes now counted as regional lymph nodes and included in the N part for staging?

*Answer*

If a tumour involves more than one site or subsite, e.g. contiguous extension to another site or subsite, the regional lymph nodes include those of all involved sites or subsites. Thus, the peripancreatic lymph node should be considered regional and counted for the pN classification.

*Question*

Rectal cancer: how should invasion of the internal sphincter and/or external sphincter be staged?

*Answer*

Direct invasion of the musculus sphincter ani internus and/or externus and/or levator ani is considered invasion of adjacent organs or structures and should be classified as pT4b.

## Anal Canal
*Question*

A surgical resection of a squamous cell anal cancer (14 cm diameter) with extensive infiltration of perianal skin, reaching scrotal skin. Should this be classified as pT4?

*Answer*

It should be considered a T3/pT3 tumour. The note in the 8th TNM edition (page 78) states that 'Direct invasion of the rectal wall, perianal skin, subcutaneous tissue or the sphincter muscle(s) alone is not classified as T4' but according to the size of the tumour (T1–T3).

*Question*

I have a case of an anal carcinoma that falls into the ypT2 category. There is one mesorectal and one external iliac lymph node positive. How should we classify the N category?

*Answer*

The definition of the regional lymph nodes of the anal canal cancers has been changed in the 8th edition. N2 and N3 categories were removed and new categories N1a, N1b and N1c are defined. Metastases in external iliac and mesorectal lymph nodes should be classified as pN1c (see UICC TNM 8th edition booklet, pages 77–78).

## Liver (Hepatocellular Carcinoma) – Intrahepatic Bile Ducts
*Question*

If there is a nodule of HCC measuring 1.1 cm and a larger nodule showing features of MRN, high grade dysplasia and area of early HCC. The whole nodule measures 4.4 cm. Is this a pT1 or pT2?

*Answer*

The case should be classified as pT2 because both HCCs are less than 5 cm.

*Question*

How should the following case be staged? An 8 cm hepatocellular lesion showing areas of adenoma and others suggesting well-differentiated hepatocellular carcinoma (sometimes there is no clear demarcation between the adenoma and hepatocarcinoma areas). There is no vascular invasion or tumour involving a major branch of the portal or hepatic vein(s). The lesion is confined to the liver.

*Answer*

We would consider the 8 cm tumour a hepatocellular carcinoma. According to the 8th edition of the UICC TNM classification, this case should be classified as pT1b.

*Question*

A patient with intrahepatic cholangiocarcinoma has metastasis in para-aortic lymph nodes. Is this finding classified as N1, N2 or M1?

*Answer*

The definition of the regional lymph nodes for right-liver and left-liver intrahepatic cholangiocarcinoma is shown on page 83 of the TNM 8th edition booklet. It does not include para-aortic lymph nodes, involvement of which should therefore be classified as M1 or pM1 if histologically proven. Neither in the UICC [1] nor in the AJCC classification [2] is a definition of N2 lymph nodes provided.

*Question*

Intrahepatic cholangiocarcinoma: if the tumour invades the gallbladder directly from the liver, should this be classified as pT4? In the list of adjacent organs gallbladder is not mentioned in the UICC/AJCC 8th editions.

*Answer*

This question underlines the difficulty of applying the TNM classification in clinical practice. Gallbladder is indeed not considered in the T classification of intrahepatic cholangiocarcinoma. Examples for extrahepatic structures are duodenum or colon. We recommend this to be classified as T3/pT3.

*Question*

Is there an in-situ classification for intrahepatic bile duct carcinoma? Tis is deemed a category, but there is no corresponding stage in the booklet. Is a T1 category still valid or should there only be T1a and T1b?

*Answer*

The TNM 8th edition indeed includes Tis carcinoma in situ (intraductal tumour) for intrahepatic bile duct tumours. Lesions classified as carcinoma in situ should meet histologic criteria for biliary intraepithelial neoplasia grade 3 (BilIN-3) or for high-grade dysplasia in an intraductal papillary lesion or mucinous cystic lesion. Stage 0, although initially not listed in the stage group for intrahepatic bile duct neoplasms, is appropriate. Page 11 of the UICC classification states that carcinoma in situ is categorized as Stage 0.

For the T classification: only T1a and T1b are included. If there is uncertainty about the size of a solitary lesion without vascular invasion T1a is appropriate, following rule 4 p4 of the UICC TNM classification; if in doubt then the lower category should be chosen.

## Gallbladder

*Question*

In the case of a gallbladder carcinoma, a partial hepatectomy specimen was submitted, which showed an invasion of liver parenchyma and about 1.5 cm away from the invasion a 0.4 cm nodule without macroscopic or microscopic connection to the invasive tumour. How should this nodule be classified?

*Answer*

This nodule should be classified as pM1.

*Question*

How to classify an intracystic papillary neoplasm of gallbladder with focal invasion into the wall. Unable to stage it as the wall is markedly thinned out and fibrosed and the various layers are not made out. How do I classify this case? The neoplasm, however, is limited to the gallbladder wall.

*Answer*

Identifying substructures of the gallbladder wall can be difficult. We would recommend this case to be classified as a carcinoma and stage as pT1 'Tumour invades lamina propria or muscular layer' with a comment that a subdivision in pT1a and pT1b is not possible.

## Bile Ducts – Perihilar Bile Ducts

*Question*

In a case of perihilar cholangiocarcinoma (Klatskin tumour) with direct (per continuitatem) invasion of the pancreas, how is this finding classified?

*Answer*

Although the invasion of the pancreas is not explicitly mentioned in the T categories of perihilar tumours, it is recommended to use the definition of T3 of the distal bile duct tumours and thus this case should be classified as pT3.

*Question*

Perihilar bile ducts: pT3 is defined by tumour invasion of unilateral branches of the portal vein or hepatic artery. My question is: does invasion of the external layer (tunica adventitia) of the blood vessels count as pT3 or is direct invasion of the muscle layer (tunica media) necessary?

*Answer*

Invasion of the external layer (tunica adventitia) is sufficient to classify as vascular invasion, pT3.

## Bile Ducts – Distal Extrahepatic Bile Duct

*Question*

In TNM8 of distal bile ducts, T category is now in millimetres. How does this translate to invasion depth, since the wall of the bile duct is only 1–2 mm thick? We presume this millimetre category is easier for radiology, but what is the starting point of mm measurement in the histopathological evaluation? What is the TNM 8th edition T category for:

(A) a polypoid carcinoma, with a diameter of 13 mm, but that invades only 1 mm to the bile duct muscular layer;

(B) a carcinoma that has an ulcerated surface that is 1 mm below the surrounding bile duct lumen and extends 6 mm to the surrounding tissues;

(C) a lengthy tumour that grows beneath bile duct mucosa, and a deepest invasion is 6 mm measured from the intact mucosal surface, but only 4 mm if measured from the innermost tumour cell from the outermost edge of invasion?

**Answer**

The definitions of T categories by mm was changed because of poor reproducibility of the former definitions and because of better prognostic impact of the new T categories.

The thickness of the tumours has to be taken into account in the invasive area of the bile duct wall. Therefore the deepest tumour invasion (from the basal lamina of adjacent normal or dysplastic epithelium) can be identified and measured (see also the *AJCC Cancer Staging Manual*, 8th edition [2], page 321).

Example (A)    pT1
Example (B)    pT2
Example (C)    pT1

**Question**

What is the T category for a bile duct carcinoma of the extrahepatic bile ducts that infiltrate the surrounding tissue? How can the T categories be understood? What do 5 to 12 mm (pT2) or over 12 mm (pT3) infiltration mean – across or along? What about the Infiltration of the surrounding tissue?

**Answer**

The millimetres in the definition of the T categories correspond to the depth of invasion. In the definitions of T1–T3, the invasion of adjacent tissue is not considered. Some structure involvement is mentioned in T4 (coeliac axis, superior mesenteric artery and/or the common hepatic artery).

**Question**

In the case of an adenocarcinoma of the distal bile duct near the uncinate process of the pancreas, the pancreas is infiltrated for > 2 cm with peripancreatic node direct infiltration. How can the T and N categories be classified?

**Answer**

In the 8th edition of the TNM classification of malignant tumours for tumours of the distal extrahepatic bile ducts, the depth of invasion is essential in the T1–T3 categories. An invasion of the pancreas is no longer a criterion of the T category.

The direct invasion of one peripancreatic lymph node should be classified as pN1.

## Ampulla of Vater

*Question*

How can an invasive adenocarcinoma be classified that arises in an intra-ampul-
lary papillary neoplasm, extensively infiltrating the duodenum and periduodenal/
peripancreatic soft tissue with focal minimal infiltration of the pancreas? There
is no duodenal serosal involvement.

*Answer*

This case should be classified as a carcinoma of the ampulla of Vater. Following
the description of the anatomical extent of the primary tumour, we propose to
classify it as pT3b (8th edition, UICC TNM classification).

*Question*

What is the significance of subclassification of T3 in ampullary carcinomas (like
infiltration of 0.5 cm into the pancreas and more)?

*Answer*

The difference between the definitions of T3a/pT3a and T3b/pT3b in tumours of
the ampulla of Vater is based on prognostic aspects.

## Pancreatic Tumours

*Question*

My question is about the new TNM 8th edition for pancreatic adenocarcinoma
(page 94), particularly regarding a T3 tumour.

1. In the new TNM, how to classify a tumour extended beyond the pancreas (for
   example into the peripancreatic fat) but without vessel involvement?
2. A tumour of the tail, 3 cm in greatest dimension and invading the adjacent
   stomach serosa. How to classify this tumour?

*Answer*

1. A pancreatic tumour with invasion of peripancreatic tissue but without invasion of vessels (coeliac axis, superior mesenteric artery and/or common
   hepatic artery) is still classified according to size. Peripancreatic extension
   may be difficult to determine because of the absence of a pancreatic capsule
   and is no longer considered in the T category.
2. Tumour extension in the stomach, spleen, left adrenal gland and peritoneum
   for the pancreatic body or tail tumours does not affect the T category any-
   more. It is classified according to size, in this case a pT2.

*Question*

A ductal carcinoma of the pancreas measures 5 cm in greatest dimension involving
the head and body of the pancreas. It does not show extrapancreatic extension
but it invades the common bile duct within the head of the pancreas. There is one

pancreaticoduodenal and one common bile duct lymph node positive for metastatic carcinoma of 16 examined lymph nodes. Is this a T2N1 or T3N1 tumour?

**Answer**

The case is classified as pT3pN1(2/16)cM0 (see page 80 of the TNM supplement).

**Question**

A Whipple specimen containing pancreatic ductal adenocarcinoma infiltrates the duodenal wall. Size > 2 cm. No peripancreatic spread. Should this be classified pT2 or pT3?

**Answer**

According to the 8th edition of the TNM classification of pancreatic tumours, the tumour should be classified as T2/pT2 (more than 2 cm but no more than 4 cm) or T3/pT3 (more than 4 cm) depending on size. The invasion of the duodenal wall is not a criterion in the definitions for the T categories.

**Question**

There seems to be no clear definition of pancreas carcinoma of 1 cm in the TNM 8th edition:

T1b    Tumour greater than 0.5 cm and less than 1 cm

T1c    Tumour greater than 1 cm but no more than 2 cm

**Answer**

This is indeed a typographic error, it should read: T1b Tumour greater than 0.5 cm but no more than 1 cm, T1c Tumour greater than 1 cm but no more than 2 cm.

**Question**

Should a ductal carcinoma of the pancreas with invasion of the superior mesenteric vein be staged as T4/pT4? The tumour diameter is 3.4 cm.

**Answer**

In the absence of arterial involvement (coeliac axis, superior mesenteric artery, common hepatic artery), the T category is based on size, regardless of invasion of adjacent organs or veins. The vein and others are considered resectable and are therefore not explicitly mentioned in the T4 category. The case should be classified as pT2.

## Neuroendocrine Tumours of the Gastrointestinal Tract

**Question**

How do I classify a 3 cm primary well-differentiated endocrine tumour of the small bowel with a mesenteric mass (lymph node metastasis)?

*Answer*

This case is classified as pT2pN1M0, if the mesenteric mass is not larger than 2 cm and if there are no distant metastases. If the size of the mass is greater than 2 cm then stage as pT2N2M0. As the size of the mass is not indicated use the lower category (Rule No. 4).

*Question*

How should a well-differentiated neuroendocrine carcinoma of the appendix (malignant carcinoid) with spread into mesoappendix be classified? Is it pT3 (like adenocarcinomas)?

*Answer*

Carcinoids of the appendix have their own TNM classification (as from the 7th edition [9]). This case should be classified as pT3 ('tumour more than 4 cm or with subserosal invasion or involvement of the mesoappendix').

*Question*

Well-differentiated NETs (grades 1 and 2) are classified specifically as NET whereas grade 3 is classified as carcinomas in general, according to the specific organ TNM.

How should the NX or the N0 category for NETs grade 1 and 2 be used because this is only commented under the appendix tumours on page 100; '... will ordinarily include 12 or more lymph nodes. If the lymph nodes are negative, but the number ordinarily examined is not met, classify as pN0'?

*Answer*

Recommendations for lymph node numbers are only provided for neuroendocrine tumours of the appendix because data were available to make a recommendation. In other sites, no clear (evidence-based) figures were available. Irrespective of the site of the primary, if all lymph nodes in a specimen are negative, stage as pN0 whatever the number of nodes resected.

*Question*

Is there any TNM classification for neuroendocrine tumours of the urinary system (bladder, testis, kidney, prostate)?

*Answer*

To the best of our knowledge, there are no recommendations as to TNM classifications for neuroendocrine tumours of the genitourinary system. Poorly differentiated neuroendocrine carcinomas should be classified as carcinomas of the specific organ, e.g. bladder, kidney and prostate.

For well-differentiated neuroendocrine tumours (G1 and G2) neither UICC nor AJCC offer a classification because there are not enough data to base such a classification on solid findings.

**Question**
How can the following situation be classified? A grade 2 neuroendocrine tumour involves the colon and the appendix. The tumours are discontinuous, with the bulk of the tumour in the colon. The tumour has penetrated the visceral peritoneum. Does spread to the appendix count as a metastasis?
**Answer**
If the tumours were continuous, since the main part of the tumour is in the colon, we recommend to classify it as a pT4 NET grade 2 of the colon (the tumour perforates the visceral peritoneum or invades other organs) according to the TNM 8th edition, classification of neuroendocrine tumours of the colon and rectum (page 101, TNM UICC, 8th edition [1]). As the tumours are discontinuous the appendix tumour should also be staged using the schema for neuroendocrine tumours of the appendix (page 100).

**Question**
What TNM should I use for well-differentiated neuroendocrine tumours G3 of the pancreas?
**Answer**
The TNM classification of neuroendocrine tumours of the pancreas comprises well-differentiated (G1 and G2) neuroendocrine tumours and according to a recommendation of the European Neuroendocrine Tumour Society (ENETS) also the rare cases of NET G3 [10, 11].

## Lung Tumours
**Question**
Does the 8th edition of the TNM classification for lung cancer cover all lung cancers including small cell lung cancer?
**Answer**
The classification applies to carcinomas of the lung including non-small cell carcinomas, small cell carcinomas and bronchopulmonary carcinoid tumour (see page 85).

**Question**
A tumour infiltrates the main bronchus less than 2 cm from the carina, without infiltration of the carina. According to the 7th edition it would have been pT3.
   How do I classify this tumour according to the TNM 8th edition?
**Answer**
The case you describe should be classified according to the size of the tumour, as pT2a (>3 but ≤ 4 cm), pT2b (>4 but ≤ 5 cm), pT3 (>5 but ≤ 7 cm) or pT4 (>7 cm) (see TNM8, page 107).

**Question**

For lung carcinomas, does T2 invasion of visceral pleura mean perforation of the pleural membrane?

**Answer**

T2 invasion of visceral pleura includes either of the following:

- Tumour reaches the elastic membrane of the visceral pleura.
- Tumour is present on the surface of the visceral pleura.

**Question**

If a lung tumour that is < 3 cm (2.8 cm) in maximum dimension with no visceral pleural invasion involves the bronchus intermedius, is it a T1 or a T2 tumour?

**Answer**

Bronchus intermedius should not be considered as part of the right main bronchus. The correct classification for the described tumour therefore is T1b/pT1b.

**Question**

Regarding the T classification of lung carcinoma, if a tumour is 3 cm and grows by direct invasion through a fissure to involve by direct invasion the adjacent lobe, does it become a T2 or T4?

**Answer**

A tumour with local invasion of another lobe without a tumour on the pleural surface should be classified as T2, in the 8th edition T2a/pTa. This classification changes if other features such as size dictate a higher T category.

**Question**

A pleural nodule is classified as M1a. Can you provide a clear definition of 'a pleural nodule'?

**Answer**

A pleural nodule is a nodule that is in the pleura, either parietal or visceral pleura.

There can be malignant pleural effusion without pleural nodules, and vice versa there can be pleural nodules without malignant pleural effusion.

In summary, 'a pleural nodule' is a tumour nodule that is on the surface of the pleura or within its tissue. The pleura is a thin tissue, like a sheet, that covers the inside of the ribs, diaphragm and mediastinum, and also covers the surface of the lungs. Tumour implants on or in between these two surfaces are pleural nodules. The nodules are not floating in the pleural fluid and may also exist without fluid.

**Question**

Only the invasive component is used as a descriptor of the T categories. Is this a recommendation and is this concept already applied in the TNM 8th edition (2017) of lung tumours?

*Answer*

This fact is included in the 8th edition of the *TNM Classification of Lung Tumours*, and is based on recommendations of the IASLC. See also the general rule TNM supplement, page 1ff. When size is a criterion for T/pT category, it is the measurement of the invasive component.

*Question*

Recommendation IASLC: for lung non-mucinous adenocarcinoma it is recommended to determine tumour size according to the invasive size excluding the lepidic component. Question: does this also apply for mucinous tumours?

*Answer*

Invasive mucinous adenocarcinomas should be staged as other invasive adenocarcinomas, i.e. only the invasive size being used as the T descriptor (regardless of the extent of the lepidic component). In lung cancer, TNM staging traditionally has been based on total tumour size, but data are accumulating in both the radiologic and pathologic literature to support the concept that invasive size is a better predictor of survival than is total tumour size in lung adenocarcinoma.

*Question*

According to the 8th TNM edition, how should you classify a lung tumour > 7 cm that is not infiltrating any structures; in the TNM 7th edition it would be T3.

*Answer*

According to the 8th edition of the TNM classification, the case you describe should be classified as T4.

*Question*

How do I classify a patient with a 2 cm primary adenocarcinoma of the RUL of lung with multiple deposits of adenocarcinoma in the RLL, negative lymph nodes and no other metastases?

*Answer*

This is classified as T4 (separate tumour nodules in a different lobe) and since the secondary tumour was histologically confirmed, it is pT4 (see page 88).

*Question*

Can you please define 'mediastinum' in lung cancer being classified as T4 as opposed to mediastinal pleura being classified as T3. In addition, how is intrapericardial resection with tumour in the fat underneath the pericardial pericardium but not infiltrating the pericardial fibrous tissue T categorized?

*Answer*

Until the 4th edition published in 1987 and 1992 [4, 5] the highest T category was 'T3' and this included the descriptor 'mediastinal invasion'. In the 5th edition [8] the T4 category was reintroduced and invasion of the mediastinum and contents were divided between 'T3' and 'T4'. 'Mediastinal pleura and 'parietal pericardium' remained 'T3' while invasion of 'heart', 'great vessels', etc., became 'T4'. In the 8th edition, T3 and T4 categories were reconsidered, the category 'mediastinal pleura' disappeared and 'T3' is now covering direct invasion of 'parietal pleura, phrenic nerve or parietal pericardium'. The 'direct invasion of diaphragm' is considered as T4.

Direct extension to parietal pericardium is considered as T3 and direct extension to visceral pericardium is considered as T4.

My interpretation has been that 'mediastinum' was retained and assigned to the new T4 category, to cover all the contents that were not specifically assigned to 'T3' or 'T4', i.e. mediastinal fat, connective tissue, thymus, etc. We assume that by describing invasion into the fat 'underneath' the parietal pericardium you mean 'superficial' to the pericardium as this is the only context in which fat could be invaded without pericardial invasion. If this assumption is correct then the case should be classified as 'T4' (see page 87).

**Question**

If a pT2a lung tumour ruptures through the pleural surface during surgical extraction of the lobe, does this influence (upgrade) the staging of the tumour because of the risk of tumour seeding?

**Answer**

No, neither in the IASLC recommendations nor in the TNM classification, events of rupture are considered in the definitions of the T categories in lung tumours. Tumour spillage during surgery is considered a criterion only in the T classification of tumours of the ovaries, Fallopian tube and primary peritoneal carcinomas.

**Question**

For clinical staging of lung cancer: Do we need to measure the tumour size on the lung 'window' or on the mediastinal 'window' of CT scans?

**Answer**

In order to determine tumour size in its greatest dimension, all the different projections of contrast-enhanced CT scan should be studied. Lung CT window display settings should be used when assessing images for lung tumour size (see page 88).

**Question**

Second primary lung cancers should be designated with a T, N and M category for each tumour (see CHEST 2017; 151(1), page 9). Do you agree with this statement? Or could it be considered as multifocal (= pT(m)) and could it be reported as such?

*Answer*

We agree with the formulated statement. The problem of the classification of multiple lung tumours is addressed in this Supplement (see page 95) and the *AJCC Cancer Staging Manual*, 8th edition, based on the IASLC Staging and Prognostic Factors Committee that studied this problem and made recommendations regarding the uniform use of classification rules depending on the pattern of disease. Secondary primary tumours, i.e. tumours identified clinically (or grossly) or microscopically (on pathological examination) as different primary tumours, should be classified separately, with an individual TNM for each one.

*Question*

I have an acinar adenocarcinoma of the lung, which shows large areas with a bronchoalveolar growth pattern. In the resection specimens there are foci of bronchoalveolar carcinoma away from the original tumour. Should this be counted as a synchronous tumour or simply part of the first tumour?

*Answer*

Separate tumour nodules of the same histopathologic type are classified according to their lobar location:

− Provided the separate nodule(s) are in the same lobe as the primary, the tumour is classified as T3/pT3.
− If the tumour nodules occur in an ipsilateral lobe, the case would be classified as T4/pT4.
− The case should be M1a/pM1a if the separate nodule(s) is(are) in the contralateral lung.
− See page 95 of this Supplement for more details: Classification of Lung Cancers with Multiple Sites of Involvement.

*Question*

A patient had a (histologically confirmed) typical carcinoid of the middle lobe bronchus endoscopic completely removed with laser. The middle lobe was resected: it showed a severe obstructive pneumonia but not tumour tissue.

Which 'T classification' would be correct? pT0? pT2 (because of the pneumonia)? ypT0? ypT2?

*Answer*

Given the obstructive pneumonia in the resected lobe, the appropriate pT classification would be pT2. ypT is reserved for tumours resected following neoadjuvant treatment.

### Question

Lung cancer invading 'great vessels' is classified as T4. How are 'great vessels' defined and where is the 'cutoff'? Does a large pulmonary arterial branch in a lobectomy specimen qualify as a great vessel or does it refer to only the main pulmonary artery and aorta?

### Answer

The definition of the great vessels are given on page 87:

- Aorta
- Superior vena cava
- Inferior vena cava
- Main pulmonary artery (pulmonary trunk)
- Intrapericardial portions of the right and left pulmonary artery
- Intrapericardial portions of the superior and inferior right and left pulmonary veins.

Invasion of more distal branches does not qualify for classification as T4.

### Question

1. If there are 2 adenocarcinomas in the same lobe, but they have very different histologies (for example a well-diff. papillary adenocarcinoma and a poorly diff. signet ring cell carcinoma – both TTF-1+ and proven to be of lung origin), according to the guidelines in the AJCC manual, since these are both 'adenocarcinomas' they should be staged as T4. At least at the histologic (and probably genetic) level, the tumours are quite distinct. How would you stage this situation?

2. If a patient has 2 tumours in the same lobe, and one is a bronchioloalveolar carcinoma and the other is an adenocarcinoma, would these be staged as separate primaries?

### Answers to 1 and 2

The examples that you have given could all be considered separate primaries. Therefore, one would classify the more advanced in each group and indicate that there were two primaries by putting (2) after the T, e.g. T2(2).

(See page 95 of this Supplement: Classification of Lung Cancers with Multiple Sites of Involvement.)

**Question**

How is the invasion of the 'mediastinum' as a criterion for T4/pT4 defined?

**Answer**

'Mediastinum' was assigned to the T4 category to cover all of the contents that were not specifically mentioned, e.g. mediastinal fat, connective tissue, thymus, etc.

**Question**

Referring to the lung, I have a specimen with a 7 cm adenocarcinoma in which there is a separate 1 cm subpleural adenocarcinoma that is only about 1 cm from the larger mass. The lesions are in the same lobe. There is no definite contiguity between the lesions macro- or microscopically. Is this a T4 tumour?

**Answer**

The case you describe is classified as T3 or pT3.

**Question**

How does one classify a patient with a tumour obstructing the right main bronchus, in which the resultant collapse/consolidation of the middle and lower lobes obscures the margins of the tumour and one cannot assess its size?

**Answer**

The features described suggest that the tumour is at least T2 but one cannot assess size to determine if it is T2a, T2b or T3. One should apply General Rule No. 4 in such circumstances. This states that 'If there is doubt concerning the correct T, N or M category to which a particular case should be allotted, then the lower (i.e. less advanced) category should be chosen. This will be reflected in the stage grouping'. This case should be classified as cT2a and if the lymph node is negative it is stage IB.

**Question**

How should one classify a patient with a 4 cm spiculated lesion in the left lower lobe and a 2 cm lesion in the right upper lobe? A needle biopsy from the left lesion confirms adenocarcinoma. On a PET scan there is high uptake in both of the lung lesions but no uptake elsewhere in the hilum, mediastinum or at distant sites. Does one need to biopsy the right lesion to confirm that it is of a different cell type?

**Answer**

Whether or not a needle biopsy of the right lung lesion should be undertaken in this case depends upon whether the treatment approach proposed by the multidisciplinary team would be influenced by the differing interpretations of the classification on the evidence so far available. This case could be classified as cT2a N0 M1a, Stage IV if the smaller lesion is considered a metastasis. If, however, the two lesions are shown to be synchronous primary tumours they should be classified under General Rule No. 5, which states that 'in the case of multiple simultaneous tumours in one organ (the 2 lungs are considered to be a single organ for these purposes), the tumour with the highest T category should be classified and the multiplicity or the number of tumours should be indicated in parenthesis' as cT2a(m)N0M0 or cT2a(2) N0 M0, Stage IB. If treatment decisions would be influenced by knowing the cell type of the right-sided lesion, which might show a different cell type or provide morphological, immunohistochemical or molecular differences suggesting that the tumours are different subtypes of the same cell type, then a needle biopsy of the right-sided tumour would be justified for staging purposes.

### Question

How should one classify a case in which an undifferentiated carcinoma of the left upper lobe is infiltrating the soft tissues of the chest wall. There is a positive lymph node adjacent to the chest wall lesion and no intrathoracic node involvement. Is this pM1 or pN1 if one considers the soft tissue as an infiltrated organ and the local node as a regional node?

### Answer

In answering this question, one has to assume that clinical and pathological features have excluded this tumour being a soft-tissue primary (sarcoma) or a breast carcinoma. If this is so then the supplement advises (see page 8): 'In rare cases, one finds no metastases in the regional lymph nodes, but only in lymph nodes that drain an adjacent organ directly invaded by the primary tumour. The lymph nodes of the invaded site are considered as those of the primary site for N classification.' Lymph nodes in the soft tissues of the chest wall nodes are not considered 'regional' lymph nodes in lung cancer and hence the classification to be applied should be 'pM1b'.

### Question

A case of lung cancer is classified on clinical/pre-treatment assessment as cN0 or cN1. At surgery it is deemed to be irresectable because of extensive mediastinal invasion by the primary tumour. The pathologist can only confirm that resected/sampled mediastinal nodes from stations 4 and 7 are clear of disease. Should this case be classified as pNX, pN0 or pN1?

### Answer

The TNM classification sets prerequisites for the number and distribution of lymph nodes that are required to be examined histologically to establish the pN category. In lung cancer these prerequisites are: 'Histological examination of hilar and mediastinal lymphadenectomy specimen(s) will ordinarily include 6 or more lymph nodes/stations. Three of these nodes/stations should be mediastinal, including the sub-carinal nodes (#7) and three from N1 nodes/stations.' However, if all the lymph nodes examined are negative, but the number or distribution of the lymph nodes recommended to be ordinarily examined is not met, classify as pN0.

### Question

A patient underwent a wedge resection of the right upper lobe for a pT1N0M0 adenocarcinoma. Six months later a further tumour was discovered in the right upper lobe and the patient underwent completion upper lobectomy. The pathological examination of the surgical specimen showed that the new lesion was a metastasis within an intrapulmonary lymph node and lymph node tissue was clearly seen with a capsule at the periphery of the new tumour. How should one classify this case?

### Answer

This should be classified as a recurrent tumour in a lymph node and not as a new primary. It would be appropriate to classify this as rpT0pN1pM0.

### Question

A patient underwent a right upper lobectomy with systematic nodal dissection. Pathological examination showed a pT1 adenocarcinoma and confirmed that the requirements for a full pathological examination of the lymph nodes had been met. We confirmed involvement of the interlobar lymph node station found metastasis in lymph nodes (#12) with no other deposits in N1 and N2 stations, except for isolated tumour cells (ITCs) in a paratracheal station (# R4). Should we classify this case as pN1, pN0(i+) or pN2(i+)?

### Answer

The supplement only considers ITC as a subcategory of the pN0 classification. Unfortunately, if one assigned the category of pN0(i+) or created a new one of pN2(i+) the irrefutable evidence of pN1 disease would be obscured. We can only suggest that the case be classified as pN1.

### Question

Our surgeon undertook right upper lobectomy and resection of the fused apical segment of the right lower lobe in a patient following induction chemotherapy. Macroscopically, the tumour is 3.5 cm in size and appears to involve the attached segment. However, on microscopy I cannot identify the visceral pleura of the oblique fissure to confirm invasion. How should one classify this case?

### Answer

The use of an elastin stain may facilitate the identification of the visceral pleura (see page 95). However, direct invasion of an adjacent lobe, even when the fissure is deficient and there is no pleural separation at the point of invasion, is classified as T2/pT2 (see page 87). This case should be classified as ypT2a.

## Question

On pathological examination of a resection specimen there is a 6 cm tumour with direct invasion into hilar fat. Is hilar fat considered evidence of mediastinal invasion or does this qualify as invasion of the mediastinal pleura? Is this categorized as pT2b, pT3 or pT4?

## Answer

Invasion of hilar fat is not included in any of the present T descriptors and we have no data on which to give advice. In this case there needs to be a dialogue between the surgeon and the pathologist. If the surgeon undertook a lobectomy and was certain that the resection margins were clear of disease, and if the pathologist confirms an R0 resection, then one can be reasonably sure that the 'hilar' fat is truly hilar and one could assign the pT2b category to this case. If a pneumonectomy had been performed then there would be real concern that the 'hilar' fat is really 'mediastinal' fat. If the discussion between the pathologist and the surgeon concluded that this was the case then the pT4 category should be assigned. Further discussions would no doubt centre on whether this constituted an R1 resection!

## Question

Pathological examination of a resection specimen has shown a 2.5 cm peripheral adenocarcinoma that involves the visceral pleura but does not extend through to the superficial surface of the pleura. Should this be classified as pT1b or pT2?

## Answer

Invasion of the visceral pleura is a T2 descriptor and is defined as 'invasion beyond the elastic layer including invasion to the visceral pleural surface'. The use of elastic stains is recommended when this feature is not clear on evaluation of H&E sections (see page 95). If in this case the invasion extends beyond the elastic lamina the case should be classified as pT2a.

## Question

Clinical classification suggested that our patient had a T2N2M0 non-small-cell lung carcinoma (NSCLC). Pre-operative biopsy of ipsilateral mediastinal nodes confirmed N2 disease and thoracotomy was not undertaken. Should this case be classified as cN2 or pN2? Should this case now be assigned a pathological stage?

## Answer

Microscopical confirmation of the nodal disease would allow this to be classified as pN2. Pathological staging depends on the proven anatomic extent of disease. If a biopsied primary tumour technically cannot be removed, or when it is unreasonable to remove it, the criteria for pathological classification and staging are satisfied without removal of the primary cancer if:

- Biopsy has confirmed a pT category and there is microscopic confirmation of nodal disease at any level (pN1-3).
- There is microscopical confirmation of the highest N category (pN3).
- Or if there is microscopical confirmation of pM1.

## Skin Tumours
### Carcinoma of Skin
*Question*

Is the TNM classification applicable for basal cell carcinoma (basalioma) of the skin? If yes, is this a practice recommended by UICC?

*Answer*

The TNM classifications of skin tumours of different sites include basal cell carcinomas.

*Question*

If a carcinoma of the skin invades a nerve smaller than 0.1 mm will it be classified as Pn0 or Pn1?

*Answer*

We would suggest to classify it as Pn1. There is no upper or lower size limit for perineural invasion.

*Question*

In TNM for Skin Carcinoma of the Head and Neck there is not this comment. Therefore, is it right that I have to register 3 cases if I have 3 simultaneous skin tumours in head and neck? If I also had simultaneously 1 skin tumour in the thorax, 1 skin tumour in a lower limb and 2 skin tumours in the head and neck, do I have to register overall 3 cases? Or obtain the comment above for all anatomic sites in skin carcinoma?

*Answer*

Please find below a recommendation:

  Combining multiple carcinomas of the skin should be done only with subsites (C44.5–7 or C63.2). Carcinomas of the skin of the head and neck should only be combined with carcinomas of the skin of the head and neck. A carcinoma of the skin in subsite C44.3 and a synchronous one in subsites C44.6 and C44.7 should be classified as synchronous tumours.

*Question*

Skin carcinoma of the head and neck and squamous cell carcinoma of the skull (skullcap) in a young patient with Adams-Oliver Syndrome. Direct deep infiltration of the carcinoma into the brain tissue, in this location no bone due to Adams-Oliver Syndrome. Is it pT4b or pT3 or is in this situation the TNM classification not applicable?

*Answer*

Although not explicitly mentioned in the definitions of the T categories of skin carcinoma of the head and neck it seems justified to classify this case as pT4b.

## Carcinoma of Skin of the Eyelid
*Question*

What is the correct TNM stage for a carcinoma of skin of the eyelid? An invasive moderately differentiated non-keratinizing squamous cell carcinoma that originated from the medial canthus of the left eye. After numerous excisions, enucleation and debulking of the left eye has been performed. Would involvement by tumour of the optic nerve be regarded as stage T4a (ocular or intraorbital structures) or T4b (brain)?

*Answer*

I would propose to classify as pT4a. The term 'deep invasion' also includes the involvement of named nerves.

## Malignant Melanoma of Skin
*Question*

Question regarding pT classification of melanoma. How should a melanoma with a Breslow thickness of 0.8 mm and no ulceration be classified? In the AJCC manual, it is pT1b and in the UICC TNM it is pT1a; the cutoff between pT1a and pT1b does not seem to be identical.

*Answer*

This is indeed an error in the UICC booklet; the correct version is:

pT1a   Tumour less than 0.8 mm without ulceration
pT1b   Tumour less than 0.8 mm with ulceration or tumour 0.8 mm to 1.0 mm
       with or without ulceration

*Question*

p144 melanoma, clinical stage IA = pT1a, IB = pT1b or pT2a
p145 melanoma, pathological stage, IA = pT1a or pT1b, IB = pT2a

Is this discrepancy an error and which one is correct?

*Answer*

Both are correct. For melanoma clinical stage refers to the pathological T category and the clinical N category. If the N category is determined pathologically then the pathological stage is used.

*Question*

How do we classify isolated tumour cells in a sentinel biopsy of a skin melanoma correctly? Is it a pN0(0/X; sn)i+ or is it pN1 because of microscopic metastasis, clinically occult?

*Answer*

The *TNM Classification of Malignant Tumours*, 8th edition, page 8 states: 'The exceptions are in malignant melanoma of the skin and Merkel cell carcinoma, wherein ITC in a lymph node are classified as N1 (or pN1) and not as N0'.

*Question*

What is the correct pN classification for the following case? A malignant melanoma of the thumb (pT3b). With immunohistological staining, cell clusters and lines of single cells of the melanoma were detected in two axillary sentinel nodes located in the marginal sinus without infiltration of lymph node tissue and without stromal reaction. The lines of single cells are located in one sentinel node and measure 0.237 mm, 0.304 mm and 0.361 mm. In the other sentinel node lies a cluster of cells with a size of 1.6 × 0.12 mm.

*Answer*

We refer to the *TNM Classification of Malignant Tumours*, 8th edition, page 8. The exception (of classifying ITC as pN0(i+)) are in malignant melanoma of the skin and Merkel cell carcinoma. The case you describe could be classified as pN1(sn)(2/2).

*Question*

How should one categorize a patient with multiple synchronous malignant melanomas of the skin, in different sites of the body? Skin is not a paired organ, and thus I assume that only 1 clinical and 1 pathological TNM classification should be given (Rule No. 5), but one could argue that you should classify tumours in different sites separately.

*Answer*

It is recommended to classify the malignant melanomas of skin of different sites separately because they may have different regional lymph node groups. It might be acceptable to classify malignant melanomas in a region with the lymphatic drainage as multiple and for example classify 3 tumours as pT2b(3).

## Breast Tumours

*Question*

If the clinical T has been determined by physical examination as well as by mammography and ultrasonography, which measurement is used for the cT?

For instance: when tumour is palpated as 3 cm and mammography shows 2 cm, is it T2 or T1?

*Answer*

Clinical tumour size (cT category) should be based on the clinical findings that are judged to be the most accurate for a particular case. According to a proposal in the TNM Supplement, 4th edition, the size for classification in this specific case is: $0.5 \times 3.0\,cm + 0.5 \times 2.0\,cm = 2.5\,cm$ and thus T2 (see page 120). However, the clinician should state in the health record how the T category is determined.

## Question

Is there a specific TNM classification for carcinosarcomas of the breast or malignant phyllodes tumours or can we use the TNM classification of breast tumours?

## Answer

In the TNM booklet, 8th edition, page 151, it says: The classification applies only to carcinomas and concerns the male as well as the female breast.

It is therefore not applicable to carcinosarcomas or phyllodes tumours. Sarcomas of the breast including phyllodes tumours should be classified according to the 'soft tissue sarcoma of the trunk and extremities' (e.g. liposarcoma).

## Question

Is the 8th TNM classification exactly the same as the 8th AJCC staging manual?

## Answer

The TNM classifications of UICC and AJCC are basically identical in the definitions of the T, N and M categories. However, there is a small difference in the T category: the AJCC removed the lobular carcinoma in situ (LCIS) as pTis in the manual because it often behaves as a benign entity. The UICC did not remove LCIS in pTis to be consistent with current classification in the WHO blue book. We prefer to retain LIN-3, which is considered as the precursor and mostly treated like DCIS, with the following types: macroacinar, LCIS with necrosis, signet ring cell and pleomorf type should be kept.

The UICC does not include chapters on biomarkers or gene expression profiles, but offers a Prognostic Factors Grid for breast cancer, as for all other tumours, at the end of the chapter. The AJCC manual includes besides the Stage (anatomical extent) and also a clinical and pathological prognostic stage where biomarkers and gene expression profiles are taken into account (a revised breast cancer chapter in AJCC from November 2017) available upon registration on the AJCC website).

## Question

Are microscopic measurements of breast tumour size preferred to gross measurement?

## Answer

Microscopic measurement is preferred to macroscopic measurement because the estimation of a tumour margin macroscopically might not be precise enough.

## Question

Should the rules of mathematics for rounding values be used? Should a tumour measuring 10.3 mm be rounded down to 1 cm and put in the pT1b category or should this tumour be classified as pT1c?

*Answer*
The rules of mathematics should not be used. In this case as the tumour is greater than 10 mm, the tumour should be classified as pT1c.

*Question*
Breast carcinoma 2.5 cm in diameter with invasion of the dermis/corium. Is this classified as pT2 or pT4?
*Answer*
The criteria for classifying a breast tumour T4/pT4 include oedema, peau d'orange or ulceration of the skin of the breast and not invasion of the dermis. The tumour is classified as pT2 (see page 120).

*Question*
A mastectomy specimen with 2 tumours, one retroareolar and one in the upper outer quadrant measuring 3.5 cm and 2.0 cm in greatest dimension with 3 cm distance. In the case of multifocal tumours, does this case still belong to T2?
*Answer*
The tumour with the highest T category should be classified and the multiplicity of the number of tumours should be indicated in parentheses, in this case T2(m) or T2(2). The size of multiple tumours is not added (see General Rule No. 5, page 5 of the UICC TNM classification of breast tumours, 8th edition).

*Question*
Infiltrating lobular carcinoma, 3 cm × 2 cm × 1 cm, with extensive lymphovascular invasion. Pathology report: dermal lymphatics involved. Should this be classified as T4d (inflammatory carcinoma)? There was no clinical physical examination data available.
*Answer*
Inflammatory carcinoma, T4d, requires the macroscopic (clinical) features to be present. Microscopic involvement of dermal lymphatic vessels alone does not count for classification. The tumour is pT2 based on size.

*Question*
Clinically with no palpable tumour, but with a mammogram showing suspicious microcalcifications. Physical examination did not show a tumour. Surgical removal of the lesion was a diagnosed carcinoma in situ, with questionable microinvasion. How is this classified?
*Answer*
cTis   Clinically no evidence of primary tumour
pTis   Carcinoma in situ

Questionable microinvasion leaves enough doubt to apply TNM Rule No. 4; when in doubt choose the lower category.

**Question**

Breast tumour of 5 cm in size with predominant DCIS (high-grade comedocarcinoma), largest invasive focus of 0.8 cm × 0.6 cm on slide with 4 foci of microinvasion 0.2–0.3 cm in size. Is only the invasive focus considered for the pT category or is background DCIS included in tumour size? What about the microinvasive foci?

**Answer**

When classifying pT: the tumour size is a measurement of the invasive component only (see note on page 155 of the UICC TNM classification of breast tumours, 8th edition [1]). When there are multiple foci of microinvasion, only the size of the largest focus is used to classify the microinvasion (and not the sum of the foci). The presence of multiple foci of microinvasion should also be noted as it is with multiple larger invasive carcinomas. Therefore, this case should be classified as pT1b(5) (see note b on page 153).

**Question**

In tumours of the breast, how do we classify invasion of lymphatic vessels in perinodal fatty tissue of the axilla with and without involvement of the axillary lymph nodes?

**Answer**

Invasion of lymphatic vessels in the axilla is not considered in the TNM classification of breast tumours. The optional L (lymphatic) classification can be used to describe lymphatic vessel involvement (see page 24).

**Question**

Regarding an isolated tumour cell cluster definition in lymph nodes in breast carcinoma, if you have multiple clusters in a subcapsular sinus immediately adjacent to one another (spaced approximately 20 μm apart), but each measuring less than 0.2 mm, are these foci added up for the size or each considered separately in the measurement?

**Answer**

This issue has frequently been raised in the TNM help desk and raised considerable discussion. Strictly, these findings should be considered pN0(i+) and not micrometastasis. However, biology would tell us that a classification of micrometastasis is more adequate. In these rare cases we recommend to do step sections and frequently find real micrometastasis or even macrometastasis.

**Question**

How does one classify an isolated tumour nodule in the axillary fat of a patient with breast carcinoma?

*Answer*

It should be classified as a lymph node metastasis if it has the form and smooth contour of a lymph node. A tumour nodule with an irregular contour may be classified as venous axillary invasion (V classification).

*Question*

Compared to what is mentioned in the *AJCC Manual*, 8th edition, there seems to be a discordance regarding the regional lymph nodes.

The difference is that for UICC, level III seems to be distinct from the infraclavicular nodes. Does level III equal infraclavicular? Depending on the interpretation of the level III and infraclavicular lymph nodes, there can be doubt between pN2 and pN3a.

*Answer*

Infraclavicular (subclavicular) (ipsilateral) lymph nodes are listed separately as an own group in the list of regional lymph nodes (page 152, UICC TNM, 8th edition) while they are included in level III axillary nodes in the 8th edition of the AJCC staging manual. Level III and infraclavicular lymph nodes are both considered in the (p)N3 category.

The pN3a category in the UICC publication, p.156, is stated as: '…or metastasis in infraclavicular lymph nodes', which should read: 'metastasis in infraclavicular lymph nodes/level III lymph nodes'. This will be added in the next print of the TNM 8th edition and in the errata available on the UICC website.

*Question*

A 2.3 cm axillary lymph node had a small cluster of cells 0.1 cm in size. How is that classified, according to the dimensions of the metastasis or to the dimensions of the lymph node?

*Answer*

The size used for classification is the size of the measured metastasis and not the size of the lymph node that contains the metastasis. The case would be classified as a micrometastasis (0.2 cm) and coded as pN1mi.

*Question*

Is metastatic breast cancer in a cervical lymph node considered N3 or M1? And what about contralateral lymph nodes (without a primary tumour in the contralateral breast)?

*Answer*

In the definition of regional lymph nodes there is a note 'Any other lymph node metastasis than listed in the regional lymph nodes is coded as distant metastasis (M1), including cervical and contralateral internal mammary lymph nodes (see note on page 152 of the 8th edition of the UICC *TNM Classification of Malignant Tumours*). Contralateral lymph nodes and cervical lymph nodes are classified c/pM1'.

**Question**

In a case of Paget disease of the nipple with a small 0.3 cm tumour of the breast near the nipple, is this classified as pT1a or pT4?

**Answer**

This is classified as pT1a. Paget disease associated with a tumour is classified according to the size of the tumour (page 153, TNM, 8th edition [1]).

**Question**

How is microinvasive (<1 mm) breast cancer coded in the TNM?

**Answer**

It is coded as pT1mi.

**Question**

In breast carcinoma a 3 cm tumour shows invasion of the pectoralis muscle. What will be the T category?

**Answer**

In the 8th edition of the TNM classification a note on page 153 says: 'Chest wall includes ribs, intercostal muscles and serrated anterior muscle but not pectoral muscle'. Therefore, the case should be classified as T2/pT2.

**Question**

Pathological breast cancer staging: could you please comment on pT4b specifically about satellite skin nodules? if there are ipsilateral microscopic dermal satellites, is this pT4b? We are aware that direct invasion of the dermis by the index tumour does not constitute pT4 and that these tumours are staged according to their size as usual.

**Answer**

The dermal satellite skin nodules as included in the T4b/pT4b category should be macroscopically visible. Microscopically detected dermal nodules do not qualify for pT4b.

**Question**

How do we classify a breast carcinoma with 3 micrometastases in 10 axillary lymph nodes classified? As pN1mi (0/10) or pN1mi (3/10)?

**Answer**

The micrometastases in the lymph nodes (3/10) can be classified as pN1mi(3/10); see page 155 of the 8th edition of the UICC *TNM Classification of Malignant Tumours*.

**Question**

I have a mastectomy specimen with a 15 mm breast invasive ductal carcinoma and an intramammary lymph node containing a 5 mm metastasis. The sentinel lymph nodes have no metastases. Should this be classified as pT1cN1? Other colleagues suggest that intramammary nodes should not count for the N stage and that this should be N0. Could you clarify please?

**Answer**

I may refer you to the TNM classification, 8th edition, page 152, with a note saying: 'Intramammary lymph nodes are coded as axillary lymph nodes level I'. We would classify your case as pT1pN1a.

**Question**

How does one classify breast cancer after chemotherapy? Is pTpN appropriate?

**Answer**

'In those cases in which classification is performed during or following initial multimodality therapy, the cTNM or pTNM categories are identified by a y prefix' (TNM, 8th edition, page 9); for example, ycT1N0M0 or ypT1pN0M0.

**Question**

How can complete pathological response and stage of a breast tumour be assessed after neoadjuvant therapy with no residual tumour in the breast but metastatic node deposits in axilla?

**Answer**

The breast cancer case you describe should be classified as ypT0pN1-3, depending on the lymph node status of the regional lymph nodes.

**Question**

We have a question about staging specimens after diagnostic procedures. The 'y' prefix is needed only after systemic/radiant treatment, in other words not after surgery. How to stage the following case of breast cancer with cT1c(1.5 cm) N0? The first diagnosis has been made by the 'mammotome' procedure and then the patient is admitted to complete surgery and sentinel node biopsy. In the surgical specimen a bioptic focus is found with residual cancer (max. diameter 0.6 cm) and granulomatous reaction; sentinel node biopsy is negative for metastasis.

Which is the correct stage? pT1bN0(sn) or ypT1bN0(sn)?

How can the previous surgical/diagnostic procedure be taken into account in a surgical specimen?

**Answer**

The correct pathologic stage for the breast case is pT1b N0(sn). The 'y' prefix is only used when the patient received initial therapy consisting of systemic (chemo, hormone, immune) and/or radiation therapy. After this initial therapy the patient may be assigned a yc (yclinical) stage based on physical examination and imaging. If the patient then has a surgical resection, the yp (y pathologic stage) may be assigned using all of the yc stage information plus operative findings plus the pathologist's exam of the resected specimen.

**Question**

The TNM Classification of breast tumours states: 'The clinical T1 category is further subclassified into T1mic, T1a, T1b, T1c'. There was a discussion among physicians here as to why this was included in the clinical description as microscopic invasion can only be defined pathologically.

**Answer**

Histologic examination is required on all clinical classifications for 'confirmation of the disease'. Pathologic classification, pT, requires more than histologic examination. It 'requires the examination of the primary tumour with no gross tumour at the margins of resection' (TNM, 7th edition [9], see page 15).

**Question**

What is the pT category and the R status of a 1.5 cm breast carcinoma detected histologically in the resection margin?

**Answer**

The pT category is pT1c and the R status R1.

**Question**

When a patient who had a hormonal therapy for a left breast cancer has a new cancer in the right breast, should we also use the prefix 'y' with this new cancer?

**Answer**

The carcinoma of the right breast is classified without 'y'.

The y" symbol is used in those cases in which classification is performed during or following multimodality therapy (see page 9, TNM booklet [1]).

**Question**

How does one classify a breast tumour with invasion of the nipple/mamilla with or without ulceration?

**Answer**

The nipple is not considered in the definitions of the T classification. Size and ulceration are relevant criteria for the T category.

**Example**

Breast carcinoma 1.9 cm in diameter with invasion of the nipple:

With ulceration of the nipple      T4b/pT4b
Without ulceration of the nipple      T1c/pT1c

**Question**

How do we classify a lymph node metastasis of breast cancer with a size of 1.8 mm and extension beyond the lymph node capsule?

*Answer*

It should be classified as pN1mi, on the basis of its size. Extension beyond the capsule is not a criterion for pN classification.

*Question*

I have a case of breast carcinoma where the sentinel node imprint shows carcinoma cells; however, after review of multiple levels, no malignant cells could be identified in the permanent sections from the sentinel lymph node. How do I classify the N category?

*Answer*

This is indeed a difficult question. Since the cytological demonstration (if this has not been an artefact) showed the existence of isolated tumour cells I would propose to classify the case as pN0(sn)(i+) and document the case separately.

*Question*

A breast cancer patient, classified as cT2N0 with no visible skin changes had a lumpectomy and sentinel node procedure. The pathologist sees infiltration of the epidermis with minimal ulceration (only microscopic changes, macroscopically he did not see any skin involvement). Is this tumour now classified as a pT4b or is this still a pT2? And what if there is epidermal involvement but no ulceration?

*Answer*

Minimal (microscopic) ulceration does qualify for pT4b. Epidermal invasion only would not qualify for pT4b but would rather be classified as pT2 (if other criteria are fulfilled). See Notes on page 153 of the 8th edition of the UICC *TNM Classification of Malignant Tumours*.

## Gynaecological Tumours

### Cervix Uteri

*Question*

For tumours of the cervix uteri can we base the classification on the conisation to determine the clinical TNM?

*Answer*

Conisation is a procedure that can be used to establish a clinical TNM classification in tumours of the cervix uteri. For details when to use pTNM, see page 186.

*Question*

How is the maximal horizontal spread measured in the squamous cell carcinoma of the cervix in case of multifocality? Do I measure the total extent of the lesion between the two lateral margins? Do I include only the largest tumour focus?

### Answer

It is recommended to measure the total extent of the tumour foci and separately document the largest tumour focus as well as the number and size of other tumour foci.

In the TNM Supplement it says: In the rare multifocal T1a tumours for the horizontal spread FIGO classifies by the largest focus. This is in accordance with TNM Rule No. 5.

### Question

A patient has an invasive squamous cell carcinoma of the cervix. There is direct extension to the endometrium, left tube and left ovary. The parametrium and vaginal wall are free. Pelvic nodes are negative. How should we classify this tumour?

### Answer

We would suggest classifying the case as pT2. The further subdivision of pT2 depends on tumour size.

### Question

A mesonephric adenocarcinoma of the cervix was discovered incidentally on surgery for a mucinous tumour of the right ovary. There are small metastatic foci in the ovary and therefore the grossly normal cervix was entirely embedded, showing 5/16 consecutive blocks with mesonephric adenocarcinoma (approximately 1.5 cm horizontal). The uterus is uninvolved and the cervical margins are negative. There seems to be no clear guidance in the pTNM for adnexal metastasis. Is this a pT1bM1 or pT4a?

### Answer

In the 8th edition of the TNM classification of tumours of the uterine cervix it is noted: 'M1: Distant metastasis. It excludes metastasis to the vagina, pelvic serosa and adnexa'. Thus, a classification as pT2b might be appropriate.

### Question

In a radical hysterectomy for cervical cancer, is the parametrial margin with lymphovascular emboli and no direct tumour cell infiltration T1b (FIGO T1B2) or T2b (FIGO T2B)?

### Answer

In the TNM system (8th edition) neither an invasion of lymph vessels nor of veins is considered in the T categories. In the R classification, tumour cell emboli in lymph vessels or veins are considered R1 (microscopic tumour) if they are attached to the vessel endothelium or migrate through the vessel wall. If the tumour cells are in the vessel lumen without attachment, then the case should be classified as R0, provided there are no other residua at the resection margins and no distant metastasis.

### Question

Para-aortic nodes are considered 'non-regional' for cervical cancer in the UICC TNM, 8th edition. In the 8th edition of the AJCC *Cancer Staging Manual*, they are considered 'regional'.

### Answer

In the 7th edition [9] the paraaortic nodes were considered to be metastatic but to be consistent with advice from FIGO the paraaortic nodes are now classified as regional and an errata has been released (see the UICC website).

## Corpus Uteri

### Question

I have a question regarding an endometrial adenocarcinoma of the corpus uteri infiltrating beyond the inner half of the myometrium and presenting with positive cytology. How should this be classified?

### Answer

This case should be classified as pT1b c/pN0 and M0 if the lymph nodes are negative and there are no distant metastases.

Positive peritoneal cytology 'per se' does not change the stage and positive cytology should be reported separately.

### Question

A uterine corpus tumour extends into the parametrium. Should it be classified as T2 or T3a?

### Answer

It should be classified as T3b.

T2 tumours invade the cervix but do not extend beyond the uterus (pee page 172 of the TNM classification, 8th edition.

### Question

Serous adenocarcinoma of the endometrium T1b with extensive lymph vessel invasion and omental metastatic serous adenocarcinoma is present. Does this qualify as M1/pM1?

### Answer

This case is classified as pT1b pM1 and the lymph node status should be added. Note that lymphatic vessel invasion is neither considered in the T categories nor in the N categories.

### Question

A radical hysterectomy specimen shows an adenocarcinoma penetrating the serosal surface (pT3a) of the corpus uteri. All regional lymph nodes were negative, but there was metastatic adenocarcinoma in parametrial soft tissue. Does this change the stage of the tumour?

*Answer*
T3a includes 'discontinuous involvement of adnexa and serosa within the pelvis'.

*Question*
I received a hysterectomy specimen with both adnexae operated for endometrial carcinoma. The Fallopian tubes have malignant glands floating in the lumen (however, the Fallopian tubes themselves are not involved). Will the case be staged as pT3a?

*Answer*
Since the floating tumour cells may be artificial and have shown no signs of invasion they should not be considered in the TNM classification of endometrial carcinoma. Thus, the classification only depends on the extent of the carcinoma in the uterus.

*Question*
Primary endometrial carcinoma of the corpus uteri with direct invasion (per continuitatem) into the small bowel wall and the omentum majus. How is this classified, pT4 or pM1?

*Answer*
If endometrial carcinoma directly invades the bowel wall (small bowel or large bowel) as well as the omentum this is classified as pT4.

*Question*
With regard to a carcinosarcoma of the uterine corpus with invasion of more than 50% of the myometrium and only a pouch of Douglas involvement, is this T3a? Adnexa or parametria are not involved and the tumour measures 2 mm from the uterine serosa.

*Answer*
Carcinosarcomas should be classified according to tumours of the uterus – endometrium. The case you describe could be classified as T3a/pT3a.

*Question*
A case of endometrioid adenocarcinoma with metastasis into the soft tissue at the backside of the external urethra. The metastasis was pathologically identified as endometrioid adenocarcinoma and completely separated from the original location. Should we classify this case as T1bNXM1 or T3bNXM0?

*Answer*
The case you describe should be classified as pT1pNXpM1 (provided this is not a lymph node metastasis).

*Question*

Endometrial carcinoma of the corpus uteri with metastases in the omentum. Is this classified as pT4 or pM1?

*Answer*

Omental foci (discontinuous from the primary tumour) are considered distant metastasis = M1/pM1.

*Question*

A patient has an endometrial cancer with a right inguinal positive lymph node and the omentum is also involved. Should omentum be considered as distant metastasis?

*Answer*

Omental metastasis is classified as M1/pM1. You report on an endometrial carcinoma with inguinal lymph node metastasis: the latter are not listed among the regional lymph nodes and should also be considered M1/pM1.

*Question*

Inguinal lymph nodes are listed as regional lymph nodes for ovarian cancer, page 179 in the UICC TNM *Classification of Malignant Tumours*, 8th edition. However, in the M1b category p.181, it says 'including inguinal lymph nodes'. If the inguinal nodes are considered regional, how can they also qualify for distant metastases?

*Answer*

Unfortunately, this is an error in the 1st print of the 8th edition: Metastasis in the inguinal lymph nodes should be considered distant metastasis. They will be removed from the list of regional lymph nodes in a reprint of the 8th edition.

Correct Regional Lymph Nodes

The regional lymph nodes are the hypogastric (obturator), common iliac, external iliac, lateral sacral, para-aortic and retroperitoneal nodes:

**Note.**

Add: 'including the intra-abdominal node such as greater omental nodes'.

## Uterine Sarcomas

*Question*

A uterine endometrial sarcoma, high grade (10 cm) invading the myometrium with serosal involvement. Would it be still stage I according to the FIGO classification, because there is no comment about a serosal involvement T category.

*Answer*

Indeed, serosal penetration by an endometrial stromal sarcoma is not listed as a criterion in the T categories. We would suggest classifying the case as pT1b because the definitions of the T2 categories are not met.

## Ovary Versus Uterus

*Question*

A patient has a high-grade (serous and clear cell) carcinoma confined to endometrium with peritoneal implants including surface of both ovaries, a small focus in one ovary and a large omental cake. Should we stage this as an ovarian tumour (M0) or an endometrial tumour (M1)?

*Answer*

It would be very unusual for a superficial endometrial primary to produce an omental mass. Most would treat this as a primary ovarian lesion with a superficial second primary in the endometrium, making it a Stage IIIC ovarian with a Stage IA endometrial tumour.

*Question*

A patient presents with a carcinoma of the endometrium and left ovarian endometroid carcinoma. How to stage? Individually?

*Answer*

Assuming that you have two different foci in the endometrium and in the left ovary and no direct invasion of an endometrial carcinoma into the left ovary, we would suggest classifying the tumours separately. There might be further indicators to prove the different origin.

## Ovarian, Fallopian Tube and Primary Peritoneal Carcinoma

*Question*

A patient has a primary ovarian cancer. Ovaries were not removed. Laparotomy shows a 2 cm epiploic metastasis of papillary serous adenocarcinoma. Should I stage this tumour, cT3b or pT3b, or something else?

*Answer*

Even though the ovaries are not removed, if you have microscopic confirmation of a 2 cm peritoneal metastasis outside the pelvis, pT3b is correct (see Chapter 3, TNM Supplement).

*Question*

What pathologic T category does the presence of omental metastases confer in an ovarian carcinoma? What about metastases to the rectosigmoid pericolic fat?

*Answer*

The classification of omental metastasis is summarized below:

| UICC | FIGO | |
|------|------|---|
| T3 and/ or N1 | III | Tumour involves one or both ovaries with microscopically confirmed peritoneal metastasis outside the pelvis and/or to the retroperitoneal lymph nodes |
| T3a | IIIA | Microscopic peritoneal metastasis beyond pelvis |
| T3b | IIIB | Macroscopic peritoneal metastasis beyond pelvis, 2 cm or less in greatest dimension, including bowel involvement outside the pelvis with or without retroperitoneal lymph nodes |
| T3c | IIIC | Macroscopic peritoneal metastasis beyond pelvis more than 2 cm in greatest dimension and/or retroperitoneal lymph node metastasis (includes extension of tumour to capsule of liver and spleen without parenchymal involvement of either organ) |

Invasion or metastasis of the rectosigmoid pericolic fat would be classified as T2b/pT2b.

*Question*

I have a case with a bilateral ovarian serous surface borderline tumour. There are microscopic non-invasive epithelial implants in the omentum. Do these implants make the case a Stage III?

*Answer*

The TNM classification applies to malignant ovarian neoplasms of both epithelial and stromal origin, including those of borderline malignancy or of low malignant potential.

Neither the FIGO classification nor the UICC/AJCC TNM classification in their 8th editions make a difference between non-invasive or invasive implants in the omental fat.

Therefore, the case you describe should be classified as pT3a (FIGOIIIA).

It is recommended to document these cases separately to get more information on possible different outcomes.

*Question*

Why are borderline tumours of the ovary classified according to TNM, although they are not invasive carcinomas?

*Answer*

Apart from the fact that borderline tumours of the ovary can show invasive parts and rarely recur or metastasize, the classification according to TNM was considered necessary to record the anatomical extent of these cases. For practical reasons, it was decided by FIGO, AJCC and UICC to keep one staging system for all ovarian cancers (malignant neoplasms of both epithelial and stromal origin including those of borderline malignancy and germ cell tumours).

This system takes into account the most relevant prognostic parameters shared by all tumour types.

**Question**

What is the TNM stage for a unilateral ovarian immature teratoma with gliomatosis peritonei and mature glial implants in the omentum?

**Answer**

Teratomas are germ cell tumours and these tumours, particularly if they are immature, have a malignant potential. Germ cell tumours should be classified according to TNM 8 for ovarian cancer. This tumour should be classified as pT3. A further subdivision in pT3a, pT3b or pT3c depends on the size of the tumour foci in the peritoneum or omentum. Certainly, the prognosis is not comparable with common epithelial tumours of the ovary or Fallopian tube.

**Question**

How to stage a serous tubal intraepithelial carcinoma (STIC) of the Fallopian tube? Neither the WHO blue book nor the UICC TNM classification lists pTis as a possibility. Should I therefore stage STIC as pT1a, FIGO IA?

**Answer**

Indeed, in the 8th edition of the TNM classification of tumours of the ovary and Fallopian tube, a Tis is not defined and was not in the 7th edition either. High-grade serous tubal intraepithelial carcinoma (STIC) can metastasize and therefore cannot be considered in situ carcinoma. The case should be classified as pT1a, provided there are no malignant cells in ascites or peritoneal washings. Borderline tumours of the ovary are classified in the same way as 'common' epithelial ovarian tumours.

**Question**

Fallopian tube carcinoma involving right obturator node – what would be the stage?

**Answer**

According to the *TNM Classification of Malignant Tumours* (8th edition), page 179, the obturator (hypogastric) lymph nodes are considered to be regional lymph nodes. This case should be classified as pN1.

pN1 can be subdivided in pN1a or pN1b depending on the size of the metastasis.

## Gestational Trophoblast Tumours

**Question**

Choriocarcinoma of the uterus, arising from the fundus, invades the serosal layer of the uterus and directly involves the perimuscular adipose tissue of the adjacent colon. The mucosa, submucosa and the muscularis propria of the colon are free. The bilateral, ovaries, Fallopian tubes, broad ligament and cervix are free. What should be the pathological stage of the tumour – pT1/pT1M1b?

*Answer*
Invasion of the perimuscular adipose tissue would not qualify for an invasion of the colon (which would be classified as M1b). We would suggest classifying the case as pT2 (corresponding to an invasion of the broad ligament).

## Urological Tumours
### Penis
*Question*
1. How should I classify a superficial invasion of the tunica albuginea (the fibrous envelope of the corpora cavernosa penis) if the tumour invades into corpus spongiosum? As pT2 or as pT3?
2. If a tumour invades connective tissue between the epidermis and corpora and superficially invades the tunica albuginea should it be pT1 or pT3?

*Answer*
Tumour invasion in the tunica albuginea is considered as pT3.

*Question*
In cancer of glans penis, if growth continuously extends from the mucosa to he urethral opening with corpus spongiosum infiltration is this T2 or T3?

*Answer*
The case should be classified as T2/pT2: 'Tumour invades into corpus spongiosum with or without urethral invasion.'

### Prostate
*Question*
The AJCC cancer staging manual, 8th edition, for prostate cancer has collapsed pT2a, pT2b and pT2c into only one category pT2 because studies failed to demonstrate the value for these subcategories. UICC, however, maintains the pT2 subdivisions. Are we still supposed to subclassify pT2 prostate cancer?

*Answer*
The UICC does not have subcategories of pT2. In the listed errata the section has been rewritten for clarification: 'However, there is no pT1 category because there is insufficient tissue to assess the highest pT category or sub-categories of pT2' has been changed to 'However, there is no pT1 category because there is insufficient tissue to assess the highest pT category. There are no sub-categories of pT2'.

**Question**

From 2017 onwards, how can a prostatic tumour, confined within prostate, be classified that is not palpable but visible by imaging? So, 'clinically apparent' but not palpable? The same problem for interpretation is met in the TNM book published by the AJCC.

**Answer**

The tumour should be classified as T1c. The T2 tumours are palpable and hence all non-palpable tumours whether seen on imaging or not are T1c. The clinical T category should reflect DRE (digital rectal examination) findings only.

**Question**

If the biopsies are positive in both lobes (right and left) of the prostate but only in one lobe a nodule is seen on TRUS and is palpable, do I classify this as a T2a/b or T2c?

**Answer**

We would classify this as T2a or T2b since the tumour is palpable in one lobe.

**Question**

During a radical cystoprostatectomy for transitional cell carcinoma if we find a clinically unexpected bilateral prostatic adenocarcinoma should we consider it as incidental (pT1) or as a pT2 tumour?

**Answer**

pT2 (see page 133). There is no pT1 category for prostate cancer.

**Question**

How do we classify perineural spread of prostatic carcinoma in extracapsular tissue?

**Answer**

pT3a.

**Question**

If a patient has had biopsies showing different Gleason grades in different biopsy specimens, how is the overall Gleason score reported? Does the TNM system follow the 2005 International Society of Urological Pathology (ISUP) Consensus Conference on Gleason grading in prostatic adenocarcinoma recommendation, i.e. that the highest individual Gleason score is designated the overall Gleason score?

**Answer**

The TNM system recommends use of the WHO and the International Society of Urological Pathology (ISUP) standard of grade score, which has replaced the Gleason score [13, 14]. However, for information and comparison both are reproduced in the TNM classification, 8th edition [1].

**Question**

If there is adenocarcinoma of the prostate in sections of the seminal vesicle without involving the muscular wall of the seminal vesicle and without direct contact to fat, should it be classified as pT3a? Is involvement of the soft tissue surrounding the seminal vesicle muscle wall equivalent to extraprostatic extension?

**Answer**

A classification of prostate tumours with invasion of seminal vesicles as pT3b requests tumour infiltration of the muscular wall of the seminal vesicle (invasion via the periprostatic soft tissue through the capsule of the prostate; see page 192 of TNM 8). Involvement of the periseminal vesicle soft tissue should indeed be classified pT3a (equivalent to extraprostatic extension).

**Question**

How should I classify a prostate carcinoma in both lobes with positive surgical margins in the apex (5 mm): pT2c or pT3a?

**Answer**

Invasion into the prostatic apex is not classified as T3 but as T2 (in this case pT2c) (see page 192, 8th edition of the UICC TNM classification [1]) since it is considered organ confined. A positive surgical margin can be indicated by the additional R1 descriptor (residual microscopic disease).

**Question**

Does infiltration of the bladder wall by a prostate carcinoma correspond to pT3a or to pT4 (bladder is not mentioned explicitly in the T4 category)?

**Answer**

Such a bladder wall invasion should be classified as pT4.

If there is only microscopic bladder neck involvement, then pT3a would be appropriate.

## Testis

**Question**

UICC and AJCC TNM 2017 staging for testis seem to differ. Applying AJCC rules, most of the TNM pT1 will change, with possibly relevant therapy modification. Are you planning to make an addendum? I found these differences misleading and dangerous for patient management.

**Answer**

There are indeed some slight differences between the pT1 definitions of testis tumours.

After discussion and recommendation from the authors the UICC considers the proposals of a subdivision by size for pure seminoma T1 as unnecessary as survival is not affected [15].

It is important to note that the UICC TNM classification is a classification of anatomical extent of disease and not a treatment guideline.

**Question**

I have a testicular tumour that is invading into the epididymis and into the peri-hilar fat. There is lymphovascular invasion. It does not extend into the tunica vaginalis. Does the fat at the hilum count as spermatic cord or not?

**Answer**

Hilar soft tissue invasion is considered as pT2. Invasion into the perihilar fat does not account for invasion of the spermatic cord.

**Question**

A mixed germ cell tumour in the testicle of a 33-year-old man with lymphovascular invasion and the tunica vaginalis is adherent to the tunica albuginea, though definite invasion is not seen. Three sections are taken from the spermatic cord. The one at the resection margin shows a nodule of mixed germ cell tumour while the two sections taken closer to the testicle show no malignancy (i.e. the involvement of the spermatic cord is discontinuous). The focus is approximately 4 mm and round. No nodes were submitted. A number of opinions were given by colleagues: pT3 (involvement of the spermatic cord, albeit discontinuous), pT2 (possibly just intravascular) and pT2 pM1b (metastasis other than lung or non-regional nodes).

**Answer**

Invasion of the spermatic cord (pT3) refers to direct extension of the primary tumour. Discontinuous involvement of the spermatic cord by vascular/lymphatic invasion represents M1 disease (please see *TNM Supplement*, 5th edition, page 136). We propose to classify as pT2 pNX pM1b.

**Question**

An 80-year-old male patient presents with scrotal swelling and underwent high inguinal orchidectomy. Pathologic assessment confirmed a diffuse large B cell lymphoma. Imaging confirms disease confined to testis with no nodal involvement. CSF and BMA are normal.

**Answer**

According to the Lugano classification, which was taken for the 8th edition of TNM [1], your case could be staged as stage IE.

## Kidney
**Question**

Grossly invasion of the renal vein in kidney cancer is classified as pT3a in the 8th TNM edition: how is 'grossly' defined? The AJCC does not mention 'grossly' for pT3a classification in the 8th edition. How should we treat this difference?

*Answer*

In contrast to the 7th edition, in the 8th edition, the word 'grossly' has been removed in the T3a category. Unfortunately, the first print of the UICC TNM 8th edition still mentions 'grossly'. This will be corrected in the next print of the 8th edition and is listed in the errata. Extension of a tumour in the renal vein or its segmental branches is classified as pT3a. 'Grossly' previously corresponded to macroscopically visible but was omitted because it is not uncommon that tumour involvement of the renal vein and especially its branches is unrecognized at the time of macroscopic examination of the specimen.

*Question*

We resected a renal cell carcinoma. Histology showed a small focus of tumour in the peripelvic fat and tumour invasion into blood vessels. What would be the T category?

*Answer*

Invasion of the peripelvic fat (renal sinus fat) and the renal vein (or its segmental branches) would place this case into the pT3a category (see page 199, TNM, 8th edition [1]). See also the previous case for the note on 'grossly'.

*Question*

In the TNM classification for renal cell carcinoma a tumour that involves the adrenal gland is classified as T3. It is not stated, however, that this is referring to the ipsilateral kidney. Is spread to the contralateral kidney M1?

*Answer*

Contiguous extension of the tumour into the ipsilateral adrenal gland is considered as pT4 (see page 199, UICC TNM, 8th edition [1]) and M1 if not contiguous.

Involvement of the contralateral adrenal gland as well as the contralateral kidney is cM1/pM1.

*Question*

Spread of a kidney tumour to the lumen of the renal pelvis and free floating tumour tissue in the ureter – what will the T category be?

*Answer*

The described findings of tumour extension into the renal pelvis correspond with a pT3a category. In the TNM, 8th edition, extension of the tumour into the pelvicalyceal system has been additionally introduced as pT3a. Unfortunately, this was not mentioned in the 1st print of the UICC TNM, 8th edition, and will be added in the next print and it is also in the list of errata.

*Question*

Papillary renal cell carcinoma, measuring >10 cm on imaging pre-operatively and during resection, was found to be adherent to the psoas muscle. Tumour capsule was torn during resection, spilling tumour contents intraoperatively. Consequently, the tumour was now <10 cm across at grossing (although a substantial amount of retrieved tumour was sent as an additional specimen). Firstly, would this count as extracapsular spread (pT4)? Secondly, for staging purposes should the tumour be regarded as greater than or less than 10 cm (i.e. pT2a or pT2b)? Thirdly, does intraoperative spillage upstage the tumour?

*Answer*

The invasion of the psoas muscle qualifies for T4/pT4, making the reflections about size less relevant since size only matters when the tumour is limited to the kidney. (If it would have been limited to the kidney, then we would probably recommend to add the sizes of the tumour masses.) Spillage does not alter T/pT categories in kidney tumours.

*Question*

A kidney with a main tumour mass is confined to the renal parenchyma (chromophobe carcinoma, with extensive necrosis and rhabdoid morphology, 60 mm and identifiable microvascular invasion). There are two entirely separate, very well circumscribed nodules of morphologically identical tumour within the perinephric fat, with no direct communication with the main renal tumour or the kidney itself. Microscopically there are focal peripheral lymphocytes but no definite lymph node architecture, other than being very well circumscribed. Is the most appropriate stage pT3a or pN2?

*Answer*

We recommend to classify the case as pT3a because of the identifiable microvascular invasion and the two circumscribed nodules in the perinephric fat, which likely represent vascular invasion (according to the 8th edition of TNM, both situations you mention would result in a Stage III).

*Question*

A radical nephrectomy with clear cell RCC (around 4.5 cm) shows a nodular extension into the perirenal fat covered with fibrous tissue. Is this considered perirenal fat infiltration?

   There is separate cystic RCC measuring 1.0 cm, 2.5 cm away from the main tumour. How do we stage such a case?

*Answer*

The case should be classified as pT3a(2).

## Renal Pelvis and Ureter

### Question

What pT category should be considered for urothelial carcinoma of the renal pelvis and calyces with superficial invasion to parenchyma of the renal papilla?

### Answer

T3/pT3 for the renal pelvis is defined as a tumour invasion beyond muscularis into peripelvic fat or renal parenchyma. According to that definition your case is classified as pT3.

### Question

A urothelial carcinoma in the ureter extends into the outer half of the ureter muscularis propria. Do I distinguish between T2a versus T2b as in bladder? The CAP guidelines for ureter/renal pelvis seem to lump them all into T2.

### Answer

In the 8th edition of TNM as well as in the 7th edition there is no subdivision of muscular layers in tumours of the renal pelvis and ureter (see TNM, 8th edition, page 202). They are all considered as T2/pT2.

## Bladder

### Question

How is a TCC of the bladder with (exclusive) invasion of the bladder neck musculature classified? Is this pT2?

### Answer

The bladder neck muscularis could be considered as part of the inner or outer half of muscularis propria; thus it is a T2a/pT2a or T2b/pT2b depending on which part of the muscularis is involved.

### Question

If I have a urothelial carcinoma with extensive infiltration of the subepithelial tissue and a doubt of focal infiltration of the muscle what is the correct T? pTX or pT1 with a comment?

### Answer

In the case of a TUR-B, the case you describe should be classified as cT1. A questionable invasion of muscularis should be dealt with under TNM Rule No. 4. When in doubt, use the lesser category. In the case of a bladder resection specimen a pT1 would be appropriate.

A comment that there might be an invasion of muscularis propria with a recommendation to examine further might be helpful.

### Question

For carcinoma of the bladder, if there is involvement of the seminal vesicle, should it be regarded as pT4a?

*Answer*

If the wall of the seminal vesicle or stroma of the prostate is involved, it should be T4a. If there is only in situ carcinoma in the seminal vesicle, it should not be classified T4. There are data that CIS in the prostatic ducts do not adversely impact survival [16].

*Question*

For carcinoma of the bladder, if there is invasion of the prostate by extension to the urethra, is this classified as T3 or T4?

*Answer*

A T4/pT4 bladder carcinoma is diagnosed if there is a direct invasion (transmural) of the prostatic stroma (glands are not sufficient to classify as T4). The extension of an in situ component does not qualify for T4/pT4. There are data that CIS in the prostatic ducts do not adversely impact survival [16].

*Question*

How is a carcinoma of the bladder with invasion of the abdominal cavity and perhaps invasion of the small or large bowel staged?

*Answer*

I may refer you to the Supplement, page 140, Direct invasion of a bladder tumour of the large or small intestine should be classified as T4a/pT4a. The same applies to an invasion through the peritoneum covering the bladder.

*Question*

Is invasive urothelial carcinoma in but not through the muscularis propria and discontinuous extravesical venous invasion adjacent to the muscularis propria classified as pT2V1 or pT3aV1?

*Answer*

Neither venous nor lymphatic invasion are considered in the T categories of urothelial and other tumours. The case described should indeed be classified as pT2 V1 if it is a resection specimen and cT2 V1 if it is a TUR-B specimen.

*Question*

A small-cell carcinoma of the bladder occurred with metastases in common iliac and para-aortic lymph nodes. Is this case classified as pN3pM1?

*Answer*

Metastasis in common iliac lymph nodes are classified as N3/pN3 and metastasis in para-aortic lymph nodes are classified as M1/pM1.

*Question*

What is the definition (in millimetres) of an R1 margin resection versus an R0 margin resection in bladder cancer cystectomy samples?

*Answer*
In the R classification of the UICC, R1 is defined by showing cancer cells by microscope in the cut resection margin. If you have a cancer distance to resection margin of 0.5 mm this should be classified as R0. There are proposals, mainly in the literature from the UK, to classify R1 if the distance of a cancer to the cut resection margin is 1 mm or less.

## Urethra
*Question*
Urothelial carcinoma shows extension along urethral mucosa to the skin of the glans penis (pagetoid extension within epidermis of the skin of glans). What would the TNM stage be? The tumour itself was in situ within the urethra.
*Answer*
The extension as a carcinoma in situ does not change the T category of the stage. Additionally, in carcinoma in situ no regional lymph node metastases are to be expected.

**Advice on further questions may be obtained from the TNM Helpdesk by accessing the *TNM Classification of Malignant Tumours* page at the UICC website: www.uicc.org.**

# References

[1] UICC (Union for International Cancer Control) *TNM Classification of Malignant Tumours*, 8th edn, Brierley JD, Gospodarowicz MK, Wittekind C (eds). Oxford: Wiley Blackwell; 2017.
[2] American Joint Committee on Cancer (AJCC) *Cancer Staging Manual*, 8th edn, Amin MB, Edge SB, Greene FL, et al. (eds.) New York: Springer, 2017.
[3] Greene FL, Brierley JD, O'Sullivan B, et al. On the use and abuse of X in the TNM Classification. *Cancer* 2005; 103:647–649.
[4] UICC (International Union Against Cancer) *TNM Classification of Malignant Tumours*, 4th edn, Hermanek P, Sobin LH (eds). Berlin, Heidelberg, New York: Springer; 1987.
[5] UICC (International Union Against Cancer) *TNM Classification of Malignant Tumours*, 4th edn, 2nd revision, Hermanek P, Sobin LH (eds) Berlin, Heidelberg, New York: Springer; 1992.
[6] Ohkagi H, Reifenberger G, Nomura K, et al. Brain tumours: gliomas. In *UICC Prognostic Factors in Cancer*, Gospodarowicz MK, Henson DE, Hutter RVP, et al. (eds), 2nd edn. New York: Wiley; 2001.
[7] Som PM, Curtin HD. Fascia and spaces of the neck. In *Head and Neck Imaging*, Som PM, Curtin HD (eds), 4th edn. St. Louis: Mosby; 2003, pp. 1805–1827.
[8] UICC (International Union Against Cancer) *TNM Classification of Malignant Tumours*, 5th edn, Sobin LH, Wittekind Ch (eds). New York: Wiley; 1997.

[9] UICC (Union for International Cancer Control) *TNM Classification of Malignant Tumours*, 7th edn, Sobin LH, Gospodarowicz MK, Wittekind C (eds). Oxford: Wiley-Blackwell; 2009.

[10] Pavel M, Baudin E, Couvelard A, et al. ENETS Consensus Guidelines for the Management of Patients with Liver and Other Distant Metastases from Neuroendocrine Neoplasms of Foregut, Midgut, Hindgut, and Unknown Primary. *Neuroendocrinology* 2012; 95:157–176.

[11] Garcia-Carbonero R, Sorbye H, Baudin E, et al. ENETS Consensus Guidelines for High-Grade Gastroenteropancreatic Neuroendocrine Tumors and Neuroendocrine Carcinomas. *Neuroendocrinology* 2016; 103:186–194.

[12] UICC (Union for International Cancer Control) *TNM Classification of Malignant Tumours*, 6th edn, Sobin LH, Gospodarowicz MK, Wittekind C (eds). Oxford: Wiley-Blackwell; 2002.

[13] Epstein JL, Egevad L, Amin MB, et al. The 2014 International Society of Urological Pathology (ISUP) Consensus Conference on Gleason Grading of Prostatic Carcinoma: Definition of grading patterns and proposal for new grading system. *Am J Surg Pathol* 2016; 40:244–252.

[14] Humphrey PA, Egevad L, Netto GJ, et al. Tumours of the prostate. In *WHO Classification of Tumours of the Urinary System and Male Genital Organs*, Moch H, Humphrey PA, Ulbright TM, Reuter VE (eds), Lyon: IARC Press; 2015, pp. 135–183.

[15] Chung P, Daugaard G, Tyldesley S, et al. Evaluation of a prognostic model for risk of relapse in stage I seminoma surveillance. *Cancer Medicine* 2015; 4:155–160.

[16] Montie JE, Wojno K, Klein E, et al. Transitional cell carcinoma in situ of the seminal vesicles: 8 cases with discussion of pathogenesis, and clinical and biological implications. *J Urol* 1997; 158:1895–1898.

# INDEX

Page numbers in *italic* refer to figures. Page numbers in **bold** refer to tables.

*TNM Supplement: A Commentary on Uniform Use*, Fifth Edition.
Edited by Christian Wittekind, James D. Brierley, Anne Lee and Elisabeth van Eycken.
© 2019 UICC. Published 2019 by John Wiley & Sons Ltd.